CLINICAL CARE CLASSIFICATION (CCC)©
SYSTEM MANUAL

ABOUT THE AUTHOR

Virginia K. Saba, EdD, RN, FAAN, FACMI, President and CEO of SabaCare, Inc., has pioneered the integration of computer technology in the nursing profession for over 30 years. She spearheaded the nursing informatics movement; integrated computer technology in nursing; promoted distant learning technologies; and developed computer-based information systems for community health, including the Clinical Care Classification (CCC) System. She is an Informatics Consultant and has served as a faculty member in academia and as a Nurse Officer in the US Public Health Service (PHS).

Dr. Saba is a graduate of Skidmore College Baccalaureate Nursing Program and earned a Masters of Nursing Arts at Teachers College, Columbia University. She then received a Masters of Science in Computer Technology of Management and a Doctorate of Education in Educational Administration and Scientific & Technical Information Science at American University, Washington, DC. She holds Honorary Doctorates from the University of Athens, Greece (2000) and Excelsior College in New York (2005).

In 1997, Dr. Saba received the title of Distinguished Scholar from Georgetown University School of Nursing (GUSON). Dr. Saba also served as a full professor at the Uniformed Services University of the Health Sciences (USUHS), where she taught and integrated computer technology in the Graduate School of Nursing (GSN) Research Program. It was a prototype for an adult nurse practitioner (ANP) program using interactive video technology with participating VA medical centers. In the fall of 1997, students from eight VA medical centers across the nation participated in a Post-Masters ANP Certificate Program, culminating with its first virtual graduation in June 1999.

Dr. Saba is a Past Chair of the Nursing Informatics Special Interest Group (NI-SIG) of the International Medical Informatics Association (IMIA) and was Chair of the Steering Committee of the ISO/TC215 -WG3 *Reference Terminology Model for Nursing*. She served as a consultant and faculty member for the Excelsior College Distance Learning Informatics Program. Dr. Saba has authored several books, chapters, and articles, and has served on the original editorial board of *Computers in Nursing Journal* and other health care technology journals. She is a Fellow of the American Academy of Nursing (FAAN) and the American College of Medical Informatics (FACMI), and a member of the Sigma Theta Tau International Honor Society and the Academy of Medicine of Washington, DC.

CLINICAL CARE CLASSIFICATION (CCC)©
SYSTEM MANUAL

A GUIDE TO NURSING DOCUMENTATION

VIRGINIA K. SABA, EdD,
RN, FAAN, FACMI

SPRINGER PUBLISHING COMPANY
New York

Springer Publishing Company, LLC
11 West 42nd Street
New York, NY 10036

Acquisitions Editor: Sally J. Barhydt
Production Editor: Peggy M. Rote
Cover Design: Joanne E. Honigman
Composition: TechBooks

07   08   09   10/5   4   3   2   1

Library of Congress Cataloging-in-Publication Data

Saba, Virginia K.
   Clinical care classification (CCC) system manual : a guide to
nursing documentation / Virginia K. Saba.
      p. ; cm.
   Includes bibliographical references and index.
   ISBN 0-8261-0268-9 (softcover)
   1. Nursing records—Classification—Handbooks, manuals, etc.
2. Communication in nursing—Handbooks, manuals, etc.   I. Title.
   [DNLM: 1. Nursing Records—classification. 2. Forms and
Records Control—classification. 3. Medical Records Systems,
Computerized—classification.   WY 100.5 S113c 2006]
RT50.S23 2006
651.5'04261—dc22   2006022628

Printed in the United States of America by Edwards Brothers.

CONTENTS

CONTRIBUTORS

Jean M. Arnold, EdD, RN, BC, Nurse Educator, University of Phoenix—Tampa, Thomas Edison State College, Bradenton, FL

Suzanne Bakken, DNSc, RN, FAAN, FACMI, The Alumni Professor of Nursing and Professor of Biomedical Informatics, Columbia University, New York, NY

Veronica Feeg, PhD, RN, FAAN, Professor & Chair, Department of Women, Children & Family Nursing, College of Nursing, University of Florida, Gainesville, FL

William L. Holzemer, PhD, RN, FAAN, Professor and Associate Dean International Programs, University of California, San Francisco, CA

Stanley M. Huff, MD, Chief Medical Informatics Officer, Intermountain Health Care, Salt Lake City, UT

Debra J. Konicek, RN, MSN, BC, Director, Clinical Standards, SNOMED® International, College of American Pathologists, Northfield, IL

Nam-Ju Lee, DNSc, RN, Associate Research Scientist, Columbia University, New York, NY

Susan Matney, RN, MS, Clinical Informatics, Chair Nursing Clinical LOINC, Subcommittee, SIEMENS Medical Solutions—Health Services, Malvern, PA

Kathleen A. McCormick, PhD, RN, FAAN, FACMI, Senior Scientist/Vice President, Science Application International Corporation, Falls Church, VA

Sheryl L. Taylor, BSN, RN, Senior Consultant, Farrell Associates, Fairfax, VA

FOREWORD

Embedding nursing language within informatics structures is essential to make the work of nurses visible and articulate evidence about the quality and value of nursing in the care of patients, groups and populations.

Swan, Lang, & McGinley (2004)

The Clinical Care Classification (CCC) system, initially called the Home Health Care Classification (HHCC) system, was developed by Dr. Virginia K. Saba and her colleagues at Georgetown University to provide a method for predicting home care resource needs and measure patient outcomes. Having been utilized now in the acute care as well as ambulatory care areas, the nursing and patient-focused CCC system enables the capture of patient care data documented by nurses using an electronic health record (EHR) at any point in the care continuum. This manual describes the rationale behind the CCC system, as well as how to use the terminologies in the computerized plan of care and clinical documentation applications.

The need for a standard nursing terminology has been understood by nursing leaders ever since the modern nursing profession was established. In her *Notes on Nursing* (1860), Florence Nightingale wrote: "It has been said and written scores of times, that every woman makes a good nurse. I believe, on the contrary, that the very elements of nursing are all but unknown." Dr. Norma Lang stated nearly 140 years later, "If you can't name it, you can't control it, finance it, research it, teach it or put it into public policy" (Clark & Lang, 1992).

Unlike medical procedures, nursing care has never generated charges for reimbursement. Without this incentive, the U.S. health care industry has not mandated a standard coded terminology for classification of patient care provided by nurses, and the patient care data generated by nurses is invisible. As a result, the effect of nursing care actions on patient outcomes is unmeasurable, and the value of these actions remains unacknowledged. Recent studies have shown a positive relationship between the number of *direct-care hours* provided by registered nurses and quality of care for hospitalized patients, but exactly what *patient care actions* nurses are performing during those hours is still a mystery. By naming, classifying, and coding nursing diagnoses and interventions at the atomic level, CCC enables the patient care actions performed by nurses to be identified and studied.

In the 21st century, the need for a standard nursing terminology is more urgent than ever; and, with utilization of an EHR, the full benefit of a properly *coded* standard nursing terminology can be realized. Amazingly, most nursing care provided today is still based on intuition or trial and error. The profession needs to investigate nursing practices and generate *evidence* in order to improve care; prove why certain staffing levels are required; and influence the policies of institutions, states, and the federal government regarding nursing education budgets and practice requirements. Evidence-based nursing practice is key to effective nursing care, and a standard, coded nursing terminology for capturing patient care data in an EHR is essential for conducting the research necessary to generate this evidence.

This terminology has become essential to the nursing profession for another very important reason. Industry experts say a "perfect storm" situation has formed around health care in the United States with rapidly rising costs, a high percentage of Americans being uninsured, and budget crises on the federal and state levels. At the same time health care costs are soaring, U.S. health statistics show quality of care is questionable.

Reacting to these ominous signs, in 2003 the US Department of Health and Human Services (HHS) announced a "Call to Action" that included endorsement of the Institute of Medicine's (IOM) recommendations for the EHR and recognition that *standards* are key to the success of the EHR. HHS allocated $32.4 million for a 5-year contract to make the standard health care vocabulary in SNOMED CT (Systematized Nomenclature of Medical Clinical Terms) core content available free via the IOM Unified Medical Language System (UMLS) Metathesaurus, sending a message to all health care professionals that the federal government believes use of standard terminology by all disciplines is critical. The CCC system is integrated into SNOMED CT.

In addition, Phase 2 of the Health Insurance Portability and Accountability Act of 1966 (HIPAA) introduced the Patient Medical Record Information (PMRI) Uniform Data Standards—standards recommended by the National Committee on Vital and Health Statistics' (NCVHS) Subcommittee on Standards and Security for use with the EHR. The PMRI vision is that clinically specific data will be captured once by the EHR at the point of care, and that the derivatives of these data will be available for reimbursement, research, and public health. One of the dimensions of the PMRI framework is *comparability* of data—that is, consistent meaning for data as they are shared among various authorized users of the EHR—and standard coded terminology is the foundation for data comparability. In order to be included in the PMRI, the patient care data generated by nurses must be captured by a terminology that supports the comparability dimension. Only a standard nursing terminology that is classified and properly coded meets the specification for this requirement.

The federal government currently is agonizing over the twin issues of high cost and mediocre quality of health care in the United States and is determined to use health care information technology (HCIT) to help alleviate the crisis. Effective use of HCIT to address the issues requires certain elements, one of which is a standard coded terminology to support comparability of patient data. The implications for the nursing profession as the federal government acts in response to health care's perfect storm cannot be ignored. In order to obtain evidence regarding the effect of nursing care on patient outcomes, patient care data generated by nurses must be captured via the EHR using a standard coded terminology. Without this evidence, nursing will continue to be viewed by health care organizations as a cost center, leading to budget cuts and short staffing. Studies show that, when nurse staffing is inadequate, patients suffer the consequences. The CCC system described in this manual is the only standard coded nursing terminology that is based on sound research using the nursing process model framework and that meets the PMRI comparability requirement.

The CCC system allows patient care data generated by nurses to be incorporated into the PMRI database, and enables nurses' contributions to patient outcomes to be studied and acknowledged.

Sheryl L. Taylor, BSN, RN
Senior Consultant, Farrell Associates

REFERENCES

Clark, J., & Lang, N. (1992). Nursing's next advance: An international classification for nursing practice. *International Nursing Review, 39,* 109–112.

Nightingale, F. (1860). *Notes on nursing: What it is, and what it is not.* New York: D. Appleton & Company [First American Edition].

Swan, B.A., Lang, N.M., & McGinley, A.M. (2004). Access to quality health care: Links between evidence, nursing language, and informatics. *Nursing Economics, 22,* 325–332.

PREFACE

Welcome to the *Clinical Care Classification (CCC) System Manual*—which provides an overview of the CCC system Version 2.0, formerly the Home Health Care Classification (HHCC) system Version 1.0—and how to use it. The CCC system was designed to document patient care for the electronic health record (EHR) systems, regardless of health care setting. The CCC system Version 2.0 consists of two interrelated terminologies: the CCC of Nursing Diagnoses and Outcomes, and the CCC of Nursing Interventions and Action Types. Both of these terminologies are classified by 21 Care Components.

This manual addresses the many comments, questions, and concerns that have been expressed by students, researchers, vendors, and other users of the CCC system, as well as anticipates the questions of future users of the system. This manual has been created not only to provide a print version of the CCC Web site (<**http://www.sabacare.com**>), but also to offer a detailed and expanded overview of the CCC system.

Each chapter has been prepared so that it is a unit unto itself and can *stand alone*, which is why some information is presented in more than one chapter. Also, several terms have been selected to represent similar terms that have changed over time or are used by others in the field. The major terms are as follows:

- *Clinical Care Classification (CCC) system Version 2.0* is also used to refer to the HHCC system Version 1.0, the initial name and version of the system. However, the HHCC will only be used when it is specifically referenced.
- *Electronic Health Record (EHR)* system is used to refer to any computerized health care system that documents patient care, regardless of title, such as electronic medical record (EMR) system, computer-based patient record (CPR) system, patient medical record information (PMRI) system, computer-based information technology (IT) system, hospital information system (HIS), etc.
- *Plans of Care* is used to refer to the documentation of nursing practice, documentation of patient care by nurses, care process, and/or documentation of plans of care application for an EHR system.
- *Terminology* is used to refer to a classification, taxonomy, vocabulary, nomenclature, and/or language.

In the Foreword to this manual, Sheryl Taylor highlights why nursing needs a terminology such as CCC. She explains that since Nightingale's time, nursing has proposed that a nursing language was needed and essential for measuring nursing practice. The manual is divided into three parts: (1) Overview; (2) Research, Integration and Evaluation, and (3) Terminology Uses. Part I focuses on the background of the CCC system. In Chapter 1, Kathleen McCormick provides a rationale for using the CCC to document nursing practice in the emerging EHR systems. She introduces the CCC system to the reader.

The original research study from which the system was empirically developed is described in Chapter 2. It includes why the study was conducted, how it was funded, and information about the state-of-the-art of health care industry at the time. This chapter explains how and why the two terminologies—CCC of Nursing Diagnoses and Outcomes and the CCC of Nursing Interventions and Action Types—were created. Table 2.1 highlights the chronology of the critical CCC system events starting with the original research in 1988 until 2006.

Chapter 3 provides a description of the features and characteristics of the CCC as a terminology. It includes an overview of its general uses, as well as specific information about its standards, translations, maintenance policy, copyright, and trademark.

Part II of this manual focuses on the research, integration, and evaluation that have been conducted on the CCC system. It provides a theoretical overview, as well as the opinions of the CCC system by other users, researchers, educators, and implementers. Chapter 4 provides an annotated bibliography of the most critical research and evaluation studies reported by informatics experts in the literature. Chapter 5 includes selected testimonies from users in the United States and internationally. It includes comments from a vendor on the integration of the CCC system in its documentation system and a federal agency that has integrated the CCC into its national database, namely the United States Health Information Knowledgebase (USHIK).

Chapters 6 to 10 are written by nursing informatics experts and describe how they have implemented the CCC system in their specialized areas. In Chapter 6, Matney, Bakken, and Huff discuss the mapping of the CCC of Nursing Diagnoses in LOINC's (Logical Observation Identifiers, Names, and Codes) laboratory and clinical core set of EHR clinical terminology. They also discuss the messaging of the CCC system in Health Level Seven (HL7) and provide examples of HL7 messages using CCC. HL7 is a messaging standard used to transmit electronic data across health information systems. In Chapter 7, Konicek explains SNOMED CT (Systematized Nomenclature of Medical Clinical Terms) and provides examples of how CCC of Nursing Diagnoses and CCC of Nursing Interventions concepts are integrated in SNOMED CT. Bakken and colleagues have contributed two chapters, one on research and another on education. In Chapter 8, Bakken and Holzemer describe how the CCC is used in nursing research focusing on Client Adherence Profiling; and, in Chapter 10, Bakken and Lee describe how the CCC is integrated in an electronic student clinical log designed for educating students. In Chapter 9, Feeg discusses how the CCC was configured in a software package for educating nurses on electronic documentation. Part II concludes with Chapter 11. It provides a complete bibliography of the major articles and publications on the CCC system since it has been in the public domain and serves as an excellent resource. Part III of the manual focuses on the CCC system terminologies and shows how a user can document a plan of care application, using the CCC, for an EHR system. Chapter 12 by Arnold and Saba presents a theoretical model that has been tested on a few sample cases and that proposes a method for determining the cost of nursing care. Chapter 13, on documentation strategies, describes formats for documenting different plans of care applications for EHR systems. It includes not only examples of plans of care, but also a working table to be used as a tool when coding any documentation, including plans of care using the CCC system. Chapter 14 outlines the framework and structure of the CCC and describes the CCC of Nursing Diagnoses, the CCC of Nursing Outcomes (Expected and Actual), and the CCC of Nursing Interventions and Action Types. Each of these processes is not only described, but also presented with appropriate tables that serve as references for those who are configuring or documenting plans of care. These tables provide ready access to the CCC terminologies for anyone who is coding and documenting patient care manually or electronically. Fourteen tables are provided as resources.

The Appendix section includes three tables (Appendix A) that depict the revision—additions, deletions, and changes from the HHCC Version 1.0 to CCC Version 2.0; a sample permission letter (Appendix B) for anyone requesting permission to use the CCC system; and NTIS (National Technical Information Service) ordering information (Appendix C) for the final report of the original research study.

This manual is an indispensable guide and resource for anyone who is documenting patient care or configuring, coding, and implementing plans of care applications using the CCC terminologies for integration in an EHR system. It will serve you well.

Virginia K. Saba

ACKNOWLEDGMENTS

This manual has been developed to provide a printed version of the Clinical Care Classification (CCC) system Web site (<**http://www.sabacare.com**>), including a detailed overview of the CCC system Version 2.0. It is in response to the many comments, questions, and concerns that have been expressed by students, researchers, vendors, and other users of the CCC system. It is also designed to answer anticipated questions for future users of the system.

I want to thank all the contributors of chapters and informative pieces who have added the personal touch to this manual. Their contributions demonstrate the varied uses and impact the CCC system is having on nursing practice, management, research, and education. I also want to acknowledge my editor, Sally Barhydt, whose encouragement made this publication possible.

I also wish to acknowledge the original research team of the federally funded Home Care Project (1989–1991) conducted at Georgetown University School of Nursing from which the Home Health Care Classification (HHCC) system Version 1.0 emerged. It consisted of myself as Principal Investigator, Jennifer Boondas, Eugene Levine, David Oatway, Patricia O'Hare, William Scanlon, Alan E. Zuckerman, two graduate students (Irene Reyes and Sheila Nveva), and an office manager (Andrew McLaughlin).

Additionally, I want to acknowledge the ongoing work of CCC Scientific Advisory Board members: Terri Ayers, Suzanne Bakken, Ruth Galten Irwin, Sheila Sparks, myself, and ad hoc members Amy Coenen and Ann Fariss—all of whom donated their time to meet, review, and evaluate new concepts, labels, or terms for the CCC system Version 2.0.

I wish to recognize many of my nursing informatics colleagues and clinicians from around the world who have endorsed, promoted, and continue to support the CCC system. They believe, as I do, that the CCC system is the nursing language that demonstrates that nursing practice makes a difference and makes nursing visible.

Virginia K. Saba

OVERVIEW

1

WHY CLINICAL CARE CLASSIFICATION (CCC)©?

KATHLEEN A. MCCORMICK

There are books that describe the models and theories of nursing informatics and new books that focus on use cases, and implementation strategies; but, this is the first book that puts them all together for one coded classification system: the Clinical Care Classification (CCC)©. This book demonstrates the progress of nursing informatics to dedicate an entire book to a coded classification system. It further demonstrates the vision of the authors to have developed and tested such a system. What better way to learn history than to have the authors of the histories describe it? The pioneers who first developed and implemented this system are also in the best position to write the first book on implementation. They have lived the implementation for almost 30 years.

During the developmental years, the authors developed the system previously known as the Home Health Care Classification (HHCC) system. The original HHCC was one of the first four classifications recognized by the American Nurses Association (ANA) Steering Committee on Databases to Support Clinical Nursing Practice (DBSC) in 1991/1992. The original system was developed from funds provided by the Health Care Financing Administration (HCFA), now known as the Centers for Medicare and Medicaid Services (CMS). This manual provides a chronology of its history since its formal creation in 1991.

The manual could not be entering the market at a more appropriate time. The support for the electronic health record (EHR) comes all the way from the top—the President of the United States. With the EHR is the need for coded classifications to support interoperability. The coded systems are needed that can measure the quality of patient care. With more of a health information technology focus on the empowered consumer and the link of ambulatory and hospital information to the home, the mapping of classifications between those environments is an inherent part of tracking the person's encounters through the health care system. The performance of the caregiver during those encounters should be better monitored through structured documentation systems.

At this time, research is needed to validate the accuracy and reliability of the classification in different settings across the spectrum of health care. A significant piece of the workflow in health care is that delivered by the nursing profession. The CCC should be the seedling to measure how the patient/consumer moves between different types of health care professionals and whether the workflow is improved because of the CCC linked into other medical terminologies in the

EHR. Measurement of the workflow might indicate the need to link the CCC with emerging patient/consumer terminologies.

This manual does answer the question whether a coded structure is capable of measuring the impact and effectiveness of care from the use of the CCC internationally. It suggests that outcomes of care can be better measured with the use of this classification as a tool embedded in an EHR. When implemented, it supports decision making by individual nurses and could potentially be used for patients/consumers. The manual use cases describe how the nurses and systems work when the CCC is utilized. It provides testimony to how the CCC could facilitate data mining and aggregation of data for decision making at the local, regional, and national levels. Having a CCC should allow us to conduct evaluations of how nursing data are acquired and represented, retrieved, and linked to judgments about patient safety and quality outcomes.

Finally, the manual purports that data acquired through a CCC can be analyzed for cost and the economic impact of different nursing care measures toward outcomes can be understood. This manual is a legacy of treasured information related to the CCC: its development, use, implementation, evaluation, and innovative applications. It includes the stories of the pioneers. It has been an honor to work with these coding and classification experts over the years and to garner a bit of appreciation for their rigor and preciseness in development and testing. Examples of case studies using CCC are provided related to pneumonia and deep venous thrombosis. With interoperability as a goal in EHR, the CCC has the potential to provide the level of commonality for sharing information. Nursing should now be in a position to measure the impact of sharing processes and outcomes at a local or regional health care network.

Like the other textbooks and manuals for nursing students, it would be my wish that the success of this manual is someday measured by having a nurse say, "This manual changed my career and my thinking about nursing documentation systems." The documents of nurses are the window to a diary of care given to patients. It is obvious that a CCC embedded into an EHR improves the legacy of the contributions of the nurse in care.

BACKGROUND AND DEVELOPMENT OF THE CLINICAL CARE CLASSIFICATION SYSTEM

This chapter provides an overview of the Clinical Care Classification (CCC) system and highlights how the CCC—previously known as the Home Health Care Classification (HHCC)—system was empirically developed. It includes a detailed description of the research study that was conducted and used to design and develop the system. This chapter also provides its coding structure, including examples of how the coding structure is used.

RESEARCH STUDY

The CCC system was developed by Dr. Virginia K. Saba and colleagues of the Home Care Project (1988–1991) that was conducted at Georgetown University School of Nursing (Washington, DC) (see Exhibit 2.1). The CCC system can be seen at its Web site: <**http://www.sabacare.com**> (Saba, 2006). The research project—entitled "Develop and Demonstrate a Method for Classifying Home Health Patients to Predict Resource Requirements and Measure Outcomes"—was funded through a cooperative agreement (No. 17C-98983/3) with the Health Care Financing Agency (HCFA), which is currently named the Centers for Medicare and Medicaid Services (CMS) (Saba, 1991). To accomplish the research, data were collected on actual resource use that could be measured objectively. The research design was based on a conceptual framework, review of the literature, and findings from a pilot study. This study was considered to be a major national research study of this growing field.

The Georgetown Home Care Project addressed several important changes in the home health industry. With the enactment of Medicare and Medicaid legislation in 1966, care of the elderly sick at home changed drastically. Home health care was viewed as a cost-effective alternative to institutional care of an increasingly aging population. These patients were being discharged "sicker

EXHIBIT 2.1. CLINICAL CARE CLASSIFICATION SYSTEM HISTORICAL HIGHLIGHTS: 1988–2006

Date	Highlights
1988–May:	Georgetown Home Care Project. *Develop and Demonstrate a Method for Classifying Home Health Patients to Predict Resource Requirements and to Measure Outcomes*. Funded by the Health Care Financing Administration (HCFA) Cooperative Agreement No. 17-C-98983/3/01.
1991–Feb:	Final Report *Home Health Care Classification Project*. Submitted to the HCFA. Report contained Preliminary *Home Health Care Classification (HHCC) of Nursing Diagnoses and Interventions*.
1991–June:	First Published Article. Saba, V.K., O'Hare, P., Zuckerman, A.E., Boondas, J., Levine, E., & Oatway, D.M. (1991). A nursing intervention taxonomy for home health care. *Nursing and Health Care*, 12(6), 296–299.
1991–Nov:	HHCC System (Version 1.0). Recognized by the American Nurses Association (ANA) Steering Committee on Databases to Support Clinical Nursing Practice
1992–Feb:	HHCC System (Version 1.0). Recognized by American Nurses Association (ANA) Congress on Nursing Practice.
1992–Nov:	First Translation of the HHCC System (Version 1.0) in Dutch by Marlou de Fuiper, RN, MsN. Diagnose en interventie (pp. 73–82) (In Classification of Home Health Care Nursing Diagnoses and Interventions). In L. Regeer (Ed.), *Verpleegkundige Diagnostiek in Nederland* (pp. 62–82). Amsterdam, The Netherlands: LEO Verpleegkundig Management.
1992–Dec:	First Integration of HHCC System (Version 1.0) in a Nursing Terminology Database by E.R. Gabrieli *6-3-1-10 Nursing Terminology (V. Saba)*. Buffalo, NY: Gabrieli.
1993:	HHCC System (Version 1.0). Submitted to the National Library of Medicine for inclusion into the Metathesaurus of the Unified Medical Language System (UMLS) by the ANA.
1993:	First Manual Publication. *Home Health Care Classification Nursing Diagnoses and Interventions*. Washington, DC: Georgetown University Press.
1993–Feb:	US Copyright Office. Certificate of Registration: *Classification of Home Health Nursing Diagnoses and Interventions* (Reg. No. 573-483).
1993:	HHCC System (Version 1.0). Title Terms Only: Indexed in the Cumulative Index of Nursing and Allied Health Literature (CINAHL) Information Systems. *CINAHL 2004 Subject Heading List Thesaurus*. Glendale, CA: CINAHL.
1994:	Revised Manual Publication. *Home Health Care Classification Nursing Diagnoses and Interventions*. Washington, DC: Georgetown University Press.
1995:	HHCC of Nursing Diagnoses and HHCC of Nursing Interventions Indexed in the Cumulative Index of Nursing and Allied Health Literature (CINAHL) Information Systems. *CINAHL 2004 Subject Heading List Thesaurus*. Glendale, CA: CINAHL.
1995:	Initiated Web site at Georgetown University Dahlgren Medical Library, Washington, DC, for *Home Health Care Classification: Nursing Diagnoses and Interventions*. <**http://www.dml.georgetown.edu/research/hhcc.**>
1995:	HHCC of Nursing Intervention (Version 1.0). Translated into Finnish (2nd Translation).
1997–May:	Presentation entitled: *Home Health Care Classification (HHCC) of Nursing Diagnoses & Nursing Interventions*. To: Developers of Coding and Classification Systems Panel, Subcommittee on Health Data Needs, Standards, and Security, National Committee on Vital and Health Statistics (NCVHS). (In reference to the Health Insurance Portability and Accountability Act of 1966—Pub. Law No. 104-191.)
1998:	First Commercial Web site for HHCC System (Version 1.0): <**http://www.sabacare.com.**>
1998:	HHCC of Nursing Interventions (Version 1.0). Adapted by ABC Codes for Complementary and Alternative Medicine (CAM) and Conventional Nursing.
1998/1999:	*Home Health Care Classification (HHCC) of Nursing Diagnoses & Nursing Interventions*. Approved and published in: American National Standards Institute—Healthcare Informatics Standards Board (ANSI HISB). *Inventory of Clinical Information Standards*. Washington, DC: ANSI.
1998–Feb:	Presentation entitled: *Home Health Care Classification (HHCC) of Nursing Diagnoses and Nursing Interventions*. To Safety Regulations and Electronic Dissemination of Billing Data Committee, ANSI HISB. Inventory of Clinical Information Standards: Template C: Code Sets. Washington, DC: DHHS. (In reference to Health Insurance Portability and Accountability Act of 1966 (HIPAA) Pub. Law No. 104-191.)

(Continued)

EXHIBIT 2.1. (CONTINUED)

Date	Highlights
1999:	HHCC System (Version 1.0). Registered by Health Level Seven (HL7).
1999:	HHCC of Nursing Diagnoses Outcomes (Version 1.0). Integrated into Logical Observations, Identifiers, Names, and Codes (LOINC).
1999–May:	Presentation entitled: *Home Health Care Classification System (HHCC).* To Work Group on Computer-based Patient Records, National Committee on Vital and Health Statistics (NCVHS). Rockville, MD: AHCPR (In reference to Health Insurance Portability and Accountability Act of 1966—Pub. Law No. 104-191).
2000:	HHCC of Nursing Diagnoses (Version 1.0). Integrated into Systematized Nomenclature of Medical Reference Terms (SNOMED-RT). Chicago, IL.
2000–July:	*Home Health Care Classification (HHCC) System of Nursing Diagnoses and Nursing Interventions.* Submitted to the National Committee on Vital and Health Statistics. *Uniform Data Standards for Patient Medical Record Information.* Report to the Secretary of the US-DHHS as required by the Administration Simplification Provision of the Health Insurance Portability and Accountability Act of 1966—Pub. Law No. 104-191.
2003–Jan:	CCC System (Version 2.0). Updated on Web site: <**http://www.sabacare.com.**>
2003–Feb:	*Clinical Care Classification Terminology Questionnaire.* Submitted for Developers of Candidate Terminologies for PMRI Standards to Subcommittee on Standards and Security, National Committee on Vital and Health Statistics (NCVHS). Washington, DC. (In reference to Patient Medical Record Information (PMRI) required by the Administration Simplification Provision of the Health Insurance Portability and Accountability Act of 1966—Pub. Law No. 104-191.)
2003–April:	CCC System (Version 2.0). Submitted to the National Library of Medicine (NLM) for inclusion into Metathesaurus of the Unified Medical Language System (UMLS).
2003:	CCC System (Version 2.0). Indexed in Cumulative Index of Nursing and Allied Health Literature (CINAHL) Information Systems. *CINAHL 2004 Subject Heading List Thesaurus.* Glendale, CA.
2004–Feb:	CCC System (Version 2.0). New Name and Version announced at the HIMSS meeting in Orlando, FL.
2004–July:	CCC System (Version 2.0). Integrated into Systematized Nomenclature of Medical Clinical Terms (SNOMED-CT). Chicago, IL.
2004–Oct:	US Copyright Office. Certificate of Registration: *Clinical Care Classification (CCC) System* (Reg. No. 6-100-481).
2005–Oct:	CCC of Nursing Diagnoses Outcomes (Version 2.0). Integrated to Logical Observations, Identifiers, Names, and Codes (LOINC).
2005–Oct:	CCC System (Version 2.0). Registered by Health Level Seven (HL7). OID.
2005–Dec:	US Patent and Trademark Office. Certificate Logo Registration: *Clinical Care Classification System* (Reg. No. 3,019,288).
2006:	CCC System (Version 2.0). Mapped to the *International Classification of Nursing Practice (ICNP). Version 1.0.* Geneva, Switzerland.
2006:	CCC of Nursing Interventions (Version 2.0). Adapted by ABC Codes for Complementary and Alternative Medicine (CAM) and Conventional Nursing

DHHS, Department of Health and Human Services; HIMSS, Healthcare Information and Management Systems Society; OID, object identifier.

and quicker" from hospitals, thus increasing the demand for acute, complex, home health services. The number of home health agencies (HHAs) increased from 1,275 in 1966 to over 10,000 in 1997 (National Association for Home Care, 2000). As health care services have expanded, reimbursement costs and expenditures of the services have steadily increased.

The various reimbursement methods, however, did not match the patient care services, thus making the need for an approach other than cost per visit/encounter critical. At that time, there was a lack of uniform data on home health care resources, services, and reimbursement practices. Also, the ambiguities in terminology and policies, the lack of standardized definitions among fiscal intermediaries, and the lack of a usable method or classification affected the equitable reimbursement of their services.

The Home Care Project was undertaken not only to conduct a descriptive analyses of home health care patients and services, but also to develop a classification system that could predict resource requirements and measure outcomes. The research team consisted of a nursing and a medical informatics expert, two public/home health nursing experts, a statistician, and a systems analyst. Also, a national advisory committee composed of similar national experts was established to oversee the research activities. They determined that, by collecting a large volume of data (national sample) on Medicare patients and the actual resources used for their health care, a system could be developed that could predict care requirements and evaluate outcomes. The research team conducted a pilot study, designed a framework, established a methodology, and developed a form consisting of 73 pre-coded variables for abstracting the study data. They applied the methodology to a national sample of HHAs that provided services and products used to restore, maintain, and promote physical, mental, and emotional health to patients in their homes (Spradley & Dorsey, 1985).

Sample Size

Retrospective research data were collected from 8,967 patient records from a national sample of 646 Medicare-certified HHAs that were randomly stratified by staff size, type of ownership, and geographic location. The HHAs represented every state in the nation, Puerto Rico, and the District of Columbia. Five to 50 records of recently discharged Medicare patients for an entire episode of care were abstracted from each of the sample HHAs (Saba, 1991).

Research data consisted of data based on relevant variables: demographics, patient care services by nurses and other health care providers, dates of visits/encounters, and discharge data. Findings of the research study provided the largest knowledge base and one of the most complete descriptions of this expanding health care field. Also, the research study collected relevant data elements considered possible predictors of resource requirements. They were collected from actual nursing notes and from other providers' narrative notes recorded in patient records that represented the essence of the nursing care. Abstractors used these notes to collect for each sample patient two different sets of narrative statements that addressed: patient problems and/or nursing diagnoses and nursing services, treatments, interventions, and/or actions for the entire episode of care. Approximately 40,000 narrative statements were collected representing the sample patients' problems and/or nursing diagnoses, and 80,000 narrative statements were collected representing their nursing services, treatments, interventions, and/or actions.

Processing Statements

Once the narrative statements were collected, the research team had to process and code the two sets of statements. Since none of the existing coding strategies available at the time were found to be appropriate, it was decided to develop unique vocabularies that could be used to code the two sets of statements. More than a thousand sample statements were keyboarded using permuted *keyword sorts* that were processed, analyzed, and tested to develop the concepts needed to code the two sets of narrative statements. Like concepts were stated in different words with the same meaning, making it necessary to cluster them together for analysis.

Nursing Diagnosis Example

Like or similar statements of nursing diagnoses/patient problems, such as fluid intake problem, fluid volume deficiency, and fluid alteration, were merged into *fluid volume alteration.*

Nursing Intervention Example

Like or similar statements of nursing services/interventions, such as wound drainage care, wound healing, and skin wound, were merged into *wound care.*

The concepts for patient problems/nursing diagnoses and nursing services/ interventions were not only sorted separately, but also matched together by concept and by patient. By using this technique, it was possible to empirically develop a tentative list (vocabulary) of approximately 200 discrete nursing diagnoses and 800 discrete nursing interventions. It was further noted that each of these 800 discrete patient services/interventions consisted of two aspects: a single action (core concept) and a specific action type.

Action Types Example

Concepts were written as: monitor wound, provide wound care, teach family how to care for wound, or call physician regarding condition of wound. The core concept (atomic level) was *wound care,* but the action types addressed four different types of *Actions*:

1. *monitor wound care:* meaning to assess or evaluate the wound;
2. *perform wound care:* meaning to provide direct wound care;
3. *teach wound care:* meaning to instruct or educate patient or caregiver on how to administer wound care; and
4. *manage wound care:* meaning to call physician regarding condition of wound or refer patient to a consultant.

As a result, the 800 nursing services interventions were separated into two different sets: core concept (atomic) interventions and four action-type qualifiers: (1) assess or monitor, (2) direct care or perform, (3) teach or educate, and (4) manage or refer. This strategy provided a unique and flexible vocabulary-coding scheme and reduced the number of core concepts to approximately 160 nursing interventions.

The two sets of statements, once coded, had to be grouped and/or classified for ease of use and for analysis purposes. The classes had to be used for both the nursing diagnoses and nursing interventions. Several existing classification schemes were reviewed, but none met the established criteria that were to link the nursing diagnoses to the nursing interventions to the nursing outcomes.

Linkage Example

Nursing Diagnosis—Physical Mobility Impairment should link to the
Nursing Intervention—perform Mobility Therapy to achieve
Nursing Outcome—Improved Physical Mobility Impairment

Care Components

For each concept, the above rationale was used to ensure linkage of the nursing diagnoses to nursing interventions and nursing outcomes. Also, by statistical analysis of the study data, frequencies were conducted on the two sets of coded vocabularies, resulting in 20 logical and consistent groupings and categorized as Care Components. They were tested and retested to ensure that they could be used to classify and provide the framework for the two vocabulary lists. Thus, the HHCC system (Version 1.0), with two vocabularies (list of concepts arranged in a hierarchical format), was developed, making it possible to document, code, and classify the nursing diagnoses and nursing interventions, as well as map the two terminologies together and use them for the continuum of care. Care Components were found to be not only logical and clinically significant, but also measurable and could be used to predict resource requirements.

Nursing Diagnoses

The initial vocabulary list of nursing diagnoses consisted of those nursing diagnoses and/or patient problems assessed from the signs and symptoms for the entire episode of care that required nursing and other providers of health care services. The original classification was developed not only by using an adapted version of the Nursing Diagnoses Taxonomy 1 (North American Nursing Diagnoses Association, 1991), but also by expanding it with over 50 new diagnostic concepts obtained empirically from processing the keywords from the narrative statements such as *Medication Risk, Polypharmacy,* or *Dying Process.* The original HHCC of Nursing Diagnoses (Version 1.0) consisted of 145 diagnostic concepts (50 major and 95 subcategories) derived from the study data's 40,361 narrative statements.

Nursing Outcomes

The nursing diagnoses were also used to depict the outcomes of nursing care. The outcomes were considered to be the Actual Outcomes for the patients' problems/nursing diagnoses resulting from the interventions/services performed during the care process. The patients' nursing diagnoses were evaluated by the primary nurse on discharge and were labeled in the past tense using one of three conditions:

1. Improved or Resolved,
2. Not Changed, Stabilized, or Maintained, and
3. Deteriorated or Died.

The same qualifiers were also considered usable for identifying the Expected Outcomes or the goals of care. The Expected Outcomes are presented in the present tense.

Nursing Interventions

The initial vocabulary list of nursing interventions consisted of those nursing interventions, services, and/or actions performed for the entire episode of care to treat (satisfy) the identified nursing diagnoses or patient problems. The original classification was empirically developed from processing the keywords based on the narrative statements collected from each sample patient for an entire episode of care. They included: (1) 28 HCFA Skilled Treatment codes (HCFA, 1997) required by the government, (2) a core set of concepts of major categories and subcategories based on logical groupings, and (3) four types of actions qualifiers (assess, care, teach, and manage) designed to expand and enhance the list of nursing interventions. The original HHCC of Nursing Intervention (Version 1.0) consisted of 160 nursing intervention (60 major and 100 subcategories) concepts derived from the study data's 80,283 statements.

Coding Structure

The HHCC's two terminology lists required a coding structure to facilitate computer processing. It was essential that the concepts be coded following data processing standards. Each concept in the two terminology lists had to have a unique code so that the concepts could be linked to each other and mapped to other classification systems. Each concept that depicted the hierarchical structure had to be coded, defined, and classified in a standardized manner. Finally, the concept codes had to be structured so that they could be processed, retrieved, and aggregated for analysis purposes.

Because of the characteristics required to code the two vocabulary lists, it was determined that the coding strategy be based on a classification system already in existence. The format of the tenth revision of the *International Statistical Classification of Diseases and Related Health Problems* (commonly referred to as ICD-10) (World Health Organization, 1992) was selected and used as the basis for coding the two lists. The ICD-10, which consists of a five-character alphanumeric code, was used to code the HHCC (Version 1.0). The first alphabetic character represents the Care Component classes, the next two or three digits represent the core concepts, and the last digit represents the qualifiers for both the nursing diagnosis and nursing intervention vocabulary lists.

In summary, the HHCC system (Version 1.0) was developed as two integrated vocabularies/terminologies, both of which were classified by 20 Care Components. The Care Components made it possible to link the nursing diagnoses, nursing interventions, and nursing outcomes together. Furthermore, the

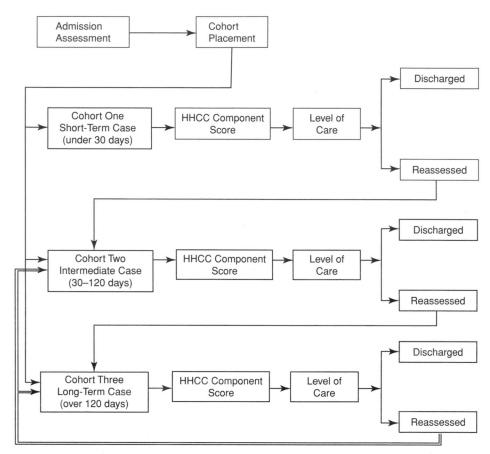

FIGURE 2.1. An example of the home health care classification method. HHCC, Home Health Care Classification.

HHCC system was designed for computer processing to document and code patient care in the computer-based patient record (CPR) systems.

Study Findings

One major finding from the research study indicated, that since the HHCC system was also based on a nursing process model, resource requirements could be predicted reliably, were clinically sound, and statistically significant. Data used to predict resource use represented one of three cohorts for a specific medical condition: (1) short term under 30 days, (2) intermediate term 30 to 120 days, and (3) long term over 120 days (see Figure 2.1). Analysis of the study findings identified that, on average, a patient with a specific medical condition generally had three to five nursing diagnoses that required eight to ten nursing interventions to treat an episode of illness. Analysis also demonstrated that the two terminologies, when combined, were found to be the most effective measure for predicting home health visits and/or encounters for an episode of illness rather than medical diagnoses. Finally, the study data demonstrated that demographics had a relatively small impact on resource use, whereas nursing diagnoses and nursing interventions combined did have an impact and could be used reliably to predict resource use (Saba, 1991, 1995; Saba & McCormick, 2001, 2006). The final report can be obtained from the National Technical Information Service as a CD-ROM. See Appendix C for ordering information.

INFLUENCING FACTORS

Clinical Nursing Practice

With the introduction of Medicare legislation, changes occurred in the documentation of clinical nursing practice as federal reporting requirements increased. For years, the American Nurses Association (ANA) has promoted the need for classification systems to support clinical nursing practice and the need for data to measure the nursing process. As CPR systems were developed, the nursing profession did not have any standardized coded classifications that information technology (IT) vendors and developers could use for nursing documentation applications. Also, because the payment of nursing services was integrated in the room rate instead of actual care cost measures, the vendors and users did not see the need to collect measurable coded nursing care data.

As early as 1980, the ANA introduced the Nursing Social Policy Statement (ANA, 1995), which recommended that the nursing process serve as the standards of care for documenting clinical nursing practice (ANA, 1998). In 1989, the ANA formed the Steering Committee on Databases to Support Clinical Nursing Practice and renamed it in 1998 as the Committee for Nursing Practice Information Infrastructure (CNPII). This committee was involved in several activities, one of which was "recognizing" classification systems to support nursing practice. In 1990, the ANA passed a resolution adopting the Nursing Minimum Data Set (NMDS) as the core data set for managing nursing data and for inclusion in national databases. In 1992, the Database Steering Committee recognized the first four classification systems under the umbrella of the NMDS and approved them as nursing data classification standards. The systems were: (1) HHCC, (2) North American Nursing Diagnoses Association Taxonomy I, (3) the Omaha System, and (4) Nursing Intervention Classification (NIC).

Since that time, nine other classification systems (13 in total) have been recognized by the ANA (Coenen et al., 2001). They include: (5) Nursing Outcomes Classification (NOC), (6) Patient Care Data Set (PCDS), (7) Perioperative Nursing Data Set (PNDS), (8) Nursing Minimum Data Set, (9) Nursing Management Minimum Data Set (NMMDS), (10) International Classification of Nursing Practice (ICNP), (11) Complete Complementary Alternative Medicine Billing and Coding Reference (ABC Codes), (12) Logical Observations, Identifiers Names, and Codes (LOINC), and (13) Systematized Nomenclature of Medicine Clinical Terms (SNOMED CT). The SNOMED CT is a terminology developed by the College of American Pathologists for health care professionals. Recently, it integrated Read Codes from the United Kingdom, as well as several nursing terminologies, including the original HHCC system and the recently renamed CCC of Nursing Diagnoses and the CCC of Nursing Interventions. The ANA continues to promote the use of nursing information, classifications, and terminologies in computer technology systems focusing on clinical nursing practice to prove that "what nurses do makes a difference" (McCormick et al., 1994).

Information Technology Systems

Since the 1950s and 1960s, computer hardware, software, and communication networks have changed radically. Computer hardware has advanced in size, speed, storage capacity, and processing capability. The multi-user mainframe computer systems of the 1960s have progressed to the single desktop (micro-computer) personal computer (PC) of the 1980s, laptop PCs of the 1990s, and handheld PDAs (personal data assistants) of the 21st century. Computer software has gone from programming languages to the Windows platform with user-friendly icons, a navigation mouse, and generic software programs. The computer communication networks have also moved from local area networks and wide area networks, to the World Wide Web (WWW) and the Internet. In addition to much progress in the local area networks and wide area networks, computer communication using the Web and the Internet offers unlimited access to WWW resources and free electronic mail (e-mail).

Information technology and electronic health record systems have had an impact on the health care delivery system, the management of clinical nursing practice, and have influenced the need to use classification systems such as the ICD-10 to document and code patient care. The classifications, vocabularies, and terminologies emerged as essential for coding and processing raw data into information and knowledge.

Nursing Vocabularies

Nursing vocabularies also emerged as critical to the advancement of the profession. They were created to name nursing phenomena and to document and code clinical nursing practice. Vocabularies have emerged as taxonomies, classifications, and nomenclatures and currently are considered terminologies. Nursing data were considered critical for documenting, coding, and measuring patient care, and were necessary for processing nursing data into information and ultimately into nursing knowledge to advance the science of nursing.

Computer-Based Patient Record

In the early 1990s, the Institute of Medicine convened a committee who determined that the CPR and CPR systems were essential for the implementation of information technology into the health care industry. This committee also recommended that a uniform structure, standardized classifications, and code sets be developed for the health care industry (Dick & Steen, 1991). The CPR systems, currently called electronic health record (EHR) systems, were designed to collect, store, process, display, retrieve, and communicate timely data and information in and across health care facilities. The need for nursing data to also be included in such systems emerged as a critical element for measuring the outcomes of patient care. Nursing data need to be collected as discrete facts (atomic-level data), stored in a relational database, processed, and transformed into meaningful information. Such systems were and continue to be needed to ensure the visibility and viability of clinical nursing practice as well as for its scientific advancement.

REFERENCES

American Nurses Association. (1995). *Nursing Social Policy Statement.* Kansas City, MO: ANA.

American Nurses Association. (1998). *Standards of Clinical Nursing Practice.* Washington, DC: ANA.

Coenen, A., McNeil, B., Bakken, S., Bickford, C., & Warren, J. J. (2001). Toward comparable nursing data: American Nursing Association criteria for data sets, classification systems, and nomenclatures. *Computers in Nursing, 19,* 240–246.

Dick, R. S., & Steen, E. B. (Eds.). (1991). *The Computer-based patient record: An essential technology for health care.* Washington, DC: Institute of Medicine–National Academy Press.

Health Care Financing Administration. (1997). *Medicare home health agency manual.* Washington, DC: HCFA, DHHS.

McCormick, K. A., Lang, N., Zielstorff, R., Milholland, D. K., Saba, V. K., & Jacox, A. (1994). Toward standard classification schemes for nursing languages: Recommendations of the American Nurses Association Steering Committee on Databases to Support Clinical Nursing Practice. *Journal of the American Medical Informatics Association, 1,* 421–427.

National Association for Home Care. (2000). *Basic statistics about home care, 2000.* Washington, DC: NAHC.

North American Nursing Diagnoses Association. (1991). *Taxonomy I: Revised—1991.* St. Louis, MO: NANDA.

Saba, V. K. (1991). *Home health care classification project.* Washington, DC: Georgetown University (NTIS No. PB 92-177013/AS).

Saba, V. K. (1995). A new paradigm for computer-based nursing information systems: Twenty care components. In R. A. Greenes, H. E. Peterson, & D. J. Proti (Eds.), *Medinfo '95 Proceedings* (pp. 1404–1406). Edmonton, Canada: IMIA.

Saba, V. K. (2006). *Clinical Care Classification.* Retrieved February 2006, from <http://www.sabacare.com>.

Saba, V. K., & McCormick, A. (2001). *Essentials of computers for nurses: Informatics in the new millennium* (3rd ed.). New York: McGraw-Hill.

Saba, V. K., & McCormick, A. (2006). *Essentials of nursing informatics* (4th ed.). New York: McGraw-Hill.

Spradley, B. W., & Dorsey, B. (1985). Home health care. In B. W. Spradley (Ed.), *Community health nursing* (pp. 528–549). Boston, MA: Little, Brown & Co.

World Health Organization. (1992). *ICD-10: International statistical classification of diseases and related health problems: Tenth revision, Volume 1.* Geneva, Switzerland: WHO.

FEATURES, USES, AND POLICIES

INTRODUCTION

This chapter focuses on the features, uses, policies, and standards that characterize the Home Health Care Classification (HHCC) system Version 1.0 and the revised and renamed Clinical Care Classification (CCC) system Version 2.0. In this manual, content that describes both versions will only name CCC, unless the content just refers to the HHCC Version 1.0.

The CCC system serves as a standardized language for nursing and other health care providers in all types of health care settings where patient care is provided. The CCC system is designed to assess, document, code, classify, track, and evaluate patient care. Vendors and implementers of information technology (IT) systems also use it to integrate patient care and nursing applications into the electronic health record (EHR).

Definitions

The CCC system consists of two interrelated terminologies: CCC of Nursing Diagnoses and Outcomes and the CCC of Nursing Interventions. The CCC system has been described in the literature and defined as a data set, code set, classification, taxonomy, terminology, and/or nomenclature (Coenen et al., 2001). The two CCC terminologies/code sets can be defined as: (1) classifications because they have a hierarchical structure, (2) taxonomies because they have relationships between levels (major categories and subcategories), (3) terminologies because they represent a system of concepts, and/or (4) nomenclatures because they follow a set of preestablished rules. Each is officially defined by the International Standards Organization (ISO) and presented in the literature by Coenen and colleagues (2001).

EXHIBIT 3.1. CORE CRITERIA FOR ANA RECOGNITION OF NURSING DATA SETS, CLASSIFICATION SYSTEMS, AND NOMENCLATURES[a]

Documentation supports evidence of:

1. Support for nursing practice by providing clinically useful terminology (e.g., nursing diagnoses, nursing interventions, etc.) and rationale for development.
2. A level of development beyond an application, adaptation, or synthesis of currently recognized ANA vocabulary/ classification schemes or presents an explicit rationale for seeking recognition for synthesis, application, or adaption of existing schemes.
3. Clear and unambiguous concepts.
4. Documented testing of reliability, validity, and utility in practice.
5. A systematic method development.
6. A named entity responsible for a formal process of documenting evolving development and maintenance, including tracking of deleted concepts terms and version control.
7. A coding scheme that provides a unique identifier for each concept.
8. Identify pertinent data elements as the variables of interest to whom and within what context.
9. Define the set of possible values for each variable.
10. Provide a clear description of a defined structure or architecture with explicit principles of division.
11. Contain terms that can be combined to represent more complex concepts.
12. Include a classification structure that supports multiple parents and multiple children as relevant.
13. Include preestablished rules for combining the concepts/terms.

[a]Printed with permission from the American Nurses Association (ANA), Washington, DC.
Notes: Criteria 8–13 are additional recognition criteria for specific systems: Data set, classification and/or nomenclature.

Classification: "An assignment of objects into groups based upon the characteristics that have common objects, e.g., origin, composition, structure, function (ISO 11179-1)" (p. 243).

Taxonomy: "Classification according to presumed natural relationships among types and their subtypes (ISO 11179-1)" (p. 243).

Terminology: "The set of terms representing a system of concepts (1SO 1087)" (p. 243).

Nomenclature: A system of designators (terms) elaborate according to preestablished rules (ISO 1087)" (p. 243).

In 1991, the HHCC Version 1.0 was initially *recognized* by the American Nursing Association (ANA) Steering Committee on Databases that Support Nursing Practice and approved by the ANA Congress on Nursing Practice in 1992 (McCormick et al., 1994). In 1998, the ANA criteria for recognizing nursing languages were updated and new features added by the renamed Committee for Nursing Practice Information Infrastructure (CNPII). The new criteria are presented in Exhibit 3.1. The CNPII reaffirmed that the CCC system continues to be recognized as a nursing taxonomy/classification that supports nursing practice.

MAJOR FEATURES

Several informatics theorists and researchers who conducted research, evaluation studies, and other analyses have evaluated the CCC system. The major informatics experts who studied the system not only evaluated different aspects of the classification, but also compared the system to several of the other ANA recognized classifications. The major studies are described in the chapter on "Research and Evaluation Studies." In their writings, the nursing informatics experts also identified the major features of the system based on their observations and conclusions and are used to characterize the CCC.

The CCC system was specifically designed for *computer processing* and computer-based systems. The concepts of the CCC terminologies are not only *granular* or *atomic*, but also are *defined* to ensure *non-ambiguity* and *non-redundancy*. Each concept has a unique identifying code that is used only once and therefore is *context-free*.

The CCC of Nursing Diagnosis terminology uses three qualifiers as **axes** for combining outcomes (expected or actual), and the CCC of Nursing Interventions uses four qualifiers for identifying types of actions, thus making them *multi-axial* and *combinatorial*. The system has a *structured framework* with *coded concepts* that are classified and usable for computer processing *input* and *retrievable for analyses*. The atomic-level concepts (data) used can be used for multiple purposes. They can be used to document nursing care process and therefore provide a *legal record* of patient care. The system also supports clinical decision making, and captures data/*concepts* that can be retrieved, aggregated, and used for analysis and research (Henry & Mead, 1997; Henry et al., 1997).

The CCC meets several of the controlled vocabulary criteria proposed by Cimino (1998) in his article entitled "Desiderata for Controlled Medical Vocabularies in the Twenty-First Century." In 2003, Cimino's nine major criteria for controlled medical vocabularies were used by Walter Sujansky, MD, as the basis for the evaluation criteria of the code sets he identified for the federal government. Dr. Sujansky developed and analyzed a Terminology Questionnaire for the National Committee on Vital and Health Statistics (NCVHS), Subcommittee on Standards and Security, to identify and recommend the standardized code sets for the Core Terminology Group for implementing the Health Insurance Portability and Accountability Act of 1966 (HIPAA) part that addressed the patient medical record information (PMRI), as well as for the electronic exchange of such information (Sujansky, 2003).

At that time, an informatics theorist indicated that the CCC did meet the four major criteria essential for a terminology, namely: (1) Concept Orientation, (2) Concept Permanence, (3) Non-Ambiquity, and (4) Explicit Version IDs that are described below:

Concept Orientation: Elements of the terminology are coded concepts with possible multiple synonymous text representation, and hierarchical or definitional relationships to the coded concepts. No redundant, ambiguous, or vague concepts exist.

Concept Permanence: The meaning of each coded concept as a terminology remains forever unchanged (permanent). If the meaning of a concept needs to be changed or refined, a new coded concept is introduced. No retired codes are deleted or reused.

Non-Ambiguity: Each coded concept in the terminology has a clear, unique meaning and definition, and each represents a single atomic (granular) concept.

Explicit Version IDs: Each coded concept has a unique identifier that is designated for it, thus making it very easy and possible to exchange data from one user to another.

Additionally, several of the other desired technical criteria were primarily met by the CCC system such as it has *No Licensing Fees*, is in the *Public Domain*, and *Responsive to Constituents*. Even though the CCC met the four essential criteria for the Core Terminology Group, it was not selected because it was already integrated into the Systematized Nomenclature of Medicine Clinical Terms (SNOMED CT), which met all the essential and desired criteria for the Core Terminology Group. SNOMED CT had integrated nursing diagnoses and nursing intervention concepts from several of the nursing classification systems into their database including CCC. Thus, the NCVHS Committee determined that SNOMED CT could support the nursing concepts for the implementation of the PMRI. It is of interest that SNOMED CT does map its codes to the CCC system on request and with permission.

MAJOR USES

The CCC system has different dimensions and is used for different purposes. The CCC system's two interrelated terminologies facilitate the electronic documentation at the point of care, permitting the analysis of nursing practices. Their concepts are defined, standardized, and classified, making it possible to link the care process—nursing diagnoses, nursing interventions, and nursing outcomes—together. The coded concepts facilitate the design of computer-based clinical pathways and protocols, decision support, and expert systems. They also make it possible to evaluate nursing practices, develop guidelines, and evidence-based practices, and advance nursing knowledge. Additionally, they facilitate the development of innovation tools for measuring workload, determining cost, and providing administrative information. Such tools can also be used to aggregate data for research on different disease conditions, population groups, and health care settings. The CCC system can improve quality, ensure safety, measure outcomes, and help determine the cost of patient care.

Several vendors are integrating the CCC terminologies in their data dictionaries or vocabulary managers, as well as using them to develop applications, depending on the architecture of the EHR, for documenting patient care. Others employ the CCC for designing plans of care applications or standardized clinical pathways that can be integrated into an EHR system. The CCC system is also being used for educational purposes by providing educators software that can be used to teach students how to document, by computer, patient care following the nursing process using a standardized coded terminology. The CCC system is being used for research by: (1) doctoral students for conducting their theses research; (2) nursing informatics analysts for analyzing aggregated data from the EHR systems to develop disease management clinical pathways, measure outcomes, and determine workload measures and costs; and (3) informatics experts for conducting meta-analysis of the electronic literature and other bibliographic materials to develop evidence-based practice guidelines.

EHR Vendor Uses

Several commercial information technology (IT) vendors have and are currently integrating the CCC Version 2.0 into their EHR systems. Some are designing plans of care applications based on the literature to integrate in their next generation of systems, and still others are coding their existing plans of care for their clients. Additionally, some commercial vendors that just design and develop freestanding applications are creating standardized plans of care pathways to market to EHR system vendors, hospitals, or other health care facilities. On the other hand, several hospitals or health care facilities are designing and coding their own plans of care for inclusion into their existing systems. The original HHCC system Version 1.0 has been integrated and implemented in several home health care computer-based systems.

Educational Uses

The CCC system has been used for several different educational applications, such as those listed below. It is being taught as part of nursing informatics courses that address the nursing classification systems recognized by the ANA and those that describe the characteristics of the nursing terminologies for documenting patient care.

- *Georgetown University:* In the late 1990s, Saba and Sparks designed and tested a method that provided a framework, based on HHCC's 20 Care Components, for nursing students to use for assessing their patients and documenting their plans of care.
- *Columbia University:* Bakken has designed and developed educational software using selected CCC coded concepts. The software has been designed for students to document their clinical nursing practice using their specially programmed PDAs (personal data assistants). Student activities are analyzed, and feedback is provided weekly to both students and faculty (2002 to present).
- *George Mason University:* Feeg has developed a PC-based software for teaching nursing students how to document clinical nursing practice following the six steps of the nursing process using the CCC system. Software is being tested by other nursing schools (2004 to present).

Research Uses

Several research studies have been conducted by nurses using the original HHCC system Version 1.0 and, more recently, the CCC system Version 2.0. Some researchers have evaluated and compared the system to other nursing classifications, such as the North American Nursing Diagnoses Association (NANDA) Diagnostic List, the Omaha System, the Nursing Intervention Classification (NIC), and/or the International Classification of Nursing Practice (ICNP). Other studies have focused on the coding of nursing care of patients in a variety of health care settings, such as the medical, psychiatric, and intensive care units, as well as home health and ambulatory care. Still others have been conducted outside the United States in Korea, the United Kingdom, Norway, and

Finland. Several of these studies are described in the chapter on "Research and Evaluation."

STANDARDS

The HHCC system Version 1.0 was recognized and accepted as a nursing standard by the ANA in 1991, 1992 and reaffirmed as *recognized* in 2000 (see Exhibit 3.1). Since the ANA is the official professional nursing organization, ANA recognition is essential and required for acceptance by governmental, other official authorized users, and/or IT vendors. The U.S. standards organization, the American National Standards Institute-Healthcare Informatics Standards Board (ANSI-HISB), approved the HHCC system Version 1.0 for inclusion in its *Inventory of Clinical Information Standards* (ANSI, 1998, 1999). Another standards organization, the International Standard Organization, Technical Committee 215 (ISO/TC-215), approved, in November 2003, the first international nursing standard entitled, "An Integrated Reference Terminology Model for Nursing" (Steering Committee, 2003). A researcher has tested the CCC system Version 2.0 and confirmed that it is configured according to the two reference terminology (RT) model structures: nursing diagnoses and nursing actions. A summary of the standards and other organizations that have recognized, registered, integrated, or indexed both versions are listed below and also presented more fully in Chapter 2 (Exhibit 2.1). They are:

- ANA: Recognized by the ANA as appropriate classification for supporting clinical nursing practice in the EHR.
- ANA: Recognized by Nursing Information Data Set Evaluation Center (NIDSEC) —as an appropriate terminology for IT vendors applying for approval to use for their nursing documentation.
- HL7: Registered as a Health Level 7 language provides the standard for the messaging communication of health care data from one system to another.
- LOINC: Integrated the CCC of Nursing Diagnosis Outcomes in the Clinical Logical Observation Identifiers, Names, and Codes nomenclature (LOINC).
- UMLS: Integrated in the Metathesaurus of the Unified Medical Language System (UMLS) of the National Library of Medicine (NLM).
- CINAHL: Indexed in the Cumulative Index of Nursing and Allied Health Literature.
- ICNP: Integrated in the International Classification of Nursing Practice (ICNP) developed by the International Council of Nurses (ICN).
- ABC: Adapted the CCC of Nursing Interventions and Actions in Complete Complementary Alternative Medical Billing and Coding Reference (ABC Codes) for Complementary and Alternative Medicine (CAM) and Conventional Nursing.
- SNOMED CT: Integrated in Systematized Nomenclature of Medicine Clinical Terms. (SNOMED CT, which offers separate mapped files of CCC Nursing Diagnoses and CCC of Nursing Interventions and Actions to their codes with permission).

■ PCDS: Adapted by Ozbolt in 1993, the 20 Care Components of HHCC Version 1.0 as the framework for the Patient Care Data Set (PCDS).

TRANSLATIONS

CCC Version 2.0 or HHCC Version 1.0 has been translated into numerous languages: Dutch, Chinese, Portuguese, Spanish, Finnish, German, Korean, and Norwegian. In Norway, it is called SabaKlass. CCC Version 2.0 continues to be translated into other languages.

MAINTENANCE POLICY

The CCC is administered by SabaCo, which is incorporated in the state of Virginia.

The office is located in Arlington, Virginia. Dr. Virginia K. Saba is the current CEO and President of SabaCo. SabaCo has an Advisory Board called the CCC Scientific Advisory Board, which consists of five or more members. The CCC Scientific Advisory Board meets each spring to review suggested concepts, terms, or labels that are proposed by users.

■ To date the HHCC has had one major revision that was finalized on November 18, 2004, and renamed at the same time as the CCC Version 2.0 system. The updated version added 37 new nursing diagnoses, 10 of which were adapted from the *NANDA: Nursing Diagnoses: Definitions & Classification 2001–2002*, and 38 new nursing interventions. See Exhibit 3.2, CCC Version 2.0 News Release, and see Exhibit 3.3 for a summary of two terminologies and core components. Additionally, the concepts that were deleted, renamed, or changed are presented in Appendix Tables A.1, A.2, and A.3.
■ See the Web site <**http://www.sabacare.com**>. It contains CCC Version 2.0 content and translations, including the terminology tables.

Revision Policy

The policy for revising the CCC system has been developed by the Scientific Advisory Board as follows:

■ Review submitted concepts, terms, or labels.
■ Approve of new concepts, terms, or labels.
■ Review the definitions and codes for new concepts, terms, or labels.
■ Determine whether the existing version needs to be revised.
    —Number of concepts has to be sufficient to warrant preparing a new revision.
■ Note that if a revision is recommended, then the developer needs to solicit professional assistance (e.g., Apelon Corporation, Ridgefield, CT) to review and assist with coding of the new, revised concepts, terms, or labels.
■ Request that Sabacare Webmaster upload the revised version on the Web site (<**http://www.sabacare.com**>).

EXHIBIT 3.2. CLINICAL CARE CLASSIFICATION SYSTEM VERSION 2.0 NEWS RELEASE OF NOVEMBER 18, 2004

For information, contact Dr. Virginia K. Saba **www.vsaba@worldnet.att.net**.

For immediate release
{tc /l2 "immediate release}

SABACARE Announces New Version of Home Health Classification System
{tc /l1 "SABACARE Announces New Version of Home Health Classification System}

Washington, DC—November 18, 2004—Sabacare is proud to announce the release of a new version of Home Health Care Classification (HHCC) System. Renamed the **Clinical Care Classification (CCC) System,** this version updates the original HHCC Version 1.0 to CCC Version 2.0. The Web site that hosts the classification remains the same (**www.sabacare.com**).

The new name, **Clinical Care Classification (CCC),** more accurately reflects the purpose of the classification. Recent research has demonstrated that the CCC could be used to document nursing and patient care in any health care environment where nurses practice such as ambulatory care, outpatient clinics, and hospital settings from medical and surgical to critical care units. The CCC can also be used by multidisciplinary teams and by other health care providers.

The updated **CCC Version 2.0** and the new name were approved by the HHCC Scientific Advisory Board who meet annually to review the terminology and make suggested revisions. Version 2.0 follows the coding guidelines of the Unified Medical Language System (UMLS) of the National Library of Medicine.

The updated **CCC Version 2.0** contains a new **Care Component** labeled **Life Cycle,** which addresses the Reproductive and Perinatal Systems, as well as Normal Growth and Development Diagnostic and Care Concepts. The updated CCC of Nursing Diagnoses contains 37 new terms, 10 of which were adapted from NANDA list of Nursing Diagnoses 2001–2002. The CCC of Nursing Interventions contains 38 new interventions that were added and renamed, and a few retired on recommendations by researchers and users of the HHCC.

Specific elements of the Clinical Care Classification (CCC) Version 2.0 include:

Care Components: contains 21 Care Components used to classify and code the taxonomies.

CCC of Nursing Diagnoses: contains 182 Nursing Diagnoses (59 major and 123 subcategories) to label and code Nursing Diagnoses.

CCC of Nursing Outcomes: derived from the CCC of Nursing Diagnoses and contains 546 of Nursing Diagnoses Outcomes using three modifiers (Improved, Stabilized, or Deteriorated) to label and code Expected and/or Actual Outcomes.

CCC of Nursing Interventions: contains 198 (72 major and 126 subcategories) using four Action Type modifiers (Assess, Care, Teach, or Manage) to label and code **792 unique Nursing Interventions.**

All of the changes (Additions, Retired, and Renamed Terms and/or Codes) from Version 1.0 to 2.0 can be found at **www.sabacare.com** in Appendices A1, A2, and A3.

About CCC
The Clinical Care Classification System emerged from the federally funded Home Care Project conducted by Saba and colleagues (1991) at Georgetown University School of Nursing in Washington, DC. The project was funded to develop a method to assess and classify patients to determine the resources required to provide home health services to the Medicare population, including measuring their outcomes of care.

For additional information visit **www.sabacare.com**.
Virginia K. Saba, EdD, DS, RN, FAAN, FACMI, LL
Developer of HHCC & CCC
Consultant: Informatics, Educational Technologies & Community Health Systems
Distinguished Scholar, Adjunct
Georgetown University
Washington, DC
Adjunct Professor
Uniformed Services University
Bethesda, MD

E-mail: **vsaba@worldnet.att.net**
Web Site: <**www.Sabacare.com**>

EXHIBIT 3.3. CLINICAL CARE CLASSIFICATION (CCC) VERSION 2.0: TWO TERMINOLOGIES AND CARE COMPONENTS

CCC of Nursing Diagnoses: 182 labels = 59 major and 123 subcategories
CCC of Nursing Outcomes: 546 labels = 182 Diagnoses and 3 Qualifiers
> **Three Expected Outcomes:**
> (1) to Improve, (2) to Stabilize, or (3) to support Deterioration
> **Actual Outcomes:**
> (1) Improved, (2) Stabilized, or (3) Deteriorated or Died

CCC of Nursing Interventions: 198 Labels = 72 major and 128 subcategories
Nursing Intervention Actions: 792 = 198 Interventions and 4 Qualifiers
> **Four Action Types:**
> (1) Assess/Monitor, (2) Direct Care/Perform, (3) Teach/Instruct, (4) Manage/Refer.

Care Component Classes: 21 Components and 4 Health Patterns
> **Four Health Patterns:**
> (1) Functional, (2) Health Behavioral, (3) Physiological, (4) Psychological
> **21 Care Component Classes:**
> (1) Activity, (2) Bowel/Gastric, (3) Cardiac, (4) Cognitive, (5) Coping, (6) Fluid Volume, (7) Health Behavior, (8) Medication, (9) Metabolic, (10) Nutritional, (11) Physical Regulation, (12) Respiratory, (13) Role Relationship, (14) Safety, (15) Self-Care, (16) Self-Concept, (17) Sensory, (18) Skin Integrity, (19) Tissue Perfusion, (20) Urinary Elimination, (21) Life Cycle

- Prepare and distribute news release regarding new version.
- Prepare new brochure describing new version.
- Distribute the new version to appropriate organizations.
- Distribute the new version to all translators of all versions.
- Notify all known individual users of revisions.

COPYRIGHT AND TRADEMARK

CCC Version 2.0 is copyrighted by Dr. Virginia K. Saba.

- CCC system Version 2.0 received an updated Certificate of Registration "Clinical Care Classification (CCC) System (Version 2.0)" issued by the US Copyright Office, The Library of Congress on October 20, 2004.
- CCC has been placed in the public domain by Dr. Virginia K. Saba, who requires a letter requesting permission from a user. (See "Sample Permission Letter" in Appendix B.)
- Anyone attempting to reproduce the CCC must get permission and must include a disclaimer indicating that the CCC cannot be sold or copyrighted by the publisher.
- CCC received a Service Mark Principal Register (logo) for the "Clinical Care Classification System" from the U.S. Patent and Trademark Office on November 29, 2005. See Exhibit 3.4 for the trademark logo.

In conclusion, the CCC system Version 2.0 is the terminology of choice for documenting nursing practice in the EHR systems. The CCC system continues

EXHIBIT 3.4. SERVICE MARK PRINCIPAL REGISTER (LOGO)

Int. Cl.: 35
Prior US Classes: 100, 101, and 102
US Patent and Trademark Office

Reg. No. 3,019,288
Registered November 29, 2005

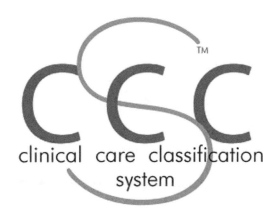

SABA, VIRGINIA K. (UNITED STATES INDIVIDUAL)
E-mail: **vsaba@worldnet.att.net**
Web Site:<**www.Sabacare.com**>

FOR: PROVIDING INFORMATION IN THE FIELD OF CLINICIAL DATA STANDARDS
FOR CODING PATIENT AND NURSING CARE DIAGNOSES, INTERVENTIONS, AND
OUTCOMES, IN CLASS 35 (US CLASSES 100, 101, AND 102).

FIRST USE: 2-0-2004; IN COMMERCE: 2-0-2004

NO CLAIM IS MADE TO THE EXCLUSIVE RIGHT TO USE "CLINICAL CARE CLASSIFICATION
SYSTEM." APART FROM THE MARK AS SHOWN.

SERIES NO.: 76-595,572; FILED: 6-4-2004

ELIZABETH PIGNATELLO, EXAMINING ATTORNEY

EXHIBIT 3.5. WHY CCC?

There are several reasons why the Clinical Care Classification (CCC) system should be
  selected for the nursing language for an electronic health record (EHR) system. It:

- Facilitates the electronic documentation of patient care at the point of care.
- Uses a framework of 21 Care Components to classify the two terminologies and
  represent four health patterns of health care focusing on a holistic approach.
- Consists of discrete atomic-level concepts using qualifiers to enhance and expand
  the concepts. Data are collected only once and are used many times for many purposes,
  and are used for aggregating the data.
- Uses a coding structure of five alphanumeric digits to link the two terminologies to
  each other, as well as map to other classification systems.
- Consists of flexible, adaptable, and expandable concepts/data elements.
- Is copyrighted, but placed in the public domain, thus making it available for anyone
  to use without cost or license, but with permission.

to expand as new concepts, terms, or labels are recommended by different nursing specialty users. Because of its structure, it can be expanded easily. Why CCC should be selected is outlined in Exhibit 3.5.

REFERENCES

ANSI-HISB. (1998/1999). Home health care classification (HHCC) of nursing diagnosis & nursing interventions. *Inventory of Clinical Information Standards*. Washington, DC: ANSI.

Cimino, J. J. (1998). Desiderata for controlled medical vocabularies in the twenty-first century. *Methods of Information in Medicine, 37,* 304–403.

Coenen, A., McNeil, B., Bakken, S., Bickford, C., & Warren, J. J. (2001). Toward comparable nursing data: American Nursing Association criteria for data sets, classification systems, and nomenclatures. *Computers in Nursing, 19,* 240–246.

Henry, S. H., & Mead, C. N. (1997). Nursing classifications systems; necessary but not sufficient for representing "what nurses do" for inclusion in computer-based patient record systems. *Journal of the American Medical Informatics Association, 4,* 222–232.

Henry, S. H., Warren, J. J., Lange, L., & Button, P. (1998). A review of major nursing vocabularies and the extent to which they have the characteristics required for implementation in computer-based systems. *Journal of the American Medical Informatics Association, 5,* 321–328.

McCormick, K. A., Lang, N., Zielstorff, R., Milholland, D. K., Saba, V. K., & Jacox, A. (1994). Toward standard classification schemes for nursing languages: Recommendations of the American Nurses Association Steering Committee on databases to support clinical nursing practice. *Journal of the American Medical Informatics Association, 1,* 421–427.

North American Nursing Diagnosis Association. (2001). *NANDA: Nursing diagnoses: Definitions & classification 2001–2002.* Philadelphia, PA: NANDA.

Ozbolt, J. (1994). Toward data standards for clinical nursing information. *Journal of American Medical Informatics Association, 1,* 175–185.

Steering Committee for ISO/FDIS 18104. (2003, September). Nursing language—Terminology models for nurses. *ISO Bulletin,* pp. 16–18.

Sujansky, W. (2003, September 1). Unpublished Report. *Summary and analysis of user testimony for PMRI terminology standards: A report to the national committee on vital and health statistics, subcommittee on standards and security: Version 3.* Washington, DC: NCVHS.

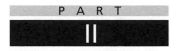

P A R T

II

RESEARCH, INTEGRATION, AND EVALUATION

4

RESEARCH AND EVALUATION STUDIES

Scope 29   Studies 30

SCOPE

During the past decade, several nursing researchers or nursing informatics theorists conducted studies on the nursing languages recognized by the American Nurses Association (ANA) or evaluated them, including the Clinical Care Classification (CCC) Version 2.0 system or the Home Health Care Classification (HHCC) Version 1.0 system (Saba, 1991). The studies focused primarily on three major areas: (1) describing the characteristics and/or features of the ANA *recognized* classifications; (2) comparing the system to other *recognized* classifications, such as the North American Nursing Diagnosis Association (NANDA) Diagnoses List; and (3) using the system to code nursing care of patients in new settings (e.g., hospitals) or patients with special conditions (e.g., depression) or patients requiring special care (e.g., postoperative coronary artery bypass graft surgery).

Several of the major studies and/or evaluations are described below. However, the researchers and/or evaluators did recognize that the CCC system uses a standardized framework to support the documentation, coding, and classification of clinical nursing practice. Several agreed that the system's two interrelated terminologies—CCC of Nursing Diagnoses and Outcomes and CCC of Nursing Interventions and Actions—were developed for computerization, making them easy to integrate into a computer-based information technology (IT) system. Others acknowledged that the system terminologies consist of granular, atomic concepts; have unique identifiers and definitions; and are coded, easily manipulated, and retrieved by the computer. Also, they concurred that the CCC system's standardized framework makes it possible to link the six steps of Nursing Process Standards of Care (ANA, 1998) together to measure outcomes. Others indicated that the standardized coded concepts and measures can be used to improve quality, ensure safety, measure outcomes, as well as determine workload and cost. The studies are annotated according to the year published.

STUDIES

1. In 1993, Zielstorff and colleagues conducted a study mapping patient problems, nursing diagnoses, or diagnostic terms from three vocabularies, classifications, or nomenclatures: (1) the Home Health Care Classification (HHCC) Version 1.0, (2) the NANDA Diagnoses List, and (3) the Omaha System. A mapping of term to term was conducted to determine commonalities and differences, as well as to determine whether it was possible to develop a single vocabulary that contained the best features of all.

Three pairs of mappings were developed: (1) NANDA Diagnoses List to HHCC of Nursing Diagnoses, Version 1.0; (2) NANDA Diagnoses List to Omaha System Problem List; and (3) HHCC of Nursing Diagnoses to the Omaha System Problem List. The terms from each of the three vocabularies were mapped to the terms in each of the other vocabularies. The terms were characterized as: (1) Same, (2) Similar, (3) Broader, (4) Narrower, and (5) No Match. Once completed, the mapping was validated by conducting reverse mappings.

In the three vocabularies, there were a total of 396 terms: (1) 128 from the NANDA Diagnoses List, (2) 146 from the HHCC of Nursing Diagnoses, and (3) 122 from the Omaha System Problem List of 40 problems with three modifiers each, which totaled 1,268 relationships. The findings from the 396 terms revealed: (1) 21 concepts accounted for 63 terms that were found to be the same or similar in all of the three vocabularies, (2) 91 terms did not match and were unique to the vocabulary in which they were found, and (3) 242 were found to have a broader or narrower match to at least one term in one other vocabulary.

The research team concluded that because of the differences in structure and incompatibilities in the three vocabularies, a master list of preferred terms was not feasible. They indicated that the Metathesaurus of the Unified Medical Language System (UMLS) of the National Library of Medicine (NLM) lacked concept matches for the majority of terms in the three vocabularies and were not labeled diagnoses or problems but findings. **The research did demonstrate that the process of mapping in a computer-based system did allow for the translation of a nursing diagnosis from one setting to another using different vocabularies.**

(Source: Zielstorff, R. D., Tronni, C., Basque, J., Griffin, L. R., & Welebob, E. M. (1998). Mapping nursing diagnosis nomenclatures for coordinated care. *Image: Journal of Nursing Scholarship, 30*, 369–373.)

2. Ozbolt and colleagues (1994) conducted a study in the early 1990s at the University of Virginia, Thomas Jefferson University Hospital, to develop standard terms and codes for documenting nursing care. Standardized care terms from the nursing units in two hospitals were compiled, classified, and coded. However, the research team determined that the first task in developing a standard vocabulary was to find a way to classify the terms. **They determined that the 20 Care Components from the Home Health Care Classification (HHCC) Version 1.0 (Saba, 1991) provide a useful organizing framework for nursing problems and interventions in the hospital setting. The HHCC also provides a conceptual meaningful structure that would assist the researchers in classifying the terms being developed.** They accepted all of the

Care Components but one (Metabolic), which they split into two separate components (Metabolic and Immunological) and also added a new component (Pre-Intra/Post-Procedure), thus resulting in 22 Components. The research team used the 22 Care Components for classifying the three separate lists of: (1) Nursing Diagnoses/Patient Care Problems, (2) Expected Patient Outcomes, and (3) Nursing Interventions/Patient Care Activities. The terms for each of the three lists were recorded only once and placed under a single Care Component, making data analysis feasible and possible. In July 1992, the resulting preliminary Patient Care Data Set (PCDS)—consisting of 209 nursing diagnoses or patient problems, 122 expected patient outcomes, and 545 patient care interventions—was created.

(Source: Ozbolt, J., Fruchtnicht, J. N., & Hayden, J. R. (1994). Toward data standards for clinical nursing information. *Journal of the American Medical Informatics Association, 1,* 175–185.)

3. In 1995, Parlocha and Henry (1998) conducted a research study that tested usefulness of the Home Health Care Classification (HHCC) Version 1.0 for coding patient problems and nursing interventions of home care elderly psychiatric patients with major depressive disorder (MDD). Closed medical records from patients with MDD were obtained from a large Visiting Nurse Association in Northern California. The sample was derived from a computer search of the patient records for the previous 5-year period and generated 193 records from which a random sample of 50 records were chosen. The patients in the sample were predominately elderly White women who lived alone or with friends or relatives.

The textual and manual data were abstracted from the nursing notes as either Problem or Intervention and were coded using the two HHCC terminologies. A total of 3,328 entries from 522 visits were collected, which represented 2,917 patient problems or nursing diagnoses and 3,243 nursing interventions. Also, using the HHCC Nursing Intervention Action Types, the data depicted that 1,391 nursing interventions were involved in teaching, 1,308 involved in assessment, 353 involved in management, and only 191 involved in direct care. **The researchers determined that the HHCC system could be used to code and classify the majority of patient problems/nursing diagnoses and nursing interventions with MDD.** They also identified that, for the MDD psychiatric population, 34 additional codes were needed for new diagnostic terms and/or problems but only two new codes were needed for the nursing interventions.

In conclusion, the HHCC system was considered to be a useful tool for many different analyses, such as quality assurance, care planning, and critical path development. Also, the coding system could be used for predicting resource requirements as well as linking nursing interventions with patient outcomes. They concluded that quantifiable nursing services could be a powerful weapon for financial support.

(Source: Parlocha, P. K., & Henry, S. B. (1998). The usefulness of the Georgetown Home Health Care Classification system for coding patient problems and nursing interventions in psychiatric home care. *Computers in Nursing, 16,* 45–52.)

4. As part of the study by Holzemer and colleagues (1997) on Quality of Nursing Care of People with AIDS, they evaluated the utility of the HHCC Version 1.0 system for classifying and coding patient problems and nursing interventions. The HHCC was selected for several reasons: (1) The research team wanted a single classification that could be used across settings, in and out of the hospital setting. They were influenced by Ozbolt and associates' acceptance of using the HHCC's Care Components for classifying patient care in the hospital setting. (2) They wanted to have the ability to code both patient problems and nursing interventions using a single classification system, including the Care Components for classifying and aggregating the data in order to potentially provide useful data analysis. (3) They also wanted the ability to differentiate between the Action Types of Nursing Interventions that would be useful in linking interventions with patient problems and outcomes, as well as with possible resource utilization. The study was undertaken to determine whether the HHCC system could be used in the hospital setting, and to identify what level (Care Component, Major Concept, or Subcategory Concept) could be used to code both the patient problem and nursing intervention data.

The study consisted of data from 600 patient encounters for 201 patients with AIDS who were hospitalized with pneumonia. The study was designed to understand the linkages between the patient problems, nursing interventions, and patient outcomes. Data were collected from three hospital settings with three different care planning systems and three different types of nursing notes. The patient terms that were collected from multiple sources resulted in 5,844 patient problems and 20,055 nursing interventions that had to be coded and classified.

They determined that patient problems and nursing interventions could be categorized using the 20 Care Components and/or Major Categories. They further demonstrated that all the classified nursing intervention terms could be coded according to the four Action Types of Nursing Interventions and concluded that the Action Type qualifiers were potentially useful attributes for the comparison of patient care among care settings. This study also demonstrated that the HHCC could be used to classify large numbers of atomic-level data into categories (Care Components) and used for meaningful analyses in the hospital as well as in home care settings.

(Source: Holzemer, W. L., Henry, S. B., Dawson, C., Sousa, K., Bain, C., & Hsieh, S.-F. (1997). An evaluation of the utility of the Home Health Care Classification for categorizing patient problems and nursing interventions from the hospital setting. In U. Gerdin, M. Tallberg, & P. Wainwright (Eds.), *NI-99: Nursing informatics: The impact of nursing knowledge on health care informatics* (pp. 21–26). Stockholm, Sweden: IOS Press.)

5. Henry and Mead (1997) prepared an article discussing the nursing intervention phase of the nursing process or the execution of the plan of care. They provided an analysis of three nursing classification systems *recognized* by the ANA, namely: (1) Home Health Care Classification (HHCC), (2) Nursing Intervention Classification (NIC), and (3) the Omaha System, for use in the computer-based patient record (CPR). They provided an overview of the

content and evaluations described in earlier studies, highlighted the formal type and structure based on the Ingenerf typology of vocabularies, and used patient records from home care patients to demonstrate examples of data transformation.

The HHCC evaluation studies presented above were highlighted. **They indicated that, according to the Ingenerf typology, the HHCC can be considered as a classification system since it possesses an attribute of a combinatorial taxonomic vocabulary in that the nursing interventions are biaxial: the core intervention focuses on the activity or service, and the second axis focuses on the modifier action types—Assess, Direct Care, Teach, or Manage.** They also determined that the HHCC's definition of a nursing intervention as a single nursing action is more granular than NIC even though in some instances they are not uniformly abstracted as a single nursing action. They indicated that there was still a need for a comprehensive controlled vocabulary for capturing atomic-level nursing action data that could be added to the existing classification systems.

(Source: Henry, S. B., & Mead, C. N. (1997). Nursing classifications systems; necessary but not sufficient for representing "A What Nurses Do" for inclusion in computer-based patient record systems. *Journal of the American Medical Informatics Association, 4* , 222–232.)

6. Henry, Warren, Lange, and Button (1998) reviewed the evaluation literature related to the six major nursing classification systems recognized by the ANA, namely the Home Health Care Classification (HHCC) system, the North American Nursing Diagnoses Association (NANDA) Diagnoses List, the Nursing Intervention Classification (NIC), the Nursing Outcome Classification (NOC), the Omaha System, and the International Classification of Nursing Practice (ICNP). Their goal was to determine the extent to which they possess the characteristics needed for implementation in computer-based systems. They presented a chronological review of studies related to nursing classification systems, several of which are described above. They presented the features and characteristics of a formal terminology as defined by Ingenerf in his typology for taxonomies and/or vocabularies that addressed concept representation.

Of the 13 features presented, only three of the six nursing classifications that classified nursing interventions—**HHCC, the Omaha System, and the ICNP—have five features needed for the computer-based systems. They include: (1) atomic and compositional character, (2) attributes (modifiers and qualifiers), (3) hierarchies and inheritance (multiple parents or children), (4) unique identifiers (codes), and (5) definitions (concise explanations of meaning).** They indicated that none of the nursing classifications contained all of the proposed features. They further described that several of the nursing classifications became a part of the Metathesaurus of the Unified Medical Language System (UMLS), in which the terms were linked and presented with other coded concepts but with minimal mappings. However, the mapping between classifications has been prepared, such as the mapping between ICNP and HHCC. They recommended that several areas for future research were needed to meet the needs of nursing for the development of vocabularies into computer-based systems.

(Source: Henry, S. B., Warren, J. J., Lange, L., & Button, P. (1998). A review of major nursing vocabularies and the extent to which they have the characteristics required for implementation in computer-based systems. *Journal of the American Medical Informatics Association, 5,* 321–328.)

7. Another study conducted by Bakken and colleagues (2000) evaluated the adequacy of the semantic structure of Clinical LOINC (Logical Observation Identifiers, Names, and Codes), originally designed to support laboratory results reporting as a terminology model for standardized clinical assessment measures. The research team dissected 1,096 items from 35 standardized assessment instruments, including the Home Health Care Classification (HHCC) system into the elements of the Clinical LOINC semantic structure.

The results supported the adequacy of the Clinical LOINC semantic structure as a terminology model for standardized assessments. Using the revised definitions, the research coders were able to dissect all the standardized assessment items in the sample instruments into the Clinical LOINC axes. This evaluation was an initial step toward the representation of standardized assessment items. Also, they determined that classification by component and dimension would make it possible to retrieve assessments.

As a result of the study, they extended Clinical LOINC to support common assessment instruments. They considered the 146 Nursing Goals/Expected Outcomes from the HHCC Classification of Nursing Diagnoses classified by 20 Care Components as a standardized nursing assessment and its three outcome qualifiers—Improved, Stabilized, or Deteriorated—as possible values to evaluate outcomes of health care. They further suggested that Care Components could be useful for the classification of standardized assessments.

(Source: Bakken, S., Cimino, J. J., Haskell, R., Kukafka, R., Matsumoto, C., Chan, G. K., & Huff, S. M. (2000). Evaluation of clinical LOINC (logical observation identifiers, names, and codes). *Journal of the American Medical Informatics Association, 7,* 529–538.)

8. In 2000, Bakken and colleagues conducted another study on concept-oriented terminologies that they defined as being used "to refer to a terminology in which the concepts are formally defined (e.g., using description logic) in a manner that renders them suitable for computer processing" (p. 83). She focused the study on the evaluation of the adequacy and utility of a type definition for a nursing activity in which the intentional service is performed by a provider to a recipient. The study focused on three attributes: Delivery Mode, Activity Focus, and Recipient. The Delivery Mode is the means or Action Types by which the activity is administered (e.g., the HHCC Action Types—Assess, Direct Care, Teach, Manage), the Activity Focus is the problem being addressed or the focus of the intervention, and Recipient is the person, family, or other to whom the activity is performed.

The study data were obtained from 1,039 nursing activity terms from 300 patients hospitalized with HIV/AIDS-related health problems. They were matched with two nursing terminologies: the HHCC of Nursing Interventions and the Omaha System Intervention List. The terms were decomposed into the three attributes for the type definition: Delivery Mode, Activity Focus, and

Recipient. Each of the three attributes was coded as present or absent for each term by several raters; the Delivery Mode was rated as Explicit or Implicit; and the Recipient was rated as Explicit, Implicit, or Ambiguous.

The results demonstrated that the three attributes of the type definition for a component of the concept-oriented terminology structure were present in 73.9% of the chart terms. **Attributes of the type definition were present in the HHCC of Nursing Interventions as follows: Delivery Mode (Assess, Direct Care, Teach, or Manage), 100%; Activity Focus, 100%; and Recipient, 78.3%. Overall, the HHCC of Nursing Interventions matched 91.3% of the chart terms compared with only 63.5% of the Omaha System Intervention List terms. Finally, based on these results, the authors suggested that since the HHCC is in the public domain, it is more readily available for convergence as a concept-oriented terminology for health care in a computer-based system than proprietary terminologies**.

(Source: Bakken, S., Cashen, M. S., Mendonca, E. A., O'Brien, A., & Sieniewicz, J. (2000). Representing nursing activities within a concept-oriented terminological system. *Journal of the American Medical Informatics Association, 7*, 81–90.)

9. In 2000, Bakken and colleagues conducted an evaluation of the International Classification of Nursing Practice (ICNP) as terminology model components of nursing actions. They wanted to determine the percentage of terms or term phrases from two terminologies—Home Health Care Classification (HHCC) and the Patient Care Data Set (PCDS)—that contained the semantic categories represented in the eight intervention axes of the ICNP. The eight nursing action axes focus on: (1) Action Type, (2) Target, (3) Beneficiary, (4) Times, (5) Means, (6) Topology, (7) Location, and (8) Route. They also wanted to compare these eight axes with those found in SNOMED (Systematized Nomenclature of Medical Clinical Terms)-reference terminology (RT) 12 high-level semantic categories.

The researchers identified the percentage of terms or term phrases in the HHCC of Nursing Interventions that could be dissected into valid ICNP axes. **They found that the HHCC of Nursing Interventions contained primarily those in three ICNP axes: (1) 100% Action Types, (2) 90% Implicit Beneficiary, and (3) 100% Target**. The results related to evaluation of the SNOMED semantic model led to the recommendation that SNOMED would have to expand their links semantic model to support the terms or term phrases from the HHCC of Nursing Interventions and other nursing intervention classification systems.

(Source: Bakken, S., Parker, J., Konicek, D., & Campbell, K. E. (2000). An evaluation of ICNP intervention axes as terminology model components. *American Medical Informatics Association 2000 Proceedings* (pp. 42–46). Washington, DC: AMIA.)

10. In 2001, Coenen et al. described the American Nurses Association (ANA) Committee for Nursing Practice Information Infrastructure (CNPII) revised criteria for recognition of nursing language systems. In 1989, the new CNPII that emerged from the ANA Steering Committee on Databases to Support Clinical Nursing Practices was formed. In 1992, the Database Committee

developed the original criteria for the first four recognized nursing classifications: the Home Health Care Classification (HHCC) System, the NANDA Diagnoses List, the Omaha System, and the Nursing Intervention Classification (NIC). They were subsequently submitted to the National Library of Medicine (NLM) for inclusion into the Metathesaurus of the Unified Medical Language System (UMLS). The Database Committee was also influential in promoting professional information on the uses of computer-based nursing data, as well as the need for professional nursing practice standards and guidelines.

The new CNPII was given new mandates that made it necessary to review and revise the ANA's original criteria used to *recognize* the nursing classification systems. The committee expanded the criteria to distinguish between the various existing classifications, such as data sets, classification systems, and/or nomenclatures. The new criteria addressed: (1) development of standardized terminologies with structure and content different from traditional classification systems; (2) improvements in methods and instruments to produce computable concepts; and (3) intent to harmonize with recognized standards, namely Health Level Seven (HL7), International Standards Organization (ISO), the European Committee on Standardization (CEN), and the American National Standards Institute-Health Information Standards Board (ANSI-HISB). They also discussed the need for different health care data standards and the role of the ANA in this effort. Even though none of the original criteria was omitted, an additional core criterion was established recommending that developers build on existing systems.

The CNPII reaffirmed that the HHCC system was recognized as one of the original classification systems. Furthermore, they indicated that, according to the International Standards Organization (ISO) standards, the HHCC of Nursing Diagnoses and the HHCC of Nursing Interventions are each considered to be a taxonomy. The ISO definition for a taxonomy is a "Classification according to presumed natural relationship among types and their subtypes" (ISO 11179-1). Also, the ISO definition of a classification is: "An assignment of objects into groups based upon characteristics that have common objects, e.g. origin, composition, structure, function" (ISO 11179-1). Thus, the work of ANA's CNPII is responsible for continued assistance to vocabulary developers and users to ensure that nursing practice data can be collected at the point of care and reused for cost, quality, decision support, and health care policy development.

(Source: Coenen, A., McNeil, B., Bakken, S., Bickford, C., & Warren, J. J. (2001). Toward comparable nursing data: American Nursing Association criteria for data sets, classification systems, and nomenclatures. *Computers in Nursing, 19,* 240–246.)

11. In 2001, Hardiker, from the United Kingdom, conducted a research study that compared the nursing interventions of the HHCC system of Nursing Interventions, NIC, and the Omaha System Intervention List to develop a mechanism for mediating between diverse nursing intervention terminology systems. Of the three terminology systems included in the study, the **HHCC of Nursing Interventions had the largest number of terms (640 potential**

terms through post co-ordination) and the richest taxonomic structure between nursing interventions (through the classification of minor categories as major categories). The research used a formal terminology system to expose underlying concepts, thereby making it possible to map automatically between nursing interventions drawn from the three terminology systems. The research revealed that, although there were some similarities between nursing interventions drawn from different terminology systems, differences in content and structure make direct comparison difficult.

(Source: Hardiker, N. (2001). Mediating between nursing intervention terminology systems. In S. Bakken (Ed.), *A medical informatics odyssey: Visions of the future and lessons from the past* (pp. 239–243). Philadelphia: Hanley & Belfus, Inc.)

12. In 2004, Moss and colleagues (2005) conducted a study to evaluate the ability of the revised and renamed Clinical Care Classification (CCC) Version 2.0 classified by 21 Care Components (formerly known as HHCC Version 1.0 classified by 20 Care Components) to represent data in an acute care setting, and to determine if the CCC can be utilized to examine nursing practices related to the care of cardiovascular surgical patients. They focused the study on the interventions documented by nurses in the care of 50 randomly selected adult cardiovascular surgical patients undergoing coronary artery bypass graft (CABG) surgery. The data they collected from the documentation were entered into a computerized information system during the care provided during the first 24 hours postoperatively. The patient-generated nursing interventions were entered, dissected into words and phrases corresponding to the structure of the CCC of Nursing Interventions and Actions that consist of core interventions and four different Action Types—Assess, Direct Care, Teach, and Manage.

The researchers used a variation of content analysis. Through the use of systematic rules for selecting and processing recorded content, they were able to dissect and map the majority of the 219,476 study entries—words and phrases—collected to the existing terms found in the CCC of Nursing Interventions and Actions. However, several terms related primarily to the care of specific devices concerning CABG patients were not found, such as hemodynamic monitoring, balloon pump care, chest tube care, and/or arterial line care. (They have been proposed as possible new terms in the next version of the CCC.)

Analysis of the data indicated that the documentation was related to the Physical Regulation Care Component representing 40.1% and fluid volume representing 31.4%. Furthermore, the major Action Type was Monitor with 81% and Assess with 17%, and the remaining 2% represented the Action Types: Perform or Direct Care, Teach or Instruct, and Manage or Refer. **The findings did identify and determine useful nursing practice patterns and demonstrate that the CCC is a useful terminology for itemizing nursing care, for determining nursing care costs, and providing possible reimbursement.**

(Source: Moss, J., Damrongsak, M., & Gallichio, K. (2005). Representing critical care data using the clinical care classification. In C. P. Friedman, J. Ash, & P. Tarcy-Hornoch (Eds.), *American Medical Informatics Association 2005*

Proceedings: CD-ROM (pp. 545–549). Washington, DC: OmniPress, Omnipro-CD.)

13. In 2005, a study was conducted by Choi et al. that focused on the formal representation of the Outcomes and Assessment Information Set (OASIS-B1) mandated by the federal government as a concept-oriented terminology. To accomplish this, the researchers: (1) evaluated the utility of Logical Observation Identifiers, Names, and Codes (LOINC) as a terminology model to represent OASIS-B1 terms; (2) compared the OASIS-B1 terms located in LOINC with three sets of nursing terms in LOINC, namely the Home Health Care Classification (HHCC) system, the Omaha System, and the Sign and Symptom Check List for persons with HIV/AIDS; (3) assessed the modifications needed to integrate OASIS-B1 into the LOINC structure; and (4) implemented a user-friendly interface for data entry and retrieval of OASIS-B1 terms using the Dialogix system.

Two hundred nine OASIS-B1 items were dissected into the six elements of the LOINC semantic structure. Each OASIS-B1 term was mapped to the LOINC terms in the HHCC, the Omaha System, and the Sign and Symptom Check List for persons with HIV/AIDS. They were classified as no match (0) to exact match (4). **Of the 208 terms, 204 were dissected into elements of LOINC and 151 mapped to one or more nursing terms, including the HHCC of Nursing Diagnoses with actual or expected outcomes.** The study suggested that building a hierarchical structure of nursing concepts within LOINC to facilitate information retrieval of related terms and concepts was desirable, and that LOINC could be used to provide a standard way to formally represent home health care data for integration into the electronic patient record for monitoring outcomes across sites and for retrieval of evidence-based practice.

(Source: Choi, J., Jenkins, M. L., Cimino, J. J., White, T. M., & Bakken, S. (2005). Toward semantic interoperability in home health care: Formally representing OASIS items for integration into a concept-oriented terminology. *Journal of the American Medical Informatics Association, 12,* 410–417.)

14. Bakken et al. (2005) illustrated the utility of using Home Health Care Classification (HHCC) to calculate the dosage and determine the extent of tailoring of a nurse-delivered medication adherence intervention. A sample of 117 persons with HIV/AIDS from the intervention arm of the Client Adherence Profiling-Intervention Tailoring (CAP-IT) randomized controlled trial participated in the analysis. Based on previous research, Holzemer et al. (1997) demonstrated the utility of the HHCC to categorize patient problems and nursing interventions from multiple data sources. As a result, the study team selected the HHCC renamed CCC to calculate the CAP-IT doses and determine the extent of tailoring the delivered intervention.

The patients completed the CAP to obtain their specific self-reported needs, such as medication-taking knowledge, etc. The nurse selected the appropriate nursing diagnoses from the CCC of Nursing Diagnoses based on the CAP responses. Also at the initial clinic visit, the study nurse determined and administered the tailored set of CCC nursing interventions, which were based on the CAP scores and selected nursing diagnoses. Nursing interventions were documented using the CCC of Nursing Interventions and the time spent for each category of interventions. Then booster interventions were made during three telephone calls during the first week after the initial visit. The patients returned to the clinic for follow-up at 1 and 3 months, during which the patients were reassessed and delivered interventions as needed. The findings were significant such as all patients had at least one CCC Nursing Diagnosis related to medication knowledge, adherence, and self-care management of side effects, and they also received at least one intervention addressing these same three concepts. Data demonstrated a relationship between patient CCC Nursing Diagnoses and CCC Nursing Interventions. The study demonstrated that CAP-IT was a nursing process framework for the structured documentation of nursing diagnoses and nursing interventions. Measurement of the intervention dose was calculated by the number of interventions and time associated with them, and served as the basis for the analysis of the tailored interventions.

This study concluded that the nursing process framework using the structured standardized CCC of Nursing Diagnoses and the CCC of Nursing Interventions was useful in measuring the dose and tailoring interventions. The authors recommended that using a standardized terminology such as the CCC is essential to incorporate in the study protocols to facilitate documentation of nursing diagnoses and to measure nursing interventions.

(Source: Bakken, S., Holzemer, W. L., Portillo, C. J., Grimes, R., Welch, J., & Wantland, D. (2005). Utility of a standardized nursing terminology to evaluate dosage and tailoring of an HIV/AIDS adherence intervention. *Journal of Nursing Scholarship, 37,* 251–257.)

15. In 2004, Feeg and colleagues conducted a study to develop and test a bedside personal computer (PC) Clinical Care Classification (CCC) system for nursing students using Microsoft Access. The study tested a PC-based version of the CCC system developed by Saba and colleagues on students' performance of charting patient care plans. The software application was designed as an inexpensive alternative to nurse charting for use on any laptop or PC with Windows and Microsoft Access and to serve as an instructional documentation system for students to learn and use in classroom/laboratory experiences in order to prepare for the electronic documentation of the patient care they provide in their various clinical placements. The system used the standardized CCC nursing terminology to assist students with the methodological incorporation of all aspects of the nursing process.

The project was developed to evaluate the effectiveness of electronic charting simulation using a bedside PC in the clinical skills laboratory to document patient care planning. The project had two aims: (1) to design the PC application using the standardized CCC in an off-the-shelf Microsoft Program to record care planning efficiently using a PC, and (2) to conduct an evaluation of the nursing student electronic charting using a randomized design to the PC based on using the CCC versus narrative text-only type in bedside computer in the clinical laboratory. A randomized controlled trial with the experimental group using the Microsoft Access database program of the CCC designed specifically for the study and a control group using "fillable" Acrobat table formats allowed students to type in the care provided in the text area for each of the six boxes of the nursing process.

The computer-based application using the CCC system was designed by Feeg with the assistance of a Microsoft Access programmer. They revised several iterations of the software that was tested and retested until all the required documentation was possible. The PC screen was designed so that the six steps of the nursing process appeared on one screen and were developed so that they had to be sequentially followed: (1) Assessment (Care Components), (2) Diagnosis (Nursing Diagnosis), (3) Outcome Identification (Expected Outcomes), (4) Planning (Intervention), (5) Implementation (Action Types), and (6) Evaluation (Actual Outcomes). A convenience sample of approximately 30 student volunteers were recruited and given two patient case descriptions in writing, as well as being allowed to interview two actors who portrayed the case conditions. The experimental group of students was then given a laptop with the application to record the care plan, whereas the control group was given the text-based version to document their care plan.

The study data analyses and findings demonstrated that the software application was efficient and effective in recording nursing care planning using a standardized terminology (CCC) following the nursing process in a PC computer-based system, whereas the type-in text was not standardized and the care plans varied among the students. Thus, with the growing use of the electronic health record (EHR), the need to use software applications to electronically document patient care is becoming critical and this application was determined to have great potential in teaching students of tomorrow's electronic care planning.

(Source: Feeg, V. D., Saba, V. K., & Feeg, A. (in press). Development and testing of a bedside personal computer (PC) Clinical Care Classification System (CCCS) for nursing students using Microsoft Access. *Computers In Nursing.*)

These research and/or evaluation studies all demonstrated the utility of the CCC system and its two terminologies classified by 21 Care Components. They have presented proof of the CCC's value for documenting nursing care of patients in the EHR.

REFERENCES

American Nurses Association. (1998). *Standards of clinical pursing practice.* Washington, DC: ANA.

Bakken, S., Cashen, M. S., Mendonca, E. A., O'Brien, A., & Sieniewicz, J. (2000). Representing nursing activities within a concept-oriented terminological system. *Journal of the American Medical Informatics Association, 7,* 81–90.

Bakken, S., Cimino, J. J., Haskell, R., Kukafka, R., Matsumoto, C., Chan, G. K., et al. (2000). Evaluation of clinical LOINC (logical observation identifiers, names, and codes). *Journal of the American Medical Informatics Association, 7,* 529–538.

Bakken, S., Holzemer, W. L., Portillo, C. J., Grimes, R., Welch, J., & Wantland, D. (2005). Utility of a standardized nursing terminology to evaluate dosage and tailoring of an HIV/AIDS adherence intervention. *Journal of Nursing Scholarship, 37,* 251–257.

Bakken, S., Parker, J., Konicek, D., & Campbell, K. E. (2000). An evaluation of ICNP intervention axes as terminology model components. *American Medical Informatics Association 2000 Proceedings* (pp. 42–46). Washington, DC: AMIA.

Choi, J., Jenkins, M. L., Cimino, J. J., White, T. M., & Bakken, S. (2005). Toward semantic interoperability in home health care: Formally representing OASIS items for integration into a concept-oriented terminology. *Journal of the American Medical Informatics Association, 12,* 410–417.

Coenen, A., McNeil, B., Bakken, S., Bickford, C., & Warren, J. J. (2001). Toward comparable nursing data: American Nursing Association criteria for data sets, classification systems, and nomenclatures. *Computers in Nursing, 19,* 240–246.

Feeg, V. D., Saba, V. K, & Feeg, A. (in press). Development and testing of a bedside personal computer (PC) clinical care classification system (CCCS) for nursing students using Microsoft Access. *Computers in Nursing.*

Hardiker, N. (2001). Mediating between nursing intervention terminology systems. In S. Bakken (Ed.), *A medical informatics odyssey: Visions of the future and lessons from the past* (pp. 239–243). Philadelphia: Hanley & Belfus, Inc.

Henry, S. H., & Mead, C. N. (1997). Nursing classifications systems; necessary but not sufficient for representing "what nurses do" for inclusion in computer-based patient record systems. *Journal of the American Medical Informatics Association, 4,* 222–232.

Henry, S. H., Warren, J. J., Lange, L., & Button, P. (1998). A review of major nursing vocabularies and the extent to which they have the characteristics required for implementation in computer-based systems. *Journal of the American Medical Informatics Association, 5,* 321–328.

Holzemer, W. L., Henry, S. B., Dawson, C., Sousa, K., Bain, C., & Hsieh, S.-F. (1997). An evaluation of the utility of the home health care classification for categorizing patient problems and nursing interventions from the hospital setting. In U. Gerdin, M. Tallberg, & P. Wainwright (Eds.), *NI99: Nursing informatics: The impact of nursing knowledge on health care informatics* (pp. 21–26). Stockholm, Sweden: IOS Press.

Moss, J., Damrongsak, M., & Gallichio, K. (2005). Representing critical care data using the clinical care classification. In C. P. Friedman, J. Ash, & P. Tarcy-Hornoch (Eds.), *American Medical Informatics Association 2005 Proceedings: CD-ROM* (pp. 545–549). Washington, DC: OmniPress, Omnipro-CD.

Ozbolt, J., Fruchtnicht, J. N., & Hayden, J. R. (1994). Toward data standards for clinical nursing information. *Journal of the American Medical Informatics Association, 1,* 175–185.

Parlocha, P. K., & Henry, S. B. (1998). The usefulness of the Georgetown Home Health Care Classification system for coding patient problems and nursing interventions in psychiatric home care. *Computers in Nursing, 16,* 45–52.

Saba, V. K. (1991). *Home health care classification project.* Washington, DC: Georgetown University (NTIS No. PB 92-177013/AS).

Zielstorff, R. D., Tronni, C., Basque, J., Griffin, L. R., & Welebob, E. M. (1998). Mapping nursing diagnosis nomenclatures for coordinated care. *Image: Journal of Nursing Scholarship, 30,* 369–373.

5

MAPPINGS AND TESTIMONIES

MAPPINGS

This chapter outlines the wide interest in the Clinical Care Classification (CCC) system Version 2.0 by organizations involved in many different terminology efforts. This interest is addressed in two different sections with two different approaches. The first section highlights those organizations that have mapped, imbedded, or integrated the CCC system into their structures. The second section provides the testimonies by users of the CCC system for their clinical, research, and/or educational applications.

The CCC system has been integrated in the metathesaurus of the Unified Medical Language System (UMLS), indexed in the Cumulative Index of Nursing and Allied Literature (CINAHL) bibliographic literature system, mapped to the International Classification of Nursing Practice (ICNP), imbedded in the Systematized Nomenclature of Medical Clinical Terms (SNOMED CT), imbedded in the United States Health Information Knowledgebase (USHIK) national database, as well as integrated in several clinical applications.

These applications demonstrate the versatility and the wide acceptance of the CCC system. By integrating the CCC system's two nursing terminologies—the CCC of Nursing Diagnoses and Outcomes and the CCC of Nursing Interventions and Actions—into their products, these organizations have expanded and enhanced the scope of their systems. Several of these organizations that have included the CCC system in their products are described.

Unified Medical Language System (UMLS)

The first organization to integrate the CCC system was the National Library of Medicine (NLM). In 1992, the American Nurses Association (ANA) *recognized* the CCC system (HHCC Version 1.0) as one of the first of four nursing classifications to be considered as a standardized nursing language. These four classification systems were submitted by the ANA to the NLM for integration into the Metathesaurus of the UMLS (2003). This integration made it possible for users of the Metathesaurus of the UMLS to search and retrieve the CCC of Nursing Diagnoses and the CCC of Nursing Interventions, including their definitions.

The Metathesaurus is one of three Knowledge Sources of the UMLS. It provides a uniform, integrated distribution format for more than 100 biomedical and other health-related vocabularies, classifications, and coding systems. It preserves the meanings, including synonyms, between terms from the source vocabularies. It is organized by concepts in order to link together alternative names of the same concept from other classifications. It includes vocabularies designated as standards for the electronic exchange of administrative and clinical data, including the CCC system.

Cumulative Index of Nursing and Allied Health Literature (CINAHL)

In the early 1990s, the CINAHL indexed the HHCC Version 1.0 and more recently the CCC system Version 2.0 in its online CINAHL Subject Heading Index (Pravikoff & Levy, 2005). CINAHL is a bibliographic retrieval system with a database that contains a collection of related machine-readable information for retrieval and analysis. The database contains citations with abstracts for bibliographic literature sources, such as journal articles, books, dissertations, proceedings, etc. The database is searched by using a controlled vocabulary of major or minor descriptors from its Subject Heading Thesaurus, where the CCC system terms reside.

International Classification of Nursing Practice (ICNP)

In the 1990s, the ICNP was developed by the International Council of Nurses (ICN). It included HHCC Version 1.0 concepts in its original design. Since then, the ICNP has been tested and revised into its latest ICNP Version 1.0 (Coenen, 2005). It is a classification of nursing phenomena, actions, and outcomes, and serves as a unifying framework into which existing classifications can be cross-mapped to compare nursing data. The ICNP is being mapped to the CCC, enabling nursing classification implementers to use both interchangeably.

Complete Complementary Alternative Medical Billing and Coding Reference (ABC Codes)

The ABC Codes (2003) were developed by Alternative Link, Inc., to measure, manage, and analyze the financial data and delivery of health care by all non-physician providers of health care, including nursing. Alternative Link focuses on solutions that protect and enhance health promotion and cost-effective health care interventions. Today, Complementary Alternative Medicine (CAM) includes nursing interventions with their corresponding ABC Codes to support the health care industry to keep track and make head to head comparisons of conventional, complementary, and alternative medicines. They provide support for critical business processes that can help the health industry better manage patient care, claims, and outcomes. The CCC of Nursing Interventions and codes were adapted for the ABC Codes in 2002.

U.S. Health Information Knowledgebase (USHIK)

The USHIK (<**http://www.USHIK.org**>) is an online meta-data registry of data elements and attributes used to describe health data and higher-level health meta-data (e.g., schemas, models, and meta-models) administered by the American National Standards Institute-Healthcare Informatics Standards Board (ANSI-HISB). USHIK is a strategic tool to plan, evaluate, and compare electronic health record (EHR) system requirements and supports the mission of the Office of the National Coordinator for Health Information Technology to implement the vision of interoperable electronic EHRs within 10 years (Executive Order No. 1335, issued April 2004). The goal is a common focal point for the documentation of health meta-data that is available for the cataloging and harmonizing of data elements across health Standards Development Organizations (SDOs) and other interested health care organizations. The CCC system is in USHIK.

Other Mappings

The CCC system has also been integrated into other terminology systems, such as the Systematized Nomenclature of Medicine Clinical Terms (SNOMED CT) and the Logical Observation Identifiers, Names, and Codes (LOINC) and registered as a Health Level 7 (HL7) terminology. These are described separately in Chapters 6 and 7.

Contributions

The following three contributions describe the integration of the CCC system by the actual professional who was responsible for the activity. The contributions are from the ICNP, ABC Codes, and the USHIK national database organizations. (See Exhibit 5.1 with Table 5.1, and Exhibits 5.2 and 5.3.)

The only nursing terminology that makes sense—something useful at the point-of-care that reflects nursing practice and makes sense to the entire clinical team—is CCC.

TESTIMONIES

This section of the chapter focuses on the testimonies of selected users of the CCC system in order to demonstrate its wide usage. Users include developers of EHR systems who have integrated the CCC terminologies in their nursing documentation and plans of care applications or in their data dictionaries or vocabulary managers for other documentation applications. Others are nursing

EXHIBIT 5.1. WORKING TOGETHER: CLINICAL CARE CLASSIFICATION (CCC) AND THE INTERNATIONAL CLASSIFICATION FOR NURSING PRACTICE (ICNP)

Amy Coenen, PhD, RN, FAAN
Director, ICNP Program
International Council of Nurses

The International Classification for Nursing Practice (ICNP) is a program of the International Council of Nurses (ICN). The development of the ICNP has relied on the contribution of many individuals and groups. One of the first steps in the development of the ICNP was to collect and compare all the nursing concepts in existing nursing terminologies, including the Clinical Care Classification (CCC) [previously known as Home Health Care Classification (HHCC)]. Since its inception in 1989, nurses and their professional colleagues have completed research studies, development projects, translations, critical reviews and evaluations, and strategic planning for earlier versions (alpha, beta, beta 2), which have now culminated in ICNP Version 1.0.

ICNP Version 1.0 is defined as a unified nursing language system. ICNP Version 1.0 enables nurses around the world to systematically document their work with clients, families, and communities by using standardized nursing diagnoses, interventions, and outcomes. In addition, because ICNP Version 1.0 was developed as a unified nursing language system and a compositional terminology, nurses can cross-map local, regional, or countrywide classification systems to ICNP Version 1.0. The ability to cross-map other classification systems with the ICNP means that the important contributions of existing systems can continue to advance, by both informing ICNP and being informed by ICNP development.

The primary motivation for a unified nursing language system is to be able to communicate and compare nursing data across settings, countries, and languages. These data can be used to support clinical decision-making, evaluate nursing care and patient outcomes, develop health policy, and generate knowledge through research. In addition to promoting comparable nursing data, the ICNP is intended to facilitate comparison of nursing data with data from other health disciplines.

To facilitate the goal of ICNP as a unified nursing language system, a project is underway to map the CCC to the ICNP Version 1.0. The map will identify how CCC concepts are represented using ICNP. This work will facilitate evaluation and ongoing development of both terminologies and allow ICN to compare data using CCC codes with data from other standard nursing terminologies. After a preliminary technical mapping is completed, experts in ICNP and CCC will assist in conceptual validation of the mappings. An example of preliminary mapping is displayed in Table 5.1.

CCC and ICN have initiated collaboration through the cross-mapping project. These two distinct tools serve different but complementary purposes. ICNP and CCC can work together within clinical information systems to support clinical practice and advance nursing science. Ongoing collaboration among nursing and health care terminology developers will advance the opportunities to describe, compare, and evaluate nursing practice internationally. For further information on ICNP see the ICN Web Site <www.icn.ch>

TABLE 5.1. EXAMPLE OF MAPPING CONCEPTS FROM CCC TO ICNP

CCC Care Component/Nursing Diagnosis	ICNP Version 1.0	ICNP Codes
Tissue Perfusion Component	Tissue Perfusion	(10019745)
Tissue Perfusion Alteration—S48	Ineffective Tissue Perfusion	(10001344)
Sensory Component	Perception	(10014270)
Acute Pain—Q45.1	Acute Pain	(10000454)
Activity Component	Mobility	(10012108)
Sleep Pattern Disturbance—A01.6	Impaired Sleep	(10001300)

EXHIBIT 5.2. ABC/CCC CODES FOR NURSING PROVIDE GREATER ACCESS TO QUALITY HEALTH CARE

Connie Koshewa
Practitioner Relations Director
<http://Connie.Koshewa@ABCcodes.com>

ABC Coding Solutions—Alternative Link developed ABC codes for nursing not only by adapting selected nursing interventions from the Clinical Care Classification system, but also from several other nursing terminologies. They were developed in collaboration with nursing terminology experts beginning in 1999.

Approximately 200 Complete Complementary Alternative Medical Billing and Coding References (ABC Codes) were developed to accurately document nursing and integrative health care processes, classify and track clinical care, and develop evidence-based practice models—thus filling significant gaps in older medical code sets. ABC codes provide standardized terminology to support the financing, administration, and delivery of nursing and other integrative health care practices. ABC codes are a recognized code set of the American Nurses Association (ANA).

ABC codes generate valuable outcomes data on the cost and effectiveness of health care. Better outcomes data will increase access to managed care provider networks, reduce claims processing costs and paperwork burdens, and position nurses and other practitioners to identify best practices. Policymakers and health plans need this information to make evidence-based decisions, enabling more people to gain greater access to more health care at an optimal cost.

ABC codes are published in the *ABC Coding Manual for Integrative Healthcare* available at <http://www.ABCcodes.com>, with ABC-CCC terminology mapping.

ABC/CCC Code Mapping Example:

CCC Component	CCC Terminology	ABC Code	ABC Procedure Description	Expanded Definition
A01.01	Activity therapy assessment	CDBAV	Activity therapy assessment, each 15 minutes	Assessing a client's level of interest, aptitude and/or functional level for an activity or activities in addition to his or her recreational activity history to determine if activity therapy should be incorporated into the treatment plan. Service is billed in 15-minute increments.
E12.22	Stress reduction management and control direct care	CDAET	Stress reduction assistance individual, each 15 minutes	Using counseling techniques to assist a client in identifying, reducing, and managing his or her stress. Service is billed in 15-minute increments.
G18.12	Compliance with diet management	BFBAQ	Diet compliance management individual, each 15 minutes	Managing and/or assisting a patient in complying with his or her prescribed and/or suggested dietary intake. Service is billed in 15-minute increments.
Q47.03	Pain management training individual	CDAFS	Pain coping assistance individual, each 15 minutes	Using counseling techniques to assist a client in developing a coping technique(s) to manage his or her pain. Service is billed in 15-minute increments.

ABC Coding Solutions also publishes the *Practitioner's Guide to Billable Interventions Using ABC Codes* (*The Guide*) that includes legal scope of practice information to ensure the financing, administration, and delivery of health care is in compliance with state scope of practice regulations. More than 800 versions of *The Guide* are available to all levels of nurses and other health care practitioner types. *The Guide* lists only those ABC codes within a practitioner's state scope of practice for his/her specialty.

(Continued)

EXHIBIT 5.2. (CONTINUED)

Relative Value Studies Inc., publishes corresponding relative value information that supports pricing, fee schedule development, contracting, and medical economics studies (Relative Values for Integrative Health Care Using ABC Codes available at <**http://www.rvsdata.com**>).

ABC Coding Solutions-Alternative Link hosts an open and impartial terminology and code development process. To request (1) new ABC terminology and corresponding code, (2) a change to an existing ABC code and terminology, or (3) the retirement of an existing ABC code, mail, fax, or e-mail your request to the address provided below. All Terminology and Code Requests, as well as suggestions, are appreciated and will be considered.

ABC Coding Solutions–Alternative Link, Inc.
Code Development and Maintenance
6121 Indian School Road NE
Suite 131
Albuquerque, NM 87110
<**http://CodeDevelopment@ABCcodes.com**>

EXHIBIT 5.3. UNITED STATES HEALTH INFORMATION KNOWLEDGEBASE (USHIK)[a]

LuAnn Whittenburg, RN, MSN, FNP, BC, CPHQ
Health Informatics Consultant
Department of Defense (Health Affairs)

The United States Health Information Knowledgebase (<**http://www.USHIK.org/**>) is an online meta-data registry of data elements and attributes used to describe health data and higher level health meta-data (e.g., schemas, models, and meta-models) administered by the American National Standards Institute (ANSI).

The Clinical Care Classification System (CCC) developed by Virginia K. Saba, EdD, DS, RN, FAAN, FACMI, LL, and colleagues is a nomenclature of discrete atomic-level data elements about the nursing process that encompasses nursing assessment, diagnosis, intervention, actions, and actual and expected outcomes. The CCC system is an electronic information standard to identify the contribution of nursing to patient outcomes for improved health care services.

The meta-data information displayed in the United States Health Information Knowledgebase (USHIK) contains the CCC system for use by Standards Development Organizations (SDOs) and other organizations interested in describing and communicating the electronic documentation of nursing practice. The benefits of CCC data elements in the USHIK are that it allows information technology analysts, business managers, and clinical process owners to use the common units of data in USHIK to design health information systems and applications and realize a significant and immediate return on investment for Information Technology (IT) system products.

Value of the CCC system data elements in the USHIK include the following:

1. Accelerated health software development
2. Earlier return on investment on information technology design and development costs
3. Nursing terminology increases employee productivity (standardized documentation)
4. Standardized, consistent health data for interventions and research
5. Re-usable health data for cross-organization comparisons
6. Reduced health care cost from improved, documented outcomes by intervention
7. Reduced level of effort in unnecessary computer system data element development.

For example, *a preterm risk assessment* application typically realizes a $0.34 cents per member per month (PMPM) savings on a membership with approximately 300 to 400 deliveries per month. The return on investment for an application developed using the standardized terminology in the USHIK would have a shorter application development cycle with an immediately marketable IT product.

[a]USHIK: Marco Johnson, Department of Defense Health Affairs, (703) 681-5611; Glenn Sperle, Centers for Medicare and Medicaid Services (CMS), (410) 786-4610.

EXHIBIT 5.4. SIEMENS MEDICAL SOLUTIONS

Rosemary Kennedy, MBA, RN
Chief Nursing Informatics Officer
Siemens Medical Solutions

The electronic health record, specifically nursing documentation, must support evidence-based nursing practice. The use of structured, standard terminology is necessary to express valid, comparable data that can be used across clinical applications to support point-of-care decision making and outcomes analysis. Success in capturing evidence-based practice in clinical documentation is highly dependent on having a structured format for the initial collection and representation of the data. This structured format lays the foundation for all facets of the electronic health record. In essence, this structure gives us the ability to quantify nursing care impact on outcomes and across settings, clinical specialties, and geographical locations.

Within Soarian© Clinicals, users can manage nursing problems, for any patient, using a structured list of codes that are based on the Clinical Care Classification system. This structured format supports the process of care delivery while also giving organizations the ability to measure nursing care impact on outcomes. The structure is visible to the end users through the document process, as well as all facets of workflow. Nurses can engage structured nursing terminology that reflects evidence-based practice. In addition, other disciplines can also use the problem list to reflect "what is going on" with the patient and use terminology that is mutually understood by all clinicians. The Clinical Care Classification was integrated within Soarian as a way for hospitals to immediately have standardized problems/nursing documentation to implement into their patient care, based on a standard that sets the foundation for evidence-based nursing care. It is this standardization within the electronic health record that enables health care professionals to quantify nursing practice and its impact on patient care.

---

informatics experts who have used the CCC system for research and evaluation studies, as well as for developing educational software.

The first testimony is from the Chief Nursing Informatics Officer of Siemens Medical Solutions, an international EHR vendor who is integrating the CCC Version 2.0 system into the next generation of their EHR system. Another testimony is from a nurse developer who, in the 1980s, used aspects of the Home Health Care Classification (HHCC) (Version 1.0) system for an electronic Home Care System. Two other testimonies are from doctoral students who conducted their research and evaluated the usability of the terminologies: one focusing on psychiatric patients and the other focusing on coronary artery bypass graft (CABG) patients in the Cardiovascular Intensive Care Unit (CVICU). Another testimony is from a Finnish nurse who not only translated the HHCC into Finish for her doctoral research, but also implemented the translated version for a hospital in Korpio, Finland. The last two reports are two new applications being developed in Norway with the CCC system known as SabaKlass.

Other users of the CCC system describe their specific applications of the CCC in Chapters 6 to 10. Chapter 6 addresses how the CCC of Nursing Diagnoses Outcomes is integrated into the Logical Observation Identifiers, Names, and Codes (LOINC) clinical system. Also described in that chapter is how the CCC is recognized as a standardized terminology by Health Level Seven (HL7), an organization that provides standards for the exchange, management, and integration of data that support clinical patient care. Chapter 7 focuses on how the CCC is integrated in and mapped by SNOMED CT (Systematized

EXHIBIT 5.5. APPLICATION OF HOME HEALTH CARE CLASSIFICATION (HHCC) INTO CLINICAL SOFTWARE

Kay Hollers, RN, MPH, FHHC, CHCE
President, Healthcare Executive Resources
Austin, TX

Software that allows for assessment-based documentation of the nursing process requires an organizing framework in order to assign relationships between data elements and observations collected. The task of developing such software for home health in the United States is also complicated by the mandatory integration of the OASIS (Outcomes and Assessment Information Set) items, which relate over time but do not, in themselves, correlate to any particular medical approach. The ability to incorporate the OASIS items as required, to produce an assessment-based plan of care, and to use language recognized by clinicians regardless of discipline was achieved only when we adopted the Home Health Care Classification (HHCC) system developed by Saba and Colleagues and accepted the HHCC Care Components as the organizing framework.

Using the Care Components allows us to define observed symptoms (regardless of whether the data comes from OASIS or other observations) as evidence of the manifestation of various Care Components, to guide the selection of goals appropriate to the Care Component, and to present selection interventions associated with the Care Component. Using the HHCC's Care Components in this manner, we are able to provide a powerful clinical tool that allows the clinician to focus on the manifest problems and issues presented by the patient, set measurable goals for those problems, and target interventions to the achievement of the goals. Therefore, the care plan is individualized to the specific issues identified on assessment, but benefits from the structure and organization provided by this standardized conceptual framework.

The beauty of the HHCC's Care Components system is that it can be used consciously and deliberately, as was done in the design of our software system, or it can function "in the wings" to guide clinicians into appropriate choices. Because it orders, classifies, and simplifies nursing diagnoses, it broadly encompasses all those issues addressed by the community care clinician. Like any well-designed tool, the nurse user does not have to know the details of how it functions to use it to improve the quality of the work product. Wellspring Innovations, Inc. (Austin, TX), the developer who is using the HHCC Care Components, has found that the HHCC's Care Components provide the platform required to guide the clinical decision making for its HomeCare Elements system.

HomeCare Elements is the best point-of-care clinical management system and decision support tool available. It is used to document the entire clinical process from comprehensive assessments through care planning and implementation to discharge and outcomes analysis. HomeCare Elements is the cost-effective clinical expert system to help home health agencies thrive under the OASIS Prospective Payment System (PPS).

In conclusion, without the HHCC Care Components, the HomeCare Elements software could not have produced such a usable home care system. The HHCC Care Components provide the standardized framework, and, in doing so, makes it possible for the appropriate nursing diagnoses and nursing interventions to be associated and programmed for each Care Component. This strategy makes the HomeCare Elements software not only easy for the clinicians to use, but also clinically relevant while generating meaningful required PPS reports.

Note: **HomeCare Elements** is the clinical point-of-care software system available from:

Wellspring Innovations
<http://www.winnovations.com>

EXHIBIT 5.6. TESTIMONY USING HOME HEALTH CARE CLASSIFICATION (HHCC) FOR RESEARCH ON PSYCHIATRIC HOME CARE PATIENTS

Professor Pamela Parlocha
Department of Nursing and Health Sciences
College of Science 143
California State–Hayward
Hayward, CA 94542

This is a report by Pamela Kees Parlocha, DNSc, RN, on the conduct of her research study entitled "Usefulness of the Georgetown Home Health Care Classification for Classifying Patient Problems and Nursing Interventions for Elderly Home Care Patients with Depression" (1998). She highlights the experiences that she had using the HHCC system coding the research data of home care patients with depression. A description of the study is also described in the Research Study Chapter.

Why Did I Use HHCC?

I used Version 1.0 of the Home Health Care Classification (HHCC) system. As part of a larger study attempting to empirically define a critical path for psychiatric home care patients with a diagnosis of Major Depressive Disorder. My study examined the utility of the Georgetown HHCC System for the coding of patient problems and nursing interventions in the psychiatric home care setting.

Major Advantages

Coding systems such as this provide a useful tool for many types of analysis (e.g., quality assurance, critical path and care plan development, and linking with financial data). For example, the finding that the number of interventions per visit for "acute" patients decreased much earlier in the course of treatment while the number of interventions per visit for "continuation" and "maintenance" patients tended to stay high for the entire course of treatment is an example of how the HHCC codes may be used to analyze data. In addition, they allow for prediction of patient resource requirements and linking nursing interventions with patient outcomes. Studies using these types of systems may be used to provide support for the value of nursing services and thus for the continuing reimbursement of these services by health insurance sources.

Major Disadvantages

One element of the Georgetown coding system that was less useful as applied in this study was the coding used to indicate patient outcomes. The fifth digit of the patient problem codes was meant to indicate the expected outcome/problem as "improved," "stabilized," or "deteriorated." In this study, these outcomes were not useful as applied to each problem on every visit. Often, changes in problems between visits were small and a clear distinction was not apparent. The codes were applied to the identified problems on the discharge visit, but often charting for the discharge visit was cursory and did not always address all of the previously identified patient problems. Since clearly defined measurable patient outcomes are necessary for testing the effects of nursing interventions, further prospective testing of this system on larger numbers of home care patients with depression would be useful in clarifying the issue further.

Design/Development of Software/System

Tables were created within the relational database Paradox to collect textual data describing patient problems/nursing diagnoses and nursing interventions and to encode the text entries. Paradox allows the user to collect and code textual data while preserving the data's integrity, and it was found to be the most effective and efficient software program (for its time) for both organizing and analyzing these types of data. If I were to do the same analysis today, I would use Microsoft Access. But, at that time, Paradox was the database of choice.

(Continued)

EXHIBIT 5.6. (CONTINUED)

How and Where It Was Used?

Closed medical records of patients with a diagnosis of Major Depressive Disorder were obtained from a large Visiting Nurses Association in Northern California. I audited the medical records of 32 patients. Raw data taken verbatim from the "nurses' notes" section of the charts were entered into tables in fields labeled "Problem" and "Intervention," with adjacent fields left blank for subsequent coding. Next, these entries were coded using the Georgetown system. The codes were then used to ask questions of the data, such as "Can a critical path be discerned from the data?"

In order to ensure reliability of code application by the author, two expert psychiatric home care nurses were recruited to code a subset of the data. Interrater reliability was tested by having the experts code the data after receiving training from the principal investigator. Their frequencies of agreement with the author were calculated using Cohen's kappa. For rater 1, the kappa value was 0.721 ($p = 0.0000$), and for rater 2, the kappa value was 0.498 ($p = 0.0000$). Considering that there were 20 possible categories from which to choose, interrater reliability can be considered good.

Were All Terms Used? Or, If Selected Ones Were Used, Which Ones and Why?

I'm not sure if I used all of the codes, but I know that I used most of them. The HHCC coding system was not designed specifically for psychiatric home care patients, but rather for home care patients in general. Thus, while most of the patient problems/nursing diagnoses found in the medical record audit could be coded using the established codes, the system was not specific enough to adequately address all of the problems and interventions appropriate for this population without the loss of potentially significant psychiatric data. Thirty-four new codes were developed to further describe patient problems, 27 of which were found in the data of the patient sample, and two new nursing intervention codes were created. The new patient problem codes were needed in the Activity, Cognitive, Role Relationship, and Self-Concept component categories. The new Activity component codes were needed to specify the side effects of neuroleptic medications. The new Cognitive component codes were related to confusion, memory loss, and delusional ideation. The new Role Relationship codes are descriptive of impaired communication behaviors, such as perseveration, mutism, or tangential speech. The new Self-Concept component codes characterize disordered moods, specifically dysphoria and the flat affect that often accompanies it. Two new nursing intervention codes were needed: Family/Caregiver Support and Psycho-education. These additional codes were necessary for adequate description of the specific patient problems and nursing interventions found in the population of psychiatric home care patients with Major Depressive Disorder. Although it might have been possible to fit all of the patient problems and nursing interventions into an existing category of the Georgetown system, the system lacked the specificity needed to prevent significant psychiatric data loss. New codes for the sample population that would fit into the established system were not difficult to devise. For example, when additional codes for patient problems were needed to apply to the data, sources on patient mental status examinations were consulted, and the code definitions were developed accordingly. The new codes were included in the interrater reliability testing described previously, and thus may be reliably applied in this domain.

How Long Did It Take to Develop the System? When? Where?

The system took a while for me to develop. I collected data in the summer of 1994 and entered the data into a database I created in Paradox. Today, I would take a database for granted, but then everything was new to me, and there was no one to consult on Paradox. I had to use the manual that came with the program, and its main example was of a business. I had to create my own categories within the tables and then learn to connect different fields within the database and construct pertinent queries. So, it took me several months to learn the program, develop the tables and categories, and construct the queries I needed for my data. I completed my dissertation in 1995.

Source: Parlocha, P. K., & Henry, S. B. (1998). The usefulness of the Georgetown Home Health Care Classification system for coding patient problems and nursing interventions in psychiatric home care. *Computers in Nursing, 16,* 45–52.

EXHIBIT 5.7. EVALUATION OF THE CLINICAL CARE CLASSIFICATION (CCC) IN A CRITICAL CARE SETTING

Jacqueline Moss, PhD, RN
Assistant Professor, School of Nursing Scientist
Center for Outcomes Effectiveness Research & Education
University of Alabama–Birmingham
<http://mossja@uab.edu>

This is a brief report by Jacqueline Moss, PhD, RN, on the conduct of her research study entitled "Evaluation of the Home Health Care Classification in a Critical Care Setting." She highlights the experiences that she and her research team had using the Clinical Care Classification (CCC) system coding the research data of coronary artery bypass graft (CABG) patients in a cardiovascular intensive care unit (CVICU). A compete description of the study is also described in the chapter on "Research and Evaluation Studies."

Research Overview

Classification systems are needed to serve as interface terminologies between the user and the reference terminology used to organize the computer database system. However, no nursing classification systems have been designed specifically for or evaluated in the critical care setting. We used documentation collected during the care of CABG patients to evaluate the ability of the CCC to represent data in an intensive care setting and to provide recommendations for the expansion of this classification for its use in critical care documentation.

The group that mapped the computerized documentation to the CCC were all extremely familiar with the nursing care of CABG patients, the computerized documentation system, and this particular intensive care unit (ICU). A decision was made to split the four CCC Action Type qualifiers into individual terms. Therefore, the CCC qualifier descriptors became: Assess, Monitor, Care, Perform, Teach, Instruct, Manage, and Refer.

In this ICU setting, the most important qualifier was determined to be "assess/monitor." The group decided that, in critical care nursing, there was a great deal of difference between the actions "assess" and "monitor." Nurses in critical care spend a great deal of their time watching and documenting. The group coded these behaviors under the qualifier "monitor" and determined that assessment required a judgment on the nurses' part. An example of an assessment behavior would be the determination that an intravenous line was patent. No differentiation was made between the qualifiers "instruct" and "teach." The mapping group could not see any difference between the two in this setting and chose to code both under the qualifier "teach."

The majority (79.8%) of the documented terms were mapped to the CCC. By far, most of the documentation was related to physical regulation (40.01%) and fluid volume (31.14%). Concepts from four Care Components—bowel/gastric, metabolic, self-concept, and life cycle—had no documentation that mapped to a category. To map the remaining documentation (20.18%) would require the creation of intervention codes in six areas: (1) hemodynamic monitoring, (2) balloon pump care, (3) arterial line care, (4) central line care, (5) cognitive assessment, and (6) providing information.

Title of Project

"Evaluation of the Home Health Care Classification in a Critical Care Setting" (supported by a grant from the University of Alabama, Birmingham School of Nursing)

Research References

Moss, J., & Damrongsak, M. (2005). *Evaluation of the home health care classification in a critical care setting.* Poster presented at the Southern Nursing Research Society Conference, Atlanta, GA.

Moss, J., Damrongsak, M., & Gallichio, K. (2005). Representing critical care data using the clinical care classification. In C. P. Friedman, J. Ash, & P. Tarcy-Hornoch (Eds.), *American Medical Association 2005 CD Proceedings. Annual Symposium.* Washington, DC: AMA. (CD-ROM)

EXHIBIT 5.8. THE ROLE OF HOME HEALTH CARE CLASSIFICATION (HHCC)/CLINICAL CARE CLASSIFICATION (CCC) IN FINLAND

Professor and Dr. Anneli Ensio
Kuopio University & University Hospital
70210 Kuopio, Finland
<http://anneli.ensio@kuh.fi>
<http://anneli.ensio@uku.fi>

In 1995, parts of the Home Health Care Classification (HHCC) (Care Components and HHCC of Nursing Interventions' major categories and subcategories) were translated (also back-translation) and used in research projects at Kuopio University Hospital (one surgical ward and one medical ward). After the cultural modification made by an expert group, the Finnish Classification of Nursing Intervention (FiCNI) was defined.

In North-Karelian Hospital District, a large project was launched (1999–2001). Nursing electronic structured documentation was developed as a part of electronic patient record. In the first phase, the electronic nursing referral and discharge summary system between the Central Hospital and Health Centers were carried out using the FiCNI based on HHCC.

In the second phase (2001–2003), FiCNI was implemented in the electronic patient record system, and nursing care plans were documented using FiCNI.

In the third phase (2004), the Finnish Nursing Diagnoses Classification was developed using the HHCC of Nursing Diagnoses, which were translated into Finnish in 2002.

At the end of 2004, 22 wards (total of 32) and 6 outpatient clinics (total of 11) in Central Hospital and two health centers were using an electronic-structured nursing care plan system, where HHCC/CCC of Nursing Diagnoses and HHCC/CCC of Nursing Interventions were implemented.

Development activities in the North-Karelian Hospital District were funded by the Ministry of Social Affairs and Health.

The HHCC/CCC has given the structure to document nursing care (i.e., specialized and primary care) in the North-Karelian Hospital District. Reported results of the projects can be used widely when the activities start to unify the nursing documentation at the national level.

EXHIBIT 5.9. NORWEGIAN SOFTWARE USING SABAKLASS CLINICAL CARE CLASSIFICATION (CCC)

Karl Øyri
The Interventional Centre
Rikshospitalet University Hospital
Oslo, Norway
<http://www.interventionalcentre.no>
<http://carloy@ulrik.uio.no>

I wanted to update you on a very interesting development with Sabaklass here in Norway. A Master's degree student at the Department of Computer and Information Science at the Norwegian University of Science and Technology has developed an application based on Sabaklass. His work is entitled "Topic-Based Navigation in Nursing Documentation in EPR Systems Supported by Ontology and Classification."

The application is programmed in Java, with a methodology based on a vector model, a technology known from search engines. To be more specific, this means comma-separated vectors. The sensational part of the application is that the diagnosis and interventions in the Sabaklass taxonomies are automatically extrapolated from free text nursing documentation either from an electronic patient record (EPR) or other documents. For identification of Sabaklass terms from unstructured text, a predefined thesaurus is used to map the taxonomies with the text, similar to a reference terminology concept. This technology also applies to scanned documents, enabling retrospective research on nursing documentation! The application is platform independent, so the cross platform xml-based file exchange format can be implemented in any free text based EPR system.

Unfortunately, this is only the start of an application, which is not completed. Anyway, I wanted to keep you informed with this very promising approach that we have to develop further in Norway. I will contact the National Nurses Association (NNA), the Department of Health, and the Norwegian Research Council to try and establish further development of the application next fall. I will also cowrite papers with the student for academic publication.

EXHIBIT 5.10. NORWEGIAN PROJECT USING SABAKLASS (CLINICAL CARE CLASSIFICATION): "ELECTRONIC DOCUMENTATION IN COMMUNITY CARE"

Abstract

Since 2005, the municipalities of Evje/Hornnes, Gjerstad, and Krageroe and Agder College have been collaborating on a project plan for further advancement and development of the electronic patient journal implemented in the municipalities. The aim of this project is a multi-disciplinary coordination of care plans with a combination of classification systems and inpatient length of stay (IPLOS; individual-based care statistics) to be used when assessing the patients' need for help. The project will validate the 17 IPLOS scores and compare the degree in which IPLOS measures the function level of patients. The purpose of IPLOS is to assess the individual patient; therefore, it is important that the tools measure the actual function level. The municipalities in the project will start to register and report the IPLOS statistics in the autumn of 2005 and will document care plans based on the classification system SABAKLASS in the spring of 2006.
The following aims will be realized:

1. Follow-up the use of the classification system SABAKLASS as a tool for clinicians developing care plans for patients in the municipalities.
2. Validate IPLOS as a tool for assessing the function level of the individual patient/client.

   The project shall accomplish a validating study for the second aim. The planned project is described in more detail in the project plan. The results of the study will be presented continuously through participation in national and international conferences. The project will take 2 years, from June 1, 2006 until July 1, 2008.

Nomenclature of Medical Clinical Terms). It includes examples of the cross-mappings between the two terminologies. Chapter 8 addresses how the CCC terminology is used in nursing research protocols. The last two chapters are written by designers of educational software. Chapter 9 describes a software application for teaching nursing students how to document nursing care using the CCC while following the nursing process. The last chapter focuses on the integration of the selected aspects of the CCC into a PDA (personal digital assistant)-based device that is used by students to keep a log of their clinical experiences.

Each of the individual testimonies is presented as an exhibit. (See Exhibits 5.4–5.10.)

REFERENCES

ABC Coding Solutions. (2006). *ABC coding manual.* Albuquerque, NM: ABC Coding Solutions—Alternative Link, Inc.

CINAHL Information Systems. (2005). *CINAHL 2004 Subject heading list.* Glendale, CA: CINAHL Information Systems (a subdivision of EBSCO Publishing).

Coenen, A. (2005). *International classification of nursing practice (ICNP) (Version 1.0).* Geneva, Switzerland: International Council of Nurses.

National Library of Medicine. (2003). *Unified medical language system: UMLS knowledge sources* (14th ed.). *Metathesaurus, semantic network, SPECIALIST lexicon.* Bethesda, MD: US DHHS, NIH, NLM.

Pravikoff, D. S., & Levy, J. (2005). Computerized information resources. In V. K. Saba & K. A. McCormick, *Essentials of nursing informatics* (4th ed., pp. 585–603). New York: McGraw-Hill Publishing.

6

MESSAGING THE CLINICAL CARE CLASSIFICATION (CCC) SYSTEM USING LOGICAL OBSERVATION IDENTIFIERS, NAMES, AND CODES (LOINC) AND HEALTH LEVEL 7 (HL7)

SUSAN MATNEY
SUZANNE BAKKEN
STANLEY M. HUFF

The Institute of Medicine considers electronic health records (EHRs) among the most powerful tools to improve the quality of health care (Kohn & Donaldson, 2000). Data standards, particularly clinical terminology data standards, provide the backbone for successful development and implementation of an EHR. Furthermore, standard terminologies are seen as necessary to share patient information across health care organizations by facilitating interoperability of often disparate EHR systems. David Brailer, the National Coordinator for Health Information Technology, has stated that "interoperability standards and policies require immediate attention from the Federal government and private sector participants" (Brailer, 2005). The National Committee on Vital and Health Statistics (NCVHS), an advisory board to the United States Department of Health and Human Services (HHS), has developed criteria for clinical terminology standards and recommended Systematized Nomenclature of Medical Clinical Terms (SNOMED CT) and Logical Observation Identifiers, Names, and Codes (LOINC) as a core set of EHR clinical terminology standards. Health Level 7 (HL7) is the messaging standard used to send electronic data across interfaces among health information systems, such as EHRs. Coded terminology is part of those messages.

The purpose of this chapter is to:

1. Provide the history and description of LOINC
2. Describe how Clinical Care Classification (CCC) is mapped into LOINC
3. Provide the history of HL7
4. Provide examples of HL7 messages using the CCC

LOGICAL OBSERVATION IDENTIFIERS, NAMES, AND CODES (LOINC)

History and Description

The LOINC terminology is a publicly available, no-cost database that provides a set of universal names and codes identifying laboratory and clinical test results that can be used in computer databases or transmitted in electronic messages (Forrey et al., 1996). Work on LOINC, funded by the National Library of Medicine and the Agency for Health Care Policy and Research, began in 1994 at the Regenstrief Institute, a research foundation affiliated with the Indiana University School of Medicine (Huff et al., 1998). The rationale for the development of LOINC was to create universal names and codes for measurements used in medicine. Since there were a growing number of laboratory systems using internally defined names and codes that were unique to the laboratory equipment vendor or the specific institution, the first focus of the committee was the creation of names and codes for clinical laboratory observations. The goal of the LOINC committee was to create codes that are universally used by all systems and thus could facilitate clinical data exchange and use across health care organizations. Another objective in the development of LOINC was to structure the names in a format that could facilitate rapid matching, either automated or manual, between local vocabularies and the universal LOINC codes. The different LOINC axes described herein enable rapid matching.

LOINC formal names and codes are created for laboratory results and clinical variables with numeric, coded, or narrative text results. The current version has more than 31,000 lab codes and 10,000 clinical codes. The LOINC codes are not intended to transmit all possible information about an observation; they are only intended to identify the clinical observation. The LOINC names are used in resulting specific patient observations during patient care. Although LOINC does not contain the coded values for the names, there are suggested answer lists for each ordinal (e.g., 1+, 2+, 3+, 4+) and nominal code [e.g., clear, rhonchi, rales, and wheezes for breath sounds (McDonald, Huff, Vreeman, & Mercer, 2005)].

The American Nurses Association (ANA) has officially designated LOINC as an ANA-recognized nomenclature (Matney, Bakken, & Huff, 2003). A nomenclature is a system of terms composed according to pre-established composition rules (de Keizer, Abu-Hanna, & Zwetslook-Schonk, 2000). Nomenclatures provide a common reference point so that data can be communicated between health care systems (Payne, Sengupta, & Sittig, 1999). LOINC semantic structure is modeled using a multi-axial representational approach. Multi-axial means that the LOINC name is a combination of six different axes, or attributes, that are combined to create an aggregate or precoordinated expression. Each LOINC record corresponds to a single result (e.g., pain level on a scale of 1–10) or collection (e.g., pain assessment battery). The LOINC axes include component, kind of property, time aspect, system, precision, and type of method (Table 6.1).

TABLE 6.1. LOINC AXES[a]

LOINC Axis	Description
Component	The substance or entity that is measured, evaluated, or observed (e.g., systolic blood pressure, pain onset, and sodium).
Property	The characteristic or attribute of the analyte that is measured, evaluated, or observed (e.g., length, volume, time stamp, mass, ratio, number, temperature). CCC[a] codes only use the property of "finding."
Timing	The interval of time over which the observation or measurement was made (e.g., point in time, 24 hours).
System	The system (context) or specimen type within which the observation was made (e.g., urine, serum, fetus, patient, family, caregiver, respiratory system).
Type of Scale	The scale of the measure (e.g., quantitative–a true measurement), ordinal (a ranked set of options), nominal (e.g., *Escherichia coli*; *Staphylococcus aureus*), or narrative (e.g., dictation results from x-rays).
Type of Method	The procedure used to make the measurement or observation. Method is only used when it makes an important distinction in sensitivity or specificity. Method is the only axis that is optional. Observed is the method used for the CCC codes.

[a]CCC, Clinical Care Classification; LOINC, Logical Observation Identifiers, Names, and Codes

The fully specified name for a CCC diagnosis as illustrated by activity intolerance at a specific point in time looks like the following in the database and is specified according to axes as shown in Table 6.2.

The LOINC database includes columns for each of the six parts (axes) of the name. In addition, it also contains short names, related words, synonyms, and comments for all observations. Related words ("synonyms") are included to facilitate searches for individual laboratory test and clinical observation results. The table also contains information about the amount, route, and timing of physiological or pharmacological challenges.

The LOINC database is presented as an electronic document grouped by "common sense" categories to make it easier to find general areas of interest. It is divided first into two main categories: "lab" and "clinical." Lab and clinical

TABLE 6.2. AN EXAMPLE OF A FULLY SPECIFIED LOINC NAME[a]

Axis	Value
Component	Activity Intolerance
Property	Find (Finding)
Timing	PT (Point in time)
System	Patient
Scale	Ord (Ordinal)
Method	Observed using CCC[a]

[a]CCC, Clinical Care Classification; LOINC, Logical Observation Identifiers, Names, and Codes

TABLE 6.3. EXAMPLES OF CCC CODE MAPPINGS[a]

LN Code	Component	Property	Timing	System	Scale	CCC Code
28088-3	DENIAL	FIND	PT[a]	^PATIENT	ORD[a]	E12.4
	FAMILY COPING					
28098-2	IMPAIRMENT	FIND	PT	^FAMILY	ORD	E11.0
28114-7	GUSTATORY ALTERATION	FIND	PT	MOUTH	ORD	Q44.2
28119-6	HYPOTHERMIA	FIND	PT	^PATIENT	ORD	K25.3
28120-4	HYPERTHERMIA	FIND	PT	^PATIENT	ORD	K25.2
28135-2	ANXIETY	FIND	PT	^PATIENT	ORD	P40.0
28207-9	SKIN INCISION	FIND	PT	SKIN	ORD	R46.4
42819-3	FAILURE TO THRIVE	FIND	PT	^PATIENT	ORD	G17.1
42821-9	CAREGIVER ROLE STRAIN	FIND	PT	^CAREGIVER	ORD	M27.4
	COMMUNITY COPING					
42854-0	IMPAIRMENT	FIND	PT	^COMMUNITY	ORD	E52.0

[a]CCC, Clinical Care Classification; ORD, ordinal; PT, point in time.

are further divided into classes. The lab portion of the LOINC database contains classes such as chemistry, coagulation tests, blood bank tests, etc. The clinical portion contains classes that are pertinent for nursing, such as body measurement, intake and output, neonatal Apgar measures, obstetrical studies and measures, respiratory measures and ventilator management, nursing survey instruments, vaccination records, vital signs, and intake and output volumes. The LOINC database includes fully specified names for the diagnoses from the CCC system (Saba & Zuckerman, 1992).

CCC Mapped to LOINC

The primary focus of LOINC has been to support the names for data elements when data are represented as name-value pairs or using an entity-attribute-value model (Bakken et al., 2002; Huff, Hammond, & Williams, 2002). The name is the observation identifier, the question, or the "what" and the value is the answer (Table 6.3). Name-value pairs provide a mechanism to describe patient care attributes and the values assigned to those attributes. Name-value pairs are bundled and stored together (Malet, Munoz, Appleyard, & Hersh, 2000). "What are the lung sounds" has a value of "Wheezes" for one particular instance.

In the CCC, the expected (i.e., goal) or actual outcome (improved, stabilized, deteriorated) is selected for each nursing diagnosis. LOINC codes were created for these terms because goal and outcome evaluation statements are considered observations (Bakken, Cimino, Haskell, et al., 2000). The name in the method column is always "OBSERVED.CCC." The distinction between expected and actual outcomes is handled through the mood code in the model for HL7 messages.

HL7 OVERVIEW AND HISTORY

Health Level Seven (HL7) is a not-for-profit standards development organization. They provide standards for the exchange, management, and integration of data that support clinical patient care (HL7, 2005b). In 1988, Version 1.0 of the HL7 messaging standard was produced. In 1994, the HL7 organization became an accredited American National Standards Institute (ANSI) Standards Development Organization (SDO). This means that HL7 follows the ANSI guidelines for developing open consensus standards. Following an open consensus process means that any interested party is free to join HL7 and participate in the creation of standards, and that specific rules are followed to ensure that there is balanced participation between software vendors, software users, and academicians. Version 2.2 of the HL7 messaging standard and all subsequent versions of the standard have been approved as ANSI standards.

The first hospital information systems (HIS) were based on having a single large computer that serviced all the information needs of a hospital and its associated clinics and departments. The single, large "mainframe" systems had applications for entering and reviewing many kinds of clinical data, as well as other applications for functions like registering patients and billing. The codes used within the systems were usually created locally without any standardization.

Beginning in the mid-1980s, local area networks became generally available, and people began to propose systems composed of network modules (McDonald, 1984; McDonald & Hammond, 1989). This led to the development of modular, stand-alone departmental computer systems for many departments in a hospital, of which the laboratory, radiology, and pharmacy department systems were the largest. However, these systems were not initially created to "talk" to each other or the hospital-wide HIS. In order for the systems to work together as an integrated whole, information needed to be passed between them. For example, a patient's demographic data acquired using the HIS registration module were also needed by the laboratory system so that the proper patient name and visit number could be attached to all tests performed for that patient in the laboratory. Likewise, the results from laboratory testing needed to be sent back to the clinical system so they could be used to direct care of the patient. Today, the HL7 standard specifies standard messages so that departmental systems can communicate with each other and with the local HIS. The way this communication occurs on a technical level is by software interfaces that are part of the systems. The interfaces package, send or receive, and unpackage messages.

Interfaces serve a number of purposes, including data exchange within a given enterprise to reduce redundant data entry and data shared with other computers on the network. For example, the demographic data entered as part of patient registration via the HIS are then sent to the pharmacy, radiology, and laboratory systems as needed. The overall effect is that patients are given better clinical care because data are available when and where they are needed with less required redundant data entry.

Standardized interfaces are now being used for reporting public health data between local laboratories and local, state, and federal public health agencies. Effler et al. (1999) demonstrated that using standardized electronic interfaces increases the accuracy, completeness, and timeliness of reports sent to health departments.

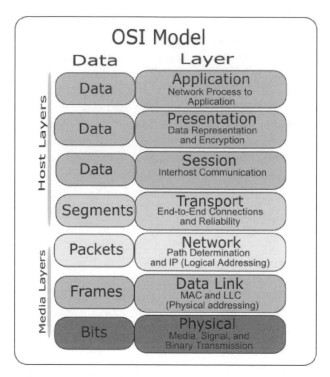

FIGURE 6.1. OSI model. OSI, open systems interconnection. IP = Internet Protocol, LLC = Logical Link Control, MAC = Media Access Control.

Interoperability and Vocabulary Use With HL7

The Institute of Electrical and Electronics Engineers (IEEE) defines interoperability as "The ability of two or more systems or components to exchange information and to use the information that has been exchanged" (Institute of Electronics Engineers, 1990). Successful communication among disparate systems requires interoperability at many levels. Computers communicate with each other using a set of rules or a protocol. Multiple levels of communication protocols are required to support messaging between a sending application on one system and a receiving application on a second system. ISO (International Standards Organization) has defined a suite of protocols to facilitate this type of messaging between computers. This suite is called the Open Systems Interconnection (OSI) Standard and provides the basis for full interoperability. The seven-layer protocol deals with the stacking of communication levels, beginning at the applications level of a sending system down to the physical level of the sending system, across to the physical level of the receiving system and up to the applications level of the receiving system.

The HL7 standard deals with the application level (what needs to be sent to fulfill the business need?) and deals partially with the presentation level (what is the syntax of the data that are sent?) of the OSI model. HL7 derives its name from the seventh (application) level of the OSI stack. Figure 6.1 describes the OSI model.

Terminology Use in HL7 Messages

HL7 recommends the use of standardized terminologies in messages. Each field in a message is assigned to a vocabulary domain. The domain is the semantic type of the attribute; or, alternatively, it can be thought of as the set of concepts that are the allowed values for that field. If a message instance contains a CCC outcome field, then the vocabulary domain for that field would consist of the allowed values, which are improved, stabilized, and deteriorated. The reason for defining a vocabulary domain "is to strengthen the semantic understanding and computability of the coded information that is passed in HL7 messages" (Bakken, Campbell, Cimino, et al., 2000, p. 334).

The HL7 Vocabulary Technical Committee recognizes that organizations need information in messages to help them determine which terminology systems the code came from. They developed a process by which any terminology system may be registered by a sponsor. The process includes recording the name and contact information about the registering organization. After the registration process, an Object Identifier (OID) is assigned to the terminology system (Table 6.4). OIDs are the preferred scheme for unique identifiers in HL7. A single message can use OIDs from various sources, and a single scheme can be identified by more than one OID (e.g., by an OID from more than one organization). Once issued, an OID is never withdrawn and always identifies the same scheme or object (HL7, 2005a).

HL7 uses coded terminology in health care message interfaces. The codes are identified by using the OID and/or the abbreviation as shown in Table 6.4.

The HL7 messaging standard, version 2.x is the most widely used HL7 standard at this time. All HL7 Version 2 messages have some similar characteristics. As shown in Figure 6.2, each message is composed of segments. Each segment starts with a specific label, which is followed by the contents of fields that have been defined for that segment. Each segment ends with a carriage return "<cr>" character. The various fields within a segment are delimited by the vertical bar character ("|"). For example, in Figure 6.2, the first segment in the message is a "MSH" or message header segment. The first field in the MSH segment shows the set of field delimiters that are allowed in the message. Subsequent fields indicate the name of the sending facility, the name of the sending application, the name of the receiving facility, the name of the receiving application, the date and time of the message, security information (left blank in the example), and the message type. These fields are used to direct the message to the correct

TABLE 6.4. OBJECT IDENTIFIERS

Terminology[a]	OID	Abbreviation[a]
CCC	2.16.840.1.113883.6.236	CCC
LOINC	2.16.840.1.113883.6.1	LN
SNOMED	2.16.840.1.113883.6.5	SNM

[a]CCC, Clinical Care Classification; LOINC, Logical Observation Identifiers, Names, and Codes (LN); OID, object identifier; SNOMED, Systematized Nomenclature of Medical Clinical Terms (SNM).

```
MSH|^~\&|SABA SENDING APPLICATION|ANY CARE CENTER|SABA RECEIVING
APPLICATION|RECEIVING FACILITY|200602150930||ORU^R01 |CNTRL-3456|P|2.5<cr>

PID|||555-44-4444||EVERYWOMAN^EVE^E^^^L|JONES |196203520|F|||126 ELFS
LANE.^^ANYWHERE^UT^84444| (206)555-5555||||| AC262644||67-
A4335^UT^20030520<cr>

OBR|1|845439^SABACARE|1045813^SABACARE|CARE COMPONENT
OUTCOME^CCC|||200202150730||||||| 555-55-5555^PRIMARY^PATRICIA
P^^^MD^JANE DOE HEALTHCARE, INC. ||||||F|||||444-44-4444^JONES^JOHN
H^^^MD<cr>

OBX|1|CE|42849-0^ CONFUSION^LN||^IMPROVED^CCC|1||||F<cr>
```

FIGURE 6.2. Health Level 7 Version 2.5 message.

destination, and to indicate to the receiving system what kind of message it is (HL7, 2003).

In the example, the message type has been set to "ORU^R01." A message type of ORU means that this is an unsolicited result message, that is, a result message sent when the results are available. The standard defines the data type (strings, formatted text, numbers, time stamps, codes, addresses, and person name, etc.) of each field in a message. The second segment in Figure 6.2 is a PID (person identification) segment. This segment contains information that identifies the particular patient to whom this message pertains.

The next segment shown is an OBR (observation request) segment, which contains information about the context in which the data being reported were collected—in this case a clinical observation. An ORU message can contain one or more OBR segments, and each OBR segment is followed by one or more OBX (observation) segments. Each OBX segment contains the details of a clinical observation or measurement. In the example, a message from the Sabacare system shows the care component nursing diagnosis of CONFUSION, code 42849-0, has an actual outcome of "IMPROVED."

The HL7 messaging standard, Version 3, like V2.x, is a standard for exchanging clinical data. One of the key elements of the HL7 Version 3 standard is the inclusion of a formal model of clinical data. The model they developed is the Reference Information Model, commonly referred to as "The RIM."

The RIM is comprised of six "back-bone" classes (see Table 6.5).

Three of these classes—Act, Entity, and Role—are further represented by a set of specialized classes, or subtypes. In the HL7 representation, a subtype is only added to the RIM if it requires one or more attributes or associations that are not inherited from its parents. Classes that represent distinct concepts, but that need no further attributes or associations, are represented solely as a unique code in the controlled terminology. Therefore, these three classes include coded attributes that serve to further define the concept being modeled (Matney, Bakken, & Huff, 2003).

In the HL7 Version 3 standard, clinical observations are represented by a RIM class named Observation. Clinical observations are represented in the patient's record using attribute-value pairs or name-value pairs. Like many HL7

TABLE 6.5. RIM CLASSES

Class	Description	Comments
Act	The actions that are executed and must be documented as health care. An intentional action.	Contains subtype classes (examples): Observation, Procedure, Supply, etc.
Participation	An association between an act and a role.	For example, a nurse (**role**) authors (**participation**) a plan of care.
Entity	The physical things and beings that are of interest to, and take part in health care acts.	Person, place, organization, material, device, etc.
Role	The roles that entities play as they participate in health care acts.	A role is played by one entity, but an entity can have more than one role (patient, nurse, author).
Act Relationship	The binding of one act to another.	Such as the relationship between expected outcome and an actual outcome or an order for an observation and the observation event as it occurs.
Role Link	The relationships between individual roles.	The relationship between roles, not between people. An organization (**entity**) employs (**role link**) a nurse (**entity**).

attributes, an Observation has a code, a value, and a TargetSiteCode that is optional. A TargetSiteCode can occur more than once. An example instance of data in this form that represent "nursing diagnosis of confusion" can be represented in the following way:

```
<assessment classCode="OBS">
  <code
    code="86644006"
    codeSystem="2.16.840.1.113883.6.96"
    codeSystemName="SNOMED CT"/>
  <value
    xsi:type="CE"
    code="D07.1"
    displayName="Confusion"
    codeSystem="2.16.840.1.113883.6.236"
    codeSystemName="CCC"/>
</assessment>
```

This example is shown as an XML encoding of an assessment. Each part of the example has been placed on a separate line to make explanation easier. The first line of the example states that the content to follow is an "assessment" and that the assessment is an observation (OBS). The subsequent four lines of the example indicate that the name part of the name-value pair is represented by a SNOMED CT code of 86644006. Following the code section, the subsequent six lines of the value section indicate that the value is expressed as a CE (coded with equivalence) data type and that the actual coded value of the observation is Confusion (code D07.1) from the CCC code system.

Data types are the basic building blocks of observations. They define the structural format, or rules, of the data carried in the observation and influence the set of allowable values an observation may assume. The previous example shows that coded concepts can play at least two different roles in a name-value pair strategy: (1) as the name of the kind of observation being made, or (2) as the value of the observation being made (Table 6.6). LOINC codes are specifically designed to be used as observation identifiers, but there are also a set of "observable" entities within SNOMED CT that can play the same role. However, LOINC does not currently create codes for items that can be the values of coded observations. The values for coded items are traditionally held in a terminology like SNOMED CT.

The attribute measures in a plan of care using CCC—Care Component, Nursing Diagnosis, Expected Outcome, Nursing Intervention, Action Type,

TABLE 6.6. SAMPLE NAME-VALUE DATA TYPES

Data Type	Definition	Observation (Name) Example	Value Example
Physical Quantity (PQ)	A dimensioned quantity expressing the result of measurement. It consists of a real number value and a physical unit. Physical quantities are often constrained to a certain dimension by specifying a unit representing the dimension (e.g., m, kg, s, kcal/d, etc.). However, physical quantities should not be constrained to any particular unit (e.g., should not be constrained to centimeter instead of meter or inch).	Serum Potassium	3.8 mg/dL
Coded Value (CV)	Coded data, consist of a code, display name, code system, and original text. Used when a single code value must be sent.	Breath sounds	Wheezing
Integer Number (INT)	Positive and negative whole numbers typically the results of counting and enumerating. The standard imposes no bounds on the size of integer numbers.	Number of intubations	Three
Time Stamp (TS)	A time stamp.	Admission time	November 1, 2005, 5:09:10 PM GMT[a]

[a]GMT, Greenwich Mean Time.

and Actual Outcome—are all messaged using the Coded Value datatype. For CCC, only expected or actual outcomes related to specific nursing diagnoses are represented in LOINC.

CONCLUSIONS

In summary, EHRs have mandated the use of standardized terminologies in applications and messaging interfaces. Using standardized terminologies will help systems become interoperable. LOINC and CCC are both publicly available terminologies that can be used.

HL7 is the messaging standard for health care data. LOINC codes, CCC codes, and other standardized terminology codes can be inserted into specific fields in Version 2.x and Version 3 HL7 messages. HL7 continues to support the Version 2 standard and to develop the Version 3 RIM. LOINC and the HL7 message structure provide an essential approach that enables the sharing of nursing data such as CCC expected or actual outcomes among a variety of information systems. Such strategies are vital to support the delivery and evaluation of nursing care.

REFERENCES

Bakken, S., Campbell, K. E., Cimino, J. J., Huff, S. M., & Hammond, W. E. (2000). Toward vocabulary domain specifications for health level 7-coded data elements. *Journal of the American Medical Informatics Association, 7*, 333–342.

Bakken, S., Cimino, J. J., Haskell, R., Kukafka, R., Matsumoto, C., Chan, G. K., et al. (2000). Evaluation of the clinical LOINC (logical observation identifiers, names, and codes) semantic structure as a terminology model for standardized assessment measures. *Journal of the American Medical Informatics Association, 7*, 529–538.

Bakken, S., Warren, J. J., Casey, A., Konicek, D., Lundberg, C., & Pooke, M. (2002). Information model and terminology model issues related to goals. *Proceedings of the AMIA 2002 Annual Symposium*, 17–21.

Brailer, D. (2005). *Office of the national coordinator for health information technology (ONC) remarks*. Paper presented at Health Information and Management Systems Society, Dallas, TX.

de Keizer, N. F., Abu-Hanna, A., & Zwetslook-Schonk, J. H. M. (2000). Understanding terminological systems, I: Terminology and typology. *Methods of Information in Medicine, 39*, 16–21.

Effler, P., Ching-Lee, M., Bogard, A., Leong, M. C., Nekomoto, T., & Jernigan, D. (1999). Statewide system of electronic notifiable disease reporting from clinical laboratories: comparing automated reporting with conventional methods. *Journal of the American Medical Informatics Association, 282*, 1845–1850.

Forrey, A. W., McDonald, C. J., DeMoor, G., Huff, S. M., Leavelle, D., Leland, D., et al. (1996). Logical observation identifier names and codes (LOINC) database: A public use set of codes and names for electronic reporting of clinical laboratory test results. *Clinical Chemistry, 42*, 81–90.

HL7. (2003). *Health level seven standard, version 2.5: An application protocol for electronic data exchange in healthcare environments*. Ann Arbor, MI: Health Level Seven, Inc.

HL7. (2005a). *Introduction for the HL7 object odentifier (OID) registry.* Retrieved January 13, 2006, from <http://www.hl7.org/oid/index.cfm>

HL7. (2005b). *What is HL7?* Retrieved January 19, 2006, from <http://www.hl7.org/.>

Huff, S. M., Hammond, W. E., & Williams, W. B. (2002). Clinical information interchange with health level seven. In J. S. Silva, M. J. Ball, C. G. Chute, J. V. Douglas, C. P. Langlotz, J. C. Niland, & W. L. Scherlis (Eds.), *Cancer informatics: Essential technologies for clinical trials* (pp. 176–193). New York: Springer-Verlag.

Huff, S. M., Rocha, R. A., McDonald, C. J., De Moor, G. J. E., Fiers, T., Bidgood, W. D. Jr., et al. (1998). Development of the LOINC (logical observation identifier names and codes) vocabulary. *Journal of the American Medical Informatics Association, 5,* 276–292.

Institute of Electronics Engineers. (1990). *IEEE standard computer dictionary: A compilation of IEEE standard computer glossaries.* New York: IEEE.

Kohn, L. T., & Donaldson, M. S. (Eds.). (2000). *To err is human: Building a safer health system.* Washington, DC: Institute of Medicine: National Academy Press.

Malet, G., Munoz, F., Appleyard, R., & Hersh, W. R. (2000). A model for enhancing Internet medical document retrieval with "medical core metadata." *Journal of the American Medical Informatics Association, 7,* 108–109.

Matney, S., Bakken, S., & Huff, S. M. (2003). Representing nursing assessments in clinical information systems using the logical observation identifiers, names, and codes database. *Journal of Biomedical Informatics, 36,* 287–293.

McDonald, C. J. (1984). The search for national standards for medical data exchange. *MD Computing, 1,* 3–4.

McDonald, C. J., & Hammond, W. E. (1989). Standard formats for electronic transfer of clinical data. *Annals of Internal Medicine, 110,* 333–335.

McDonald, C. J., Huff, S. M., Vreeman, D. J., & Mercer, K. (Eds.). (2005). *Logical observation identifier names and codes (LOINC®) users' guide.* Indianapolis, IN: Regenstrief Institute.

Payne, T. H., Sengupta, S., & Sittig, D. F. (1999). Electronic exchange of patient information: The infrastructure for electronic health records. In G. F. Murphy, M. A. Hanken, & K. A. Water (Eds.), *Electronic health records: Changing the vision* (pp. 129–130). Philadelphia: W B Saunders.

Saba, V. K., & Zuckerman, A. E. (1992). A new home health classification method. *Caring Magazine, 11,* 27–34.

WHAT IS SNOMED CT?

DEBRA KONICEK

The Systematized Nomenclature of Medical Clinical Terms© (SNOMED CT©) is a comprehensive clinical terminology that provides clinical content and expressivity for clinical documentation and reporting. It can be used to code, retrieve, and analyze clinical data. SNOMED CT resulted from the merger of SNOMED Reference Terminology© (SNOMED RT©) developed by the College of American Pathologists (CAP) and Clinical Terms Version 3 (CTV3) developed by the National Health Service (NHS) of the United Kingdom. SNOMED CT was integrated into the Metathesaurus of the Unified Medical Language System (UMLS) of the National Library of Medicine (NLM) in 2003.

The SNOMED CT terminology is comprised of concepts, terms, and relationships with the objective of precisely representing clinical information across the scope of health care. Content coverage is divided into hierarchies that include:

Clinical finding
Procedure
Observable entity
Body structure
Organism
Substance
Pharmaceutical/biological product
Specimen
Special concept
Physical object

Physical force
Events
Environments/geographical locations
Social context
Context-dependent categories
Staging and scales
Linkage concept
Qualifier value
Record artifact

SNOMED CT USES

Health care software applications focus on the collection of clinical data, linking to clinical knowledge bases, information retrieval, as well as data aggregation and exchange. Information may be recorded in different ways at different times and different sites of care.

Standardized information improves data analysis. SNOMED CT provides a standard for implementing clinical information. Software applications can use the concepts, hierarchies, and relationships as a common reference point for data analysis. SNOMED CT serves as a foundation upon which health care organizations can develop effective data analysis applications to conduct outcomes research, evaluate the quality and cost of care, and design effective treatment guidelines.

Standardized terminology can provide benefits to clinicians, patients, administrators, software developers, and payers. A clinical terminology can aid in providing health care providers with more accessible and complete information pertaining to the health care process (medical history, illnesses, treatments, laboratory results, etc.) and thereby result in improved patient outcomes. Clinical terminology can allow a health care provider to identify patients based on specific coded information within their records and thereby facilitate enhanced follow-up and treatment (SNOMED, 2006a).

NURSING TERMINOLOGY CONTENT INTEGRATIONS

Convergence of Standardized Nursing Languages Within SNOMED CT

The SNOMED CT structure allows for the convergence of nursing content from a variety of standardized nursing language sources currently recognized by the American Nurses Association (ANA). Nursing concepts with similar meaning are placed within the same hierarchies. Nursing diagnoses are located within Clinical findings, Nursing interventions are found within Procedures, and Nursing outcomes concepts are modeled within the Observable entity hierarchy. Frequently, nursing concepts become synonyms of existing SNOMED CT concepts. Occasionally, concepts from two different nursing terminologies will exist within SNOMED CT as complementary synonyms of each other. It is important to understand how nursing concepts from a variety of existing classification systems converge and interrelate to one another within SNOMED CT.

NURSING CONTENT INTEGRATION PROCESS

The basic underlying principles for the addition of nursing concepts are described below. Nursing concepts are integrated into SNOMED CT via several mechanisms:

1. A nursing concept may be identical to an existing SNOMED CT concept (exact match).
2. A nursing concept may be a synonym of an existing SNOMED CT concept and is added as such.
3. A nursing concept may be new (not currently contained within the SNOMED CT terminology). These concepts are added as new given a SNOMED CT code, modeled using current attributes, and assigned a specific IS A (parent–child) relationship, placing it within the appropriate hierarchy.

TABLE 7.1. SNOMED CT/CCC NURSING DIAGNOSES INTEGRATION EXAMPLES[a]

	SNOMED CT Clinical Finding	CCC	Problem
77427003	Activity intolerance	A01.1	Activity intolerance
73879007	Nausea	B51	Nausea
129866007	Deficient knowledge: medication regimen	D08.5	Knowledge deficit of medication regimen
18676001	Ineffective family coping: disabling	E11.2	Disabled family coping
7058009	Noncompliance	G20	Noncompliance
161838002	Infant feeding problem	J54	Infant feeding pattern impairment
78648007	At risk for infection	K25.5	Infection risk
70944005	Impaired gas exchange	L26.3	Gas exchange impairment
373191003	Self-toileting deficit	O39.0	Toileting deficit

[a]CCC, Clinical Care Classification; SNOMED CT, Systematized Nomenclature of Medical Clinical Terms.

In each of the above examples, the concept is also assigned an internal (not released) identifier representing the source nursing terminology. This "marker" then allows for these concepts to be uniquely identified in order to populate the mapping tables that will be generated. These mapping tables provide the linkages between the specific nursing terminologies and SNOMED CT. For example, the Clinical Care Classification (CCC) mapping table identifies the relationship links between the CCC source terminology and SNOMED CT.

CCC NURSING MAP

The CCC map to SNOMED CT contains nursing diagnoses, outcome qualifiers, and intervention concepts that can be utilized to document patient care in any health care setting. This content provides a rich variety of nursing concepts that will enhance and expand the SNOMED efforts toward being a "health care" terminology. Future nursing content efforts will be focused on assessing end-user nursing documentation needs. SNOMED looks to the users and developers of electronic health record systems both within the United States and

TABLE 7.2. SNOMED CT/CCC OF NURSING INTERVENTIONS INTEGRATION EXAMPLES[a]

SNOMED	SNOMED CT Procedure	CCC	Intervention
385884006	Bedrest care	A61.02	Bedbound care
370871008	Ambulation therapy	A03.12	Ambulation therapy
37799002	Urinary bladder training	T58.22	Bladder training
408885009	Breast feeding support education	J66.03	Breast feeding support (teach)
50723001	Blood pressure taking education	K33.13	Blood pressure (teach)
385980003	Cardiac rehabilitation management	C08.14	Cardiac rehabilitation (manage)
408957008	Chronic pain control management	Q47.24	Chronic pain control (manage)
385725001	Emotional support assessment	E13.01	Emotional support (assess)
410223002	Mental health care assessment	P45.01	Mental health care (assess)

[a]CCC, Clinical Care Classification; SNOMED CT, Systematized Nomenclature of Medical Clinical Terms.

internationally to provide guidance in terms of possible sources of additional nursing content (SNOMED, 2006b).

Examples of the mapping between SNOMED CT and CCC of Nursing Diagnoses and CCC of Nursing Interventions are shown in Tables 7.1 and 7.2. The mapping table can be obtained directly from SNOMED.

SUMMARY

When structured nursing documentation utilizes a clinical health care terminology, the documentation creates data that can be used to reveal both the nursing process and patient outcomes. **The outcome relationships within CCC can be represented via post-coordination by combining a nursing problem with a qualifier such as Improved, Stabilized, or Deteriorated**. Combining the influence of the CCC for documentation at the point of care with the power of SNOMED CT terminology within various electronic health care record applications enhances the ability of clinicians to share data with CCC users and others.

REFERENCES

SNOMED Clinical Terms®. (2006a). *User Guide January, 2006 Release.* Chicago, IL.
SNOMED®. International College of American Pathologists.
SNOMED®. (2006b). International College of American Pathologists' Web site. Retrieved February 25, 2006, from <http://www.snomed.org>.

8

USE OF THE CLINICIAL CARE CLASSIFICATION (CCC) IN NURSING RESEARCH PROTOCOLS: A CASE STUDY OF THE CLIENT ADHERENCE PROFILING-INTERVENTION TAILORING (CAP-IT) INTERVENTION PROTOCOL

SUZANNE BAKKEN
WILLIAM L. HOLZEMER

Standardized nursing terminologies are not routinely incorporated into nursing intervention research protocols. Only a few nurse researchers have used standardized nursing terminologies to retrospectively abstract patient problems or nursing interventions from research logs or other documents collected for nursing research (Bowles, 2000; Holzemer et al., 1997; Naylor, Bowles, & Brooten, 2000). The prospective use of standardized nursing terminologies is even less frequently reported. One exception is Bakken et al. (2005), who recently reported the prospective use of the Home Health Care Classification (HHCC [now Clinical Care Classification]) to calculate the dose of the nursing intervention for the Client Adherence Profiling-Intervention Tailoring (CAP-IT) randomized controlled trial (RCT) (R01 NR004849, William L. Holzemer, Principal Investigator) and to determine the extent to which the HIV+ patients in the intervention arm of the RCT received a tailored intervention. In this chapter, we provide specific details about how we used HHCC to guide and document the delivery of the CAP-IT intervention. The following steps and associated examples provide a model that can be applied by other researchers: (1) match elements (e.g., diagnoses, interventions, outcomes) of the standardized nursing terminology to the framework of the intervention protocol; (2) specify individual components of the intervention protocol; (3) determine which components of the intervention protocol have matching terms in the standardized nursing terminology; (4) create additional terms as needed in the semantic style of the standardized nursing terminology; (5) organize into a documentation format for completion by the interventionist; and (6) analyze data.

MATCH ELEMENTS OF THE STANDARDIZED NURSING TERMINOLOGY TO THE FRAMEWORK OF THE INTERVENTION PROTOCOL

The substantive content of CAP-IT was based on the multi-factorial framework for adherence in clinical research and clinical care proposed by Ickovics and Meisler (1997). The framework includes five categories of characteristics affecting adherence: (1) client characteristics, (2) complexity of treatment regimen, (3) client–provider relationship, (4) clinical setting, and (5) disease status. Documentation of the CAP-IT process was conceptually based in the nursing process: assessment, diagnosis, outcome identification, planning, implementation, and evaluation (American Nurses Association, 1991; Yura & Walsh, 1978).

We used nursing diagnoses and nursing interventions from HHCC to guide and to document CAP-IT substance and process. Medication knowledge, adherence, and side effect management were subcategories of the complexity of treatment regimen from the Ickovics and Meisler framework. **Non-compliance with medication regimen (G20.4)** is an example of one HHCC diagnosis that was available for selection in that category of the CAP-IT intervention protocol, and **Compliance with medication regimen: Teach (G18.43)** was a potential intervention that could be delivered and subsequently documented by the nurse interventionist.

SPECIFY INDIVIDUAL COMPONENTS OF THE INTERVENTION PROTOCOL

Table 8.1 displays the components of the CAP-IT protocol for intervening in instances of medication-related nursing diagnoses. Because the main study outcome variable for the CAP-IT RCT was medication adherence, the list is extensive and detailed to reflect potentially effective interventions based on the adherence literature and preliminary work (Holzemer, Henry, Portillo, & Miramontes, 2000). In this way, the specifics of the intervention could be captured along with the associated time to enable calculation of the dose of the intervention.

DETERMINE WHICH COMPONENTS OF THE INTERVENTION PROTOCOL HAVE MATCHING TERMS IN THE STANDARDIZED NURSING TERMINOLOGY

After we specified the components (i.e., nursing diagnoses and nursing interventions) for the CAP-IT intervention protocol, we examined HHCC to find matching terms. Table 8.2 displays HHCC codes for those intervention components for which we found a match (e.g., **Coping support: Teach (E12.13)**).

CREATE ADDITIONAL TERMS AS NEEDED IN THE SEMANTIC STYLE OF THE STANDARDIZED NURSING TERMINOLOGY

Tables 8.1 and 8.2 include terms for intervention components that are not associated with a HHCC code. In these instances, in which no HHCC term existed for the intervention component, we created a term in the semantic

TABLE 8.1. MEDICATION-RELATED NURSING INTERVENTION EXAMPLES FROM THE CAP-IT[a] PROTOCOL

Compliance with medication regimen: Teach (G18.43)
   Missing doses: Teach
   Viral resistance: Teach
   Absorption: Teach
   Dose/timing: Teach
   Special instructions: Teach
   Adherence: Teach
Personal medication regimen: Teach
Integration of medications into daily life: Teach
Integration of medications into daily life: Manage/coordinate
Memory devices: Teach
Memory devices: Manage/coordinate
Self-care management of perceived medication side effects: Teach
Self-care management of perceived medication side effects: Provide self-care symptom
   management guidelines
Self-care management of perceived medication side effects: Other
Primary care provider contact: Manage/coordinate

[a]CAP-IT, Client Adherence Profiling-Intervention Tailoring.

TABLE 8.2. ROLE OF PERFORMANCE-RELATED NURSING INTERVENTION EXAMPLES FROM THE CAP-IT[a] PROTOCOL

Role performance actions
   Communication care: Teach (M38.03)
   Other: Teach
   Home situation analysis: Assess (M39.11)
   Interpersonal dynamics analysis: Assess (M39.21)
   Case manager: Manage/coordinate
   Other: Manage/coordinate

Coping impairment actions
   Coping support: Teach (E12.13)
   Stress control: Teach (E12.23)
   Other: Teach
   Coping support: Manage/coordinate (E12.14)

IADL[a] assistance
   Energy conservation: Teach (A01.23)
   Meals on wheels or other food service: Manage/coordinate (G17.34)

[a]CAP-IT, Client Adherence Profiling-Intervention Tailoring; IADL, instrumental activities of daily living.

EXHIBIT 8.1. DOCUMENTATION OF CAP-IT PROTOCOL USING HHCC[a]

Nursing Diagnoses	Coping	Minutes		
	Nursing Interventions	Telephone	1 Month	3 Months
__Individual coping impairment [12.0] related to (*please specify*): __Disease process __Medication regimen __Other (*please specify*)	__Interventions related to coping impairment			
	Teach __Coping support [12.13] (*please specify*) (e.g., enlisting help from others when needed) __Stress control [12.23] (*please specify*) (e.g., guided imagery, deep breathing, exercise) __Other (*please specify*)			
	Manage/Coordinate __Coping support [12.14], (*please specify*) (e.g., provide information about support group) __Other (*please specify*)			

[a]CAP-IT, Client Adherence Profiling-Intervention Tailoring; HHCC, Home Health Care Classification.

style of HHCC in which the target of the intervention—a noun phrase—is modified by a verb that specifies one of the four types of action. **Case manager: Manage/coordinate** is an example of an additional intervention that we created to display the same semantics as HHCC interventions.

ORGANIZE INTO A DOCUMENTATION FORMAT FOR THE COMPLETION BY THE INTERVENTIONIST

Once the diagnosis and intervention terms were specified, we organized them into a document that guided the delivery and documentation of the CAP-IT protocol. A section of the document is displayed in Exhibit 8.1.

ANALYZE DATA

As shown in Table 8.3, collecting data in this manner allowed us to describe the nursing diagnoses assigned and interventions delivered for the HIV+ persons in the intervention arm of the RCT and facilitated calculation of the dose of the intervention from types of interventions delivered (Bakken et al., 2005). As a measure of how much of a particular intervention category the client received, the nurse interventionist also documented time.

CONCLUSION

The integration of a standardized nursing terminology, specifically HHCC, into the CAP-IT intervention protocol allowed us to capture data in a reliable manner, to describe the nursing diagnoses assigned and interventions delivered as part of the protocol, and enabled calculation of the dose of the intervention for

TABLE 8.3. SUMMARY OF ROLE PERFORMANCE-RELATED ASPECTS OF CAP-IT[a] PROTOCOL

Assignment of Nursing Diagnoses	N (%)
Role performance alteration	52 (44.4)
Good partner/spouse	8 (6.8)
Parenting	15 (12.7)
Problem-solving	41 (35.0)
Inability to seek help when needed	38 (32.5)
Individual coping impairment (E12.0)	32 (27.4)
Instrumental Activities of Daily Living alteration	5 (4.3)
	Mean (SD)
Total number of diagnoses per client in this category	2.0 (2.2)

Delivery of Nursing Interventions	N (%)
Role performance actions	52 (44.4)
Communication care: Teach (M38.03)	49 (41.9)
Other: Teach	17 (14.5)
Case manager: Manage/coordinate	14 (12.0)
Home situation analysis: Assess (M39.11)	6 (5.1)
Interpersonal dynamics analysis: Assess (M39.21)	5 (4.3)
Other: Manage/coordinate	3 (2.5)
Coping impairment actions	31 (26.7)
Coping support: Teach (E12.13)	26 (22.2)
Stress control: Teach (E12.23)	10 (8.5)
Other: Teach	11 (9.4)
Coping support: Manage/coordinate (E12.14)	22 (18.8)
Instrumental activities of daily living assistance	5 (4.3)
Energy conservation: Teach (A01.23)	3 (2.6)
Meals on wheels or other food service: Manage/coordinate (G17.34)	2 (1.7)
	Mean (SD)
Total number of interventions per client in this category	0.8 (0.8)

IT (Time in Minutes)	Mean (SD)
Initial visit	4.5 (10.7)
Telephone calls	0.04 (0.4)
1- and 3-month follow-up	3.9 (6.7)
Total dose	8.4 (15.4)

[a]CAP-IT, Client Adherence Profiling-Intervention Tailoring.

entry into a variety of data analyses for the RCT. Use of standardized nursing terminologies in research protocols has the potential to facilitate data aggregation across research studies and facilitate synthesis of the evidence related to particular interventions or clusters of interventions. In addition, use of the same standardized terminologies in both research and clinical practice has the potential to enable building evidence from practice and application of evidence gained through research studies to practice.

REFERENCES

American Nurses Association. (1991). *Standards of clinical nursing practice* (2nd ed.). Washington, DC: American Nurses Publishing.

Bakken, S., Holzemer, W. L., Portillo, C. J., Grimes, R., Welch, J., & Wantland, D. (2005). Utility of a standardized nursing terminology to evaluate dosage and tailoring of an HIV/AIDS adherence intervention. *Journal of Nursing Scholarship, 37,* 251–257.

Bowles, K. (2000). Patient problems and nursing interventions during acute care and discharge planning. *Journal of Cardiovascular Nursing, 14,* 29–41.

Holzemer, W. L., Henry, S., Portillo, C., & Miramontes, H. (2000). The Client adherence profiling-intervention tailoring (CAP-IT) intervention for enhancing adherence to HIV/AIDS medications: A pilot study. *Journal of the Association of Nurses in AIDS Care, 11,* 36–44.

Holzemer, W. L., Henry, S. B., Dawson, C., Sousa, K., Bain, C., & Hsieh, S. F. (1997). An evaluation of the utility of the home health care classification for categorizing patient problems and nursing interventions from the hospital setting. *Studies in Health Technology & Informatics, 46,* 21–26.

Ickovics, J., & Meisler, A. (1997). Adherence in AIDS clinical trials: A framework for clinical research and clinical care. *Clinical Epidemiology, 50,* 385–391.

Naylor, M., Bowles, K., & Brooten, D. (2000). Patient problems and advanced practice nurse interventions during transitional care. *Public Health Nursing, 72,* 94–102.

Yura, H., & Walsh, M. (1978). *The nursing process: Assessing, planning, implementing, evaluating* (3rd ed.). New York: Appleton-Century Crofts.

9

APPROACHES TO IMPLEMENTING THE CCC: EDUCATING NURSES IN ELECTRONIC DOCUMENTATION

VERONICA D. FEEG

As the nation moves toward a fully operational electronic health record (EHR) in the hospital and health care systems of the future, nurses will need the capability to capture salient information about their patients and record the health service they provide efficiently and in a manner that it can be aggregated for reports. Computerized records will need to evolve that demonstrate evidence of nursing care, and nurses will need to know how the systems articulate with other electronic data elements that are necessary for documentation. With widespread efforts to synthesize information and improve the quality of care provided to patients through analysis, it will be expected that health care communication and record-keeping be automated and standardized. As measures become more precise for medicine and allied health, nursing care documentation will also need a combination of precision with efficiency via electronic means.

To move from paper care planning to an automated process of documentation will require significant efforts to educate nurses about documentation in general and electronic methods specifically. This education should include both the social engagement of the nurse and patient that forms the basis of the health assessment and planning process, followed by the logical sequence of recording the results of the interaction. Recording the findings of the assessment and noting the subsequent steps of care planning is the next deliberate action of the nurse in documentation. Paper versions of charts have long served the hospital with a physical place to store relevant information, and the nursing process has served nurses with a methodology to systematically document nursing care. This process is now being transformed by the digital age and mandates a more focused action on essential data so that they can be recorded easily and reported fully. The transition from paper to computer screen can occur in a structured learning environment with tools to teach the steps to nurses in the workplace and nursing students who will be the workers of the future.

Schools of nursing and hospital education departments need to commit to developing programs to support nurses in demonstrating the care they provide to their patients and the outcomes of that care in addition to the purely technical documentation related to activities, such as medication administration, that they do now. Nurses should be encouraged to show evidence of the health service they give to justify the substantive social and therapeutic interaction between patient and nurse that result in improved health. The Clinical Care Classification (CCC) as an organized and standardized nursing terminology offers a structure for capturing information in a way that lends itself to analysis of care provided. As the Joint Commission on Accrediting Hospitals and Organizations (JCAHO) increases its expectations that clinical care must be documented in order to be evaluated, the CCC provides the language of nursing, and the computer gives it life.

TEACHING TERMINOLOGY AND LANGUAGE

The American Nurses Association, in their *Scope and Standards of Practice for Nursing Informatics*, made explicit that nurses today must have competencies in information technologies. "Informatics competencies are needed by all nurses whether or not they specialize in nursing informatics. As nursing settings become ubiquitous computing environments, all nurses must be both information and computer literate" (American Nurses Association, 2001, p. 24). The new standards emphasize the central role that information plays in the practice of nursing. Within general nursing, nurses must be highly skilled in information management and communication. According to Staggers, Gassert, and Curran (2001), nurses should be able to see relationships among data elements, make judgments based on trends, and use informatics solutions. But, where are these skills developed and how can nurse educators prepare the graduate nurse with the underlying knowledge to become technically equipped to adapt and thrive in the diverse work world where health information technology (IT) systems vary in functionality and operations?

The answer lies in emphasizing the data structures of nursing concepts within the nursing curriculum while providing opportunity to use computer applications to manage nursing clinical data, thereby demonstrating the principles of integration of standardized language and format conventions. Nurse educators need to teach the foundations of nursing classification and terminologies using the nursing process that is inherent in curriculum, while at the same time providing opportunities to document clinical care electronically.

Our current education environments have evolved to incorporate into the instructional activities a variety of opportunities for students to engage in the knowledge material they are expected to learn. From case scenarios, role-plays, and interactive media with the information presented in textbooks, process books, and journals to clinical simulations with mannequins, models, and activities with other students, educating students has become a multi-modal approach. Students practice technical skills in laboratories, but have fewer opportunities to integrate the knowledge and decision-making skills with the psychomotor skills of "doing" nursing.

There are an increasing number of books available and written materials that present the nursing process and incorporate a systematic way to communicate information from the assessment to evaluation of care. Flash cards, lists, and electronic documents exist with dictionary definitions, sequential examples, and potentially customizable forms. However, the concepts of diagnosis, intervention, and evaluation within the domain of nursing are parallel ideas if not assimilated into the learning of caring for patients.

A standardized nursing terminology forms the base of clinical decision making in operationalizing nursing care. Teaching students the standardized terms absent of real application or even simulated interaction falls short of the educational goal of having students truly understand the seamless process that is concurrent with critical thinking, problem solving, and formulating care plans. What is needed for education environments is an inexpensive method for students to engage in clinical decision making relevant to nursing where they can document efficiently via computer (laptop, handheld, or tablet) using standardized nursing terms that are exemplary of potential systems in whatever hospital or clinic environment they may work in the future.

RECENT STUDIES AND EDUCATIONAL APPLICATIONS

There have been several recent efforts to develop applications for students to document patient care using electronic methods. One recent system has been designed and built by Klein and Bakken (2001) at Columbia University as a student clinical log database and knowledge system that supports the aggregation, analysis, and reporting of graduate students in advance practice. The University of Kansas has partnered with Cerner Corporation to develop a Simulated E-hEalth Delivery System (SEEDS) that enables students to practice using a live production information system designed for care delivery (Connors, Weaver, Warren, & Miller, 2002). Another project underway by Bakken and colleagues (2002) is the development of a standardized terminology-based database with Palm interface for documentation and analysis of student clinical experiences and Web-based information retrieval at the point of care (POC) (Bakken et al., 2002). These programs ambitiously include a variety of coding dictionaries that advance practice nurses need (i.e., the International Classification of Diseases-Version 9 (ICD-9), CPT, Logical Observation Identifiers, Names, and Codes (LOINC), and select Clinical Care Classification (CCC) codes), but are not available, cost-effective, or appropriate for undergraduate nursing students.

The Nightingale Tracker (NT) is a computerized point of care patient information processing unit using the Omaha Patient Care Record System (OPCRS) software incorporated into a hand-held unit. In a collaborative project to evaluate student reactions to the NTs, researchers identified significant changes in positive responses in Associate Degree Nursing (ADN) group, but not the baccalaureate students over time. The researchers reported that the success of the technology was dependent on the hardware and system technological support, because it significantly affected student responses (Sutherland, Wofford, Hamilton, & Schmidt, 2003).

INTEGRATING TERMINOLOGY AND TECHNOLOGY INTO THE CURRICULUM

So, how do we approach teaching about standardized languages in conjunction with using technologies that will be ubiquitous in the student's future health care environment at a reasonable cost and within the constraints of curricular compatibility and time limits? Most hospital information systems demand an intensive learning experience with a steep learning curve, particularly when users are naive to technologies in general. Nursing students who arrive on their first clinical rotation discover that they must either invest the time in learning the system or opt for an alternative to learning documentation as their faculty accommodate to unit or agency requirements. It is almost impossible to fit into an already compact schedule the necessary hours to become proficient at charting the various functions that are required, much less to apply the content learned in documenting the nursing process. If a new terminology must be learned, it needs to flow from the experiences—much like anyone learns a foreign language—to master a proficiency in thinking in the language.

THE PC VERSION OF THE CCC (PC-CCC)

The PC-CCC system was developed to (1) accommodate nursing students in nursing education settings or teach nurses in practice settings an application of the standardized nursing terminology; (2) navigate an electronic documentation system with pull-down menus, buttons, and type-in boxes; (3) allow users to practice in non-threatening environment techniques to improve patient care charting; and (4) apply an established terminology to track patient care experiences that can be aggregated for reports of intervention frequencies and proportion of time spent in nursing actions. The application could be used on a laptop or modified in the future for a pocket PC or tablet, and it would be written in Microsoft Access—a universally available database that is generally part of most PC purchases with Microsoft Windows.

The PC version of the Sabacare CCC system (Feeg, Saba, & Feeg, 2005) was developed by the authors and a Microsoft Access programmer with several iterations in phase 1 of the project. At each session, the researchers discussed cases that could be documented, and identified and addressed screen design issues. The screens were developed in a way that allows the user to enter a patient problem and observe incremental notations added to a summary grid at the bottom of the screen as each problem is recorded. This "data-based" system was exported as an executable file to be launched from the desktop by the subjects in the experimental group.

The CCC system is entered through a switchboard (see Exhibit 9.1) after brief rudimentary information about the patient (Core Patient Information) is entered (see Exhibit 9.2). (**Note:** The patient core data require a minimal number of elements in this version so that the student or new learner is not spending significant time working with patient administrative data. It does, however,

EXHIBIT 9.1. SWITCHBOARD FOR THE PC-CCC. CCCS, CLINICAL CARE CLASSIFICATION SYSTEM

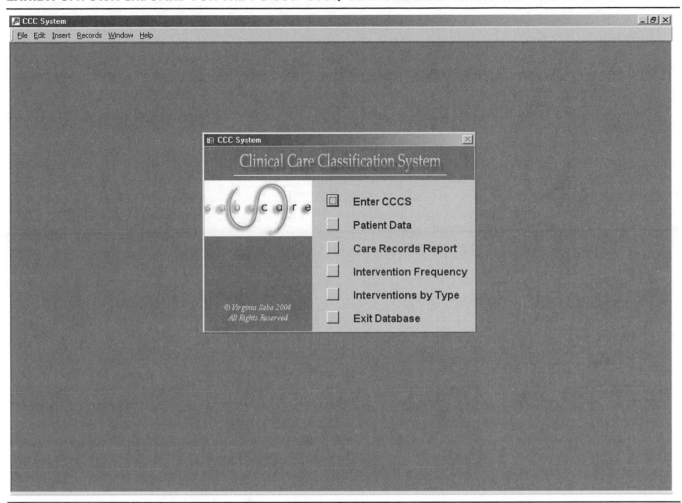

demonstrate the interactions required with radio buttons and check boxes, along with traditional type-in lines with fixed space.)

The CCC screen is organized according to the nursing process. It displays three sections with several drop-down menus and dialog boxes. The upper left side is used to record diagnosis information, and the upper right side is used to record intervention information. Each side connects to three options of outcome "modifiers": (1) **expected outcomes** of *improve, stabilize,* or *support deterioration;* and (2) **actual outcomes** of *improved, stabilized, or deteriorated.* Both sides are linked in the coding structure such that entering data on one side can populate fields on the other side automatically. The user is forced to select at least one of four types of actions (*assess, teach, care, and/or manage)* before a "record" button appears, which subsequently allows the user to view the entered problem on the summary grid (see Exhibit 9.3).

Two "notes" boxes allow the nurse to supplement the selections from the drop-down menus with clinical observations or details to the intervention. The summary grid displays the categories of information, and the user can

EXHIBIT 9.2. CORE PATIENT INFORMATION

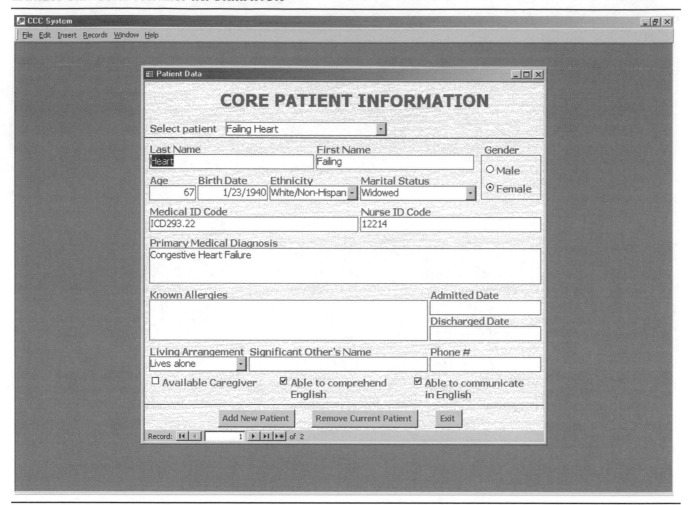

subsequently print a report of the patient's full problem list that is displayed with complete documentation, including notes and box text. The problem identified can be "resolved" with an automatic date stamp, and the user can see how adding multiple problems creates a series of areas for the nurse to focus on in providing care.

Returning to the switchboard, the user can select and learn how data can be collated and reported with a variety of organized presentations. The options included from the switchboard lead to screens of patient reports in a series (see Exhibit 9.4), aggregated frequency data of interventions that have been done for all patients in the system (see Exhibit 9.5), and a chart that provides a composite of types of actions by proportion (see Exhibit 9.6).

USING THE PC-CCC

The Microsoft application is suitable for any PC that has Microsoft Access residing on the computer. With a few necessary requirements in the set-up, the file

EXHIBIT 9.3. PC-CCC SCREEN SAMPLE. ADLS, ACTIVITIES OF DAILY LIVING

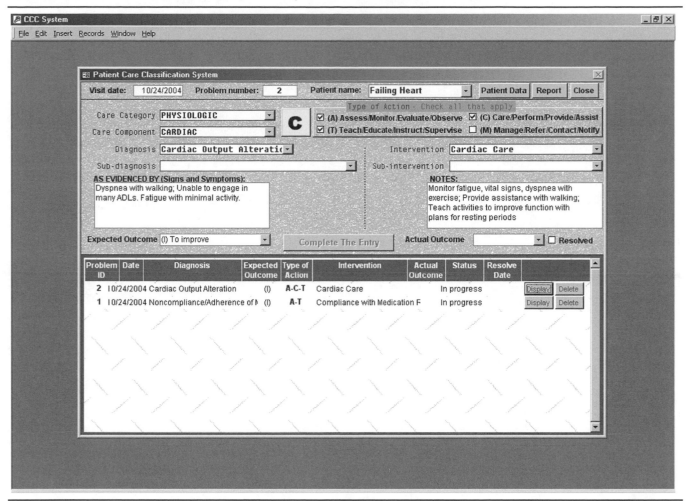

can be downloaded and made resident on each learner's PC, naming the application with a unique file name that includes ".mde" as the dot extension (see Exhibit 9.7). Each time the application is downloaded, the name can be annotated with a version or date, so that the application can calculate a series of patient entries and can be adjusted to reflect a period of documenting care. For example, in a given semester, the nursing faculty can instruct each student to download the application and use their last name as an identifier. Over a series of clinical experiences or semesters, each file can capture all the patients' care data and aggregate reports for faculty to assess the range and depth of patient encounters and interventions. (**Note:** Students should, of course, be instructed to use proxy names or some other identification code for patient names so that private patient health information (PHI) is de-identified for the purpose of learning. This should be no different than any care planning that students engage in for the purposes of learning).

EXHIBIT 9.4. PC-CCC SAMPLE PATIENT CARE REPORT. ADLS ACTIVITIES OF DAILY LIVING

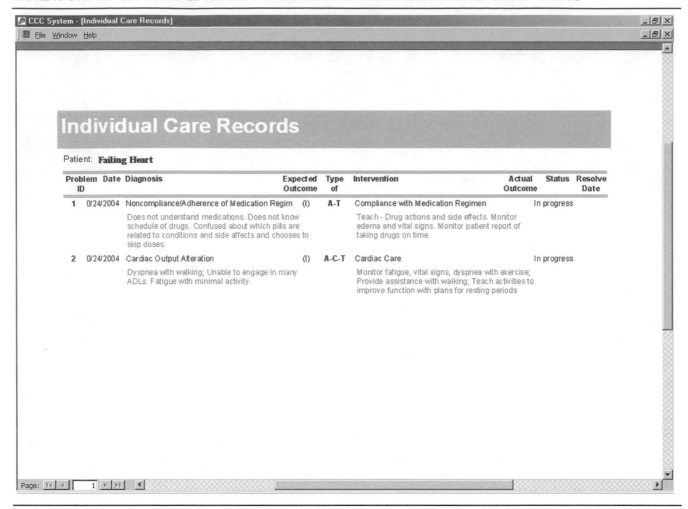

The application has been tested in student clinical lab settings (Feeg et al., 2005) and has been effective in teaching students about electronic documentation, nursing terminology, and the patient care planning process. In addition, the findings suggest that a user's care plan is significantly better than using an electronic process where free-form text is typed in to pre-set fillable boxes structured to document patient care planning.

With the growing need for educating students in the academic or laboratory setting, this study provides evidence for using the program on a laptop with a printer mounted at the bedside. The cost for each simulated "work station" is the price of an inexpensive PC and printer, less than $1,000, compared with the expensive systems being offered through vendor partnerships in only a few settings approaching $35,000 per school program. The Sabacare CCC System PC application offers a streamlined method for students to learn nursing terminologies, care planning, and electronic documentation.

EXHIBIT 9.5. PC-CCC AGGREGATE BY TYPE OF INTERVENTION

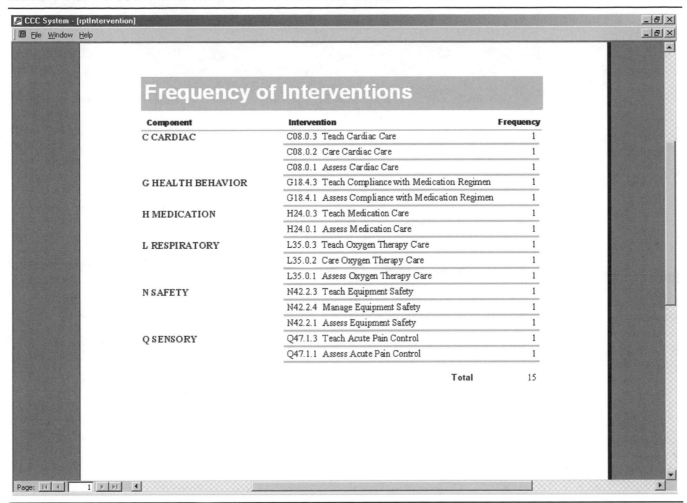

Component	Intervention	Frequency
C CARDIAC	C08.0.3 Teach Cardiac Care	1
	C08.0.2 Care Cardiac Care	1
	C08.0.1 Assess Cardiac Care	1
G HEALTH BEHAVIOR	G18.4.3 Teach Compliance with Medication Regimen	1
	G18.4.1 Assess Compliance with Medication Regimen	1
H MEDICATION	H24.0.3 Teach Medication Care	1
	H24.0.1 Assess Medication Care	1
L RESPIRATORY	L35.0.3 Teach Oxygen Therapy Care	1
	L35.0.2 Care Oxygen Therapy Care	1
	L35.0.1 Assess Oxygen Therapy Care	1
N SAFETY	N42.2.3 Teach Equipment Safety	1
	N42.2.4 Manage Equipment Safety	1
	N42.2.1 Assess Equipment Safety	1
Q SENSORY	Q47.1.3 Teach Acute Pain Control	1
	Q47.1.1 Assess Acute Pain Control	1
	Total	**15**

CONCLUSION

The Sabacare Clinical Care Classification (CCC) system is an established nursing language that has provided a base of development for numerous patient care information systems in hospitals and home care. The PC-CCC version of the system is an effective way to improve students' performance of patient care plan documentation while teaching them an application in an electronic format. The application was developed as a deliverable for any PC with Windows and Microsoft Office programs, which are ubiquitous today and readily accessible by students and faculty rather than tied to costly large mainframe "live" systems with their associated patient privacy issues that can complicate learning. The system was tested in a randomized trial with the control group using a type-in, text-based only system also mounted on the bedside computer for the study. The results demonstrated that the application is efficient and effective in recording nursing care planning information using the nursing process and

EXHIBIT 9.6. PC-CCC AGGREGATE BY TYPE OF ACTION

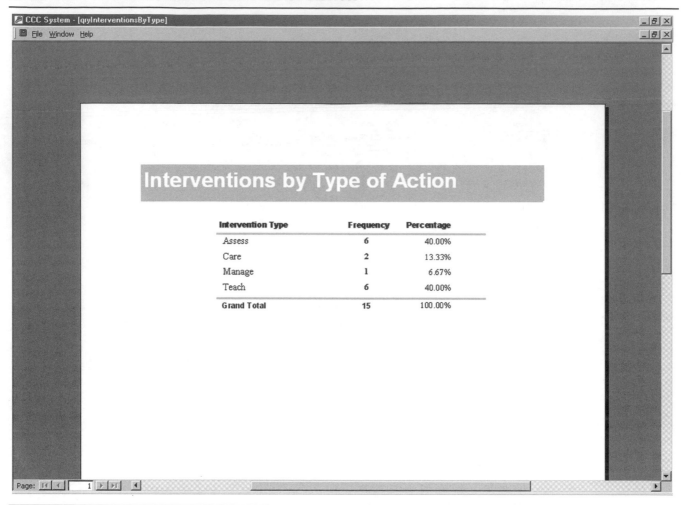

EXHIBIT 9.7. INSTRUCTIONS FOR DOWNLOADING PC-CCC EXECUTABLE FILE

To DOWNLOAD the File—http://sabacare.com

You will be directed to read background information and agree to terms to use the software. Where instructed to download the PC-CCC database, you will immediately prompted to save the file. Locate a suitable directory or desktop location and save the file. Your instructor may ask you to rename the file using your last name as part of the file name. Be sure that the dot-extension is **.mde** and that your screen display is set at 1024 x 768 pixels.

The CCCS-db is a Microsoft Access® database that will allow you to enter modest patient information, process a standard-language nursing care plan, aggregate summaries of all patients you have recorded, and print reports for individual patients, summary of all patients, or aggregates of care (interventions) performed. It is based on the Sabacare CCCS (Clinical Care Classification System) nursing language that has been used with numerous hospitals and home care information systems. This PC version gives you options to record problems and interventions from a limited operation of the system that can feasibly be stored on your own or a designated server.

capturing patient care information with a language that is standardized and ready for integration with other patient electronic medical record data. Although it needs to be tested further in real clinical environments, this study has clinical implications for developers, trainers, nursing education departments, and nursing informaticists who assist in the development and implementation of clinical systems within large enterprise hospital information systems. The simple, inexpensive, streamlined PC version can help nurses and future nurses assimilate a language while they are documenting a process. This will maximize learning and improve nursing efficiency with computerized systems, wherever they may practice.

REFERENCES

American Nurses Association. (2001). *Scope and standards of practice for nursing informatics*. Washington, DC: American Nurses Publishing.

Bakken, S., Curran, C., Delaleu-McIntosh, J., et al. (2002). Informatics for evidence-based nurse practitioner practice at the Columbia University School of Nursing. Unpublished manuscript. Klein Consulting, Inc., Ridge, NY. (Available from: kci@tklein.com.)

Connors, H., Weaver, C., Warren, J., & Miller, K. (2002). An academic-business partnership for advancing clinical informatics. *Nursing Education Perspectives, 23*, 228–233.

Feeg, V., Saba, V., & Feeg, A. (2005). Development and testing of a bedside personal computer (PC) clinical care classification system (CCCS) for nursing students using Microsoft Access®. Presented at Sigma Theta Tau International Annual Convention, Indianapolis, IN.

Klein, W., & Bakken, S. (2001). Design and implementation of a student clinical log database and knowledge base. Unpublished manuscript. Klein Consulting, Inc., Ridge, NY. (Available from: kci@tklein.com.)

Staggers, N., Gassert, C., & Curran, C. (2001). Informatics from competencies for nurses at four levels of practice. *Journal of Nursing Education, 40*, 303–316.

Sutherland, J., Wofford, D., Hamilton, M., & Schmidt, B. (2003). Application of the nightingale tracker: A collaborative research project between an associate and baccalaureate degree nursing program. *Online Journal of Nursing Informatics, 7*(3) [Online]. Retrieved November 22, 2005, from http://www.eaa-knowledge.com/ojni/ni/7_3/sutherland.htm.

10

INTEGRATION OF THE CLINICAL CARE CLASSIFICATION (CCC) INTO AN ELECTRONIC STUDENT CLINICAL LOG (ESCL)

SUZANNE BAKKEN
NAM-JU LEE

Since 2002, advanced practice nurse (APN) students at the Columbia University School of Nursing have entered de-identified clinical encounter data into a custom program on a personal digital assistant (PDA). The electronic student clinical log (ESCL) and related database and knowledgebase were designed to serve multiple purposes:

- Documentation of clinical encounters using standardized nursing terminologies and other health care-related coding systems
- Student critical examination of practice over time through benchmarking reports
- Faculty review of reports to determine if students are receiving appropriate experiences that will prepare them to deliver care safely
- Faculty feedback to students on care that is inconsistent with the best evidence or is potentially unsafe.

Key technical steps that were required to create a system that supported these multiple purposes include design of the system architecture, selection of data elements and standardized terminologies for the data elements, design and implementation of the user interface, design and implementation of the database and knowledgebase, and design and implementation of reports. These processes are documented in detail in Bakken et al. (2004); Bakken, Curran, Delaleu-McIntosh, et al. (2003); and Klein and Bakken (2003). Examples of integration into the curriculum and data use are reported in Bakken, Cook, Curtis, Soupios, and Curran (2003); Desjardins, Cook, Jenkins, and Bakken (2005); and Jenkins, Hewitt, and Bakken (2006).

In this chapter, we specifically describe our experience in integrating aspects of the Clinical Care Classification (CCC) into the PDA-based ESCL for two types of APN students: entry-to-practice (ETP) students (Year 1 of APN program for non-nurses with bachelor's degrees) and Nurse Practitioner (NP) students. In addition, we provide illustrative data about system use and discuss current strategies for expansion of the ESCL.

INTEGRATING CCC INTO THE ESCL

The process of integrating CCC into the ESCL included: (1) selection of data elements to be included in the ESCL; (2) generation of criteria for selection of standardized terminologies for representation of specific data elements, evaluation of potential terminologies, and selection of terminologies; (3) integration of terminologies into the project knowledgebase and database; and (4) organization of terms for user data entry on the PDA.

Selection of Data Elements

For the ETP program, the overarching framework for the ESCL was the nursing process and data elements were selected to represent the diagnosis, expected outcome, and intervention phases of the nursing process. Additional data elements included those related to medical diagnoses, patient demographics (e.g., age, gender, race/ethnicity), as well as student information, such as clinical site and level of independence in performing interventions.

For NP students, we selected a framework consistent with NP practice and expanded the data elements to include a broad list of medical diagnoses and treatments. The framework for the NP application is the SOAP (Subjective, Objective, Assessment, Plan) note augmented by categories of a five-part NP plan as taught in our curriculum (Diagnostics, Procedures, Prescriptions, Teaching and Counseling interventions, and Referrals). Nursing diagnoses are tied to the Assessment section of the SOAP note and nursing interventions to Teaching and Counseling and Referral sections of the NP plan of care. Data elements were reviewed by Program Directors prior to selection of the final set of data elements (Bakken et al., 2004).

Selection of Terminologies to Represent Data Elements

Our criteria for selection of the standardized terminologies for the structured data elements in the ESCL were:

- Included in the Unified Medical Language System (UMLS)
- Recognized by the American Nurses Association (ANA)
- Registered with Health Level 7 (HL7) for vocabulary domain specification
- Priority given to systems in the public domain.

Based on our evaluation, we selected International Classification of Diseases–Clinical Modification (ICD9-CM) for medical diagnoses; the National

Institutes of Health (NIH) for race/ethnicity codes; and the CCC for nursing diagnoses, nursing interventions, and expected outcomes. In some instances, no terminologies that met our criteria were available, so it was necessary to select alternatives. For example, in the ESCL for NPs, we used the Physician's Current Procedural Terminology codes for procedures and diagnostic tests. We also created custom terminologies for local concepts such as student names, clinical sites, and rotations.

Integration of Terminologies Into the Database

The Repository database is the primary location for all clinical knowledge. This database contains all coded concepts from standardized and custom terminologies, the associated meta-data, and all relationships between the concepts necessary to build each of the content tables for the PDA drop-down lists. The two main tables in the database are CODELISTS and RELATED-CODES. As shown in Exhibit 10.1, the CODELISTS table contains all terminologies,

EXHIBIT 10.1. THE CODELISTS TABLE CONTAINS ALL TERMINOLOGIES, INCLUDING CCC, CODES, DISPLAY STRINGS, AND OTHER META-DATA FOR ALL CODED CONCEPTS

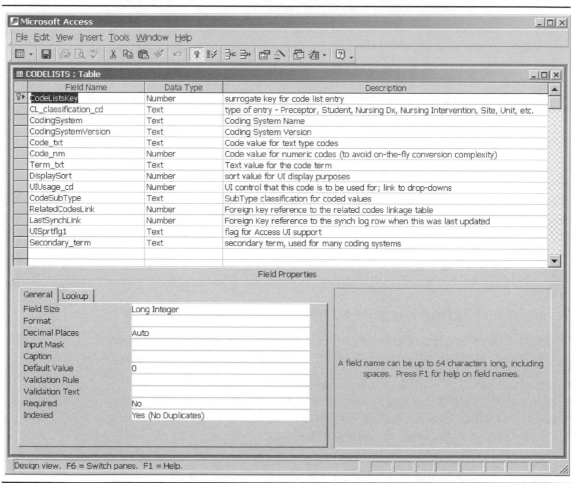

including CCC, codes, display strings, and other meta-data for all coded concepts (including aspects such as the display order of the terms for the user interface). The RELATED-CODES table maintains relationships between concepts defined in the CODELISTS table. For example, codes define the relationship between nursing diagnoses and CCC care components, and between the category of referral and CCC referral terms that are used in the interface of the ESCL for NPs.

Organization of Terms for PDA User Interface

We used several principles for organization of terms for the user interface. First, the user interface was tailored based on rotation for the ETP program and specialty for the NP program. For example, the lists of nursing diagnoses and nursing interventions differed for the medical-surgical rotation versus the community health rotation, and the types of teaching and counseling interventions were different for neonatal NPs than for gerontology NPs. Second, to minimize lengths of lists and the consequent scrolling, we used a more general term to group interventions for the user interface (Exhibit 10.2). In some instances it was a CCC care component and in other instances, we used a custom term chosen by domain experts. Third, as another strategy to limit scrolling through long lists, we linked possible nursing interventions to nursing diagnoses in the ETP ESCL (Exhibit 10.3).

USE OF THE ESCL

During approximately 2 years of data collection and analysis, ETP students documented 17,320 client encounters using the ESCL. More than 120,000 CCC nursing interventions were documented for these clients. NP students have documented 71,664 encounters since 2003. More than 38,000 CCC nursing diagnoses were entered, including: Knowledge Deficit: Safety Precautions ($n = 5,724$); Knowledge Deficit: Disease Process ($n = 4,554$); Knowledge Deficit: Therapeutic Regimen ($n = 3,450$); Knowledge Deficit: Medication Regimen ($n = 2,866$); and Noncompliance: Medication Regimen ($n = 2,482$). Most frequently occurring among the 344,132 CCC teaching and counseling interventions documented were those related to Disease Process ($n = 20,089$), Health Promotion ($n = 19,101$), Nutrition Care ($n = 18,910$), Medication Actions ($n = 14,553$), and Compliance with Therapeutic Regimen ($n = 11,835$).

EXPANSION OF THE ESCL

Currently, we are expanding the ESCL to provide decision support for clinical practice guidelines of relevance to APN practice. Through funding from the National Institute of Nursing Research, we are conducting a randomized controlled trial to examine the impact of decision support integrated into the ESCL on adherence to guideline recommendations for obesity management, depression

EXHIBIT 10.2. IN THE NP STUDENT CLINICAL LOG, ONCE THE CATEGORY OF PHYSICAL HEALTH IS SELECTED, TEACHING INTERVENTIONS CAN BE CHOSEN FROM A DROP-DOWN LIST

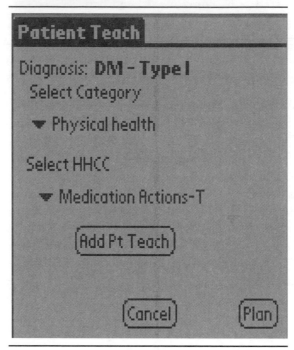

screening, and tobacco use. Where applicable, we are using CCC nursing diagnosis and nursing intervention terms to represent assessments and interventions associated with the clinical guidelines. However, in some instances, more granular intervention terms are required to represent guideline knowledge. In addition, the approaches that we used to integrate CCC and other terminologies into the ESCL are being applied in the creation of the decision support system.

CONCLUSION

The integration of CCC into the ESCL has allowed us to document the nursing diagnoses generated and nursing interventions delivered by ETP and NP students at the Columbia University School of Nursing. This provides a firm foundation in the use of nursing language in practice for ETP students. This is also important for NPs because the documentation requirements for reimbursement (medical diagnoses and procedures) often take precedence over documentation of nursing care delivered during the encounter. If we are to truly determine the impact of NPs on patient outcomes and distinguish between care delivered by NPs and physicians or between NPs prepared at the Masters degree level versus

EXHIBIT 10.3. IN THE ETP STUDENT CLINICAL LOG, THE STUDENT SELECTS NURSING INTERVENTIONS FROM A TAILORED DROP-DOWN LIST RELATED TO THE NURSING DIAGNOSIS OF RESPIRATORY ALTERATION

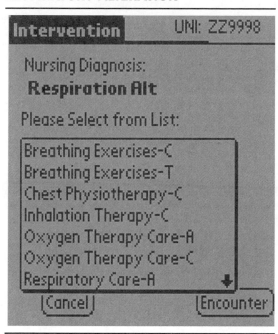

the clinical doctorate level, it is vital to document nursing judgments and nursing interventions, as well as medical diagnoses and interventions.

ACKNOWLEDGMENTS

The development of the original student clinical log was supported by an educational grant from the Health Resources and Services Administration. Mobile Decision Support for Advanced Practice Nurses is funded by the National Institute of Nursing Research (1R01 NR008903).

REFERENCES

Bakken, S., Cook, S., Curtis, L., Desjardins, K., Hyun, S., Jenkins, M., et al. (2004). Promoting patient safety through informatics-based nursing education. *International Journal of Medical Informatics, 73,* 581–589.

Bakken, S., Cook, S., Curtis, L., Soupios, M., & Curran, C. (2003). Informatics competencies pre- and post-implementation of a Palm-based student clinical log and informatics for evidence-based practice curriculum. *Proceedings of the American Medical Informatics Association Symposium,* pp. 42–46.

Bakken, S., Curran, C., Delaleu-McIntosh, J., et al. (2003). *Informatics for evidence-based nurse practitioner practice at the Columbia University School of Nursing.* Paper presented at the NI 2003, Rio de Janiero, Brazil.

Desjardins, K. S., Cook, S. S., Jenkins, M., & Bakken, S. (2005). Effect of an informatics for evidence-based practice curriculum on nursing informatics competencies. *International Journal of Medical Informatics, 74,* 1012–1020.

Jenkins, M., Hewitt, C., & Bakken, S. (2006). Women's health nursing in the context of the national health information infrastructure. *Journal of Obstetric, Gynecologic, & Neonatal Nursing, 35,* 141–150.

Klein, W. T., & Bakken, S. (2003). *Design and implementation of a student clinical log database and knowledge base.* Paper presented at the NI 2003, Rio de Janeiro, Brazil.

11

BIBLIOGRAPHY OF MAJOR CLINICAL CARE CLASSIFICATION (CCC) SYSTEM ARTICLES: 1991–2006

Purpose 95   Articles 95

PURPOSE

This chapter consists of a bibliography of the major articles written about the Clinical Care Classification (CCC) system previously known as the Home Health Care Classification (HHCC) system referred to in the context of the article by Saba and other authors. It includes articles written about the HHCC system (Version 1.0) that were first published in 1991, as well as those written about the CCC system (Version 2.0) until the publication of this manual in 2006. The articles are listed by year starting with the most current. This bibliography will serve as a reference for people interested in the CCC system.

ARTICLES

2006

Feeg, V. D., Saba, V. K., & Feeg, A. (in press). Development and testing of a bedside personal computer (PC) clinical care classification system (CCCS) for nursing students using Microsoft Access. *Computers in Nursing*.

Saba, V. K. (2006). Appendix: Clinical care classification (Version 2.0). Two terminologies: CCC of nursing diagnoses and CCC of nursing interventions classified by 21 care components. In V. K. Saba & K. A. McCormick (Eds.), *Essentials of nursing informatics* (4th ed., pp. 681–686). New York: McGraw-Hill.

Struk, C. M., Peters, D. A., & Saba, V. K. (2006). Community health applications. In V. K. Saba & K. A. McCormick, *Essentials of nursing informatics* (4th ed., pp. 391–412). New York: McGraw-Hill.

2005

Bakken, S., Holzemer, W. L., Portillo, C. J., Grimes, R., Welch, J., & Wantland, D. (2005). Utility of a standardized nursing terminology to evaluate dosage and tailoring of an HIV/AIDS adherence intervention. *Journal of Nursing Scholarship, 37,* 251–257.

Choi, J., Jenkins, M. L., Cimino, J. J., White, T. M., & Bakken, S. (2005). Toward semantic interoperability in home health care: Formally representing OASIS items for integration into a concept-oriented terminology. *Journal of the American Medical Informatics Association, 12,* 410–417.

Moss, J., Damrongsak, M., & Gallichio, K. (2005). Representing critical care data using the clinical care classification. In C. P. Friedman, J. Ash, & P. Tarcy-Hornoch (Eds.), *Proceedings of the AMIA 2005 Annual Symposium* (pp. 545–549). Washington, DC: OmniPress, Omnipro-CD. CD-ROM.

Saba, V. K. (2005). Home Health Care Classification (HHCC) system: An overview. In M. D. Harris (Ed.), *Handbook of home health care administration* (pp. 247–260). Sudbury, MA: Jones & Bartlett Publishing, Inc.

2004

Bakken, S., Cook, S. S., Curtis, L., et al. (2004). Promoting patient safety through informatics-based nursing education. *International Journal of Medical Informatics, 73,* 581–589.

Kuntze, A. (2004, November). The evaluation of the home health care classification for its practical use in German-speaking countries. *PR-Internet für die Pflege, 6,* 621–626.

Lee, N. J., Bakken, S., & Saba, V. K. (2004). Representing public health nursing information concepts with HHCC and NIC. In M. Fieschi et al. (Eds.), *MEDINFO* (pp. 525–529). Amsterdam, The Netherlands: IOS Press.

Saba, V. K. (2004). Costing nursing care using the clinical care classification systems. In *Connecting the health care continuum: 14th Annual Summer Institute in Nursing Informatics,* July 21–24, 2004 (p. 5). Baltimore, MD: University of Maryland, Summer Institute of Nursing.

Saba, V. K., & Arnold, J. M. (2004). Clinical care costing method for the clinical care classification system. *International Journal of Nursing Terminologies and Classifications, 15,* 69–77.

Saba, V. K., & Arnold, J. M. (2004). A clinical care costing method. In M. Fieschi et al. (Eds.), *MEDINFO* (pp. 1372–1373). Amsterdam, The Netherlands: IOS Press.

2003

Arnold, J. M., & Saba, V. K. (2003). Linking Home Health Care Classification System and ambulatory patient classification for nurse practitioner services. In H. Marin, E. Marques, E. Hovenga, & W. Goossen (Eds.), *NI-2003: Proceedings of the 8th International Congress in Nursing Informatics* (pp. 257–261). Rio de Janeiro, Brazil: e-Papers Services Editorials, Ltd.

Bakken, S., Cook, S. S., Curtis, L., Soupious, M., & Curran, C. (2003). Informatics competencies pre- and post-implementation of a Palm-based student clinical log and informarics for evidence-based practice curriculum. *Proceedings of the AMIA 2003 Annual Symposium* (pp. 41–45). Nashville, TN: Hanley & Belfus.

Bakken, S., Curran, C., Delaleu-McIntosh, J., et al. (2003). Informatics for evidence-based nurse practitioner practice at the Columbia University School of Nursing. In H. F. Marin, E. P. Marques, E. Hovenga, & W. Goossen (Eds.), *NI 2003: Proceedings of the 8th International Congress on Nursing Informatics* (pp. 420–424). Rio De Janeiro, Brazil: e-papers Servicos Editorials, Ltd.

Charters, K. G. (2003). Nursing informatics, outcomes, and quality improvement. *AACN Issues: Advanced Practice in Acute and Critical Care, 14,* 282–294.

Ensio, A., & Saranto, K. (2003). Finland: The Finnish classification of nursing interventions (FICNI)–Development and use in nursing documentation. In J. Clark (Ed.), *Naming nursing: Proceedings of the 1st ACENDIO Ireland/UK Conference held September 2003 in Swansea,* Wales, UK (pp. 191–195). Bern, Germany: Verlag Hans Huber.

Irwin, R. G., & Saba, V. K. (2003). An electronic 3 care tracking system. In H. Marin, E. Marques, E. Hovenga, & W. Goossen (Eds.), *NI-2003: Proceedings of the 8th International Congress in Nursing Informatics* (pp. 124–125). Rio de Janeiro, Brazil: e-Papers Services Editorials, Ltd.

Klein, W. T., & Bakken, S. (2003). Design and implementation of a student clinical log database and knowledge base. In H. F. Marin, E. P. Marques, E. Hovenga, & W. Goossen (Eds.), *NI 2003: Proceedings of the 8th International Congress on Nursing Informatics* (pp. 617–622). Rio De Janeiro, Brazil: e-papers Servicos Editorials, Ltd.

Matney, S. (2003, Fall). Nursing terminology update. *On-Line Journal of Nursing Informatics,* 7(3), 8 pp.

Saba, V. K. (2003). The Home Health Care Classification System (HHCC). In J. Clark (Ed.), *Naming nursing: Proceedings of the 1st ACENDIO Ireland/UK Conference held September 2003 in Swansea, Wales, UK* (pp. 131–138). Bern, Germany: Verlag Hans Huber.

2002

Park, H. S. (2002, June). Cross-mapping the ICNP with NANDA, HHCC, Omaha System and NIC for unified nursing language system development. *International Nursing Review, 49,* 99–110.

Saba, V. K. (2002). Nursing classifications: Home health care classification system (HHCC): An overview. *Online Journal of Issues in Nursing.* Retrieved from <http://www.nursing world.org/ojin/tpct/tpc7_7.htm.>

Saba, V. K. (2002). Nursing information technology: Classifications and management. In J. Mantas, & A. Hasman (Eds.), *Textbook in health informatics: A nursing perspective* (pp. 21–44). Amsterdam, The Netherlands: IOS Press.

Saba, V. K. (2002). Overview of home health care classification system (HHCC). In N. Oud (Ed.), *Acendio 2002: Proceedings of the Special Conference of the Association of Common European Nursing Diagnoses, Interventions and Outcomes in Vienna* (pp. 65–90). Bern: Verlag Hans Huber.

Schoneman, D. (2002). The intervention of surveillance across classification systems. *International Journal of Nursing Terminologies and Classifications, 13,* 137–147.

2001

Alfrink, V., Bakken, S., Coenen, A., McNeil, B., & Bickford, C. (2001). Standardized nursing vocabularies: A foundation for quality care. *Seminars in Oncology Nursing, 17,* 18–23.

Coenen, A., Marin, H., Park, H. A., & Bakken, S. (2001). Collaborative efforts for representing nursing concepts in computer-based systems. *Journal of the American Medical Informatics Association, 8,* 202–211.

Coenen, A., McNeil, B., Bakken, S., Bickford, C., & Warren, J. J. (2001). Toward comparable nursing data: American Nursing Association criteria for data sets, classification systems, and nomenclatures. *Computers in Nursing, 19,* 240–246.

Hardiker, N. (2001). Mediating between nursing intervention terminology systems. In S. Bakken (Ed.), *A medical informatics odyssey: Visions of the future and lessons from the past* (pp. 239–243). Philadelphia: Hanley & Belfus, Inc.

Marin, H. F., Rodriques, R. J., Delaney, C., Nielsen, G. H., & Yan, J. (Eds.). (2001). *Building standard-based nursing information systems.* Washington, DC: Pan American Health Organization.

Peters, D. A., & Saba, V. K. (2001). Community health applications. In V. K. Saba & K. A. McCormick (Eds.), *Essentials of computers for nurses: Informatics for the new millennium* (3rd ed., pp. 265–295). New York: McGraw-Hill, Inc.

Saba, V. K. (2001). Appendix A: Home health care classification (HHCC) system: Two terminologies: HHCC of nursing diagnoses and HHCC of nursing interventions classified by 20 care components. In V. K. Saba & K. A. McCormick, *Essentials of computers for nurses: Informatics for the new millennium* (3rd ed., pp. 529–533). New York: McGraw-Hill.

Saba, V. K. (2001). Evidence-based practice, language, & documentation. International Council of Nurses (ICN) 22nd Quadrennial Congress, June 10–15, 2001. *Nursing: A new era for action: Abstract for concurrent sessions and symposia.* List of Posters. Geneva, Switzerland: ICN.

Saba, V. K. (2001). Nursing's languages: International terminologies, classifications & standards. In V. L. Patel, R. Rogers, & R. Haux Medinfo (Eds.), *2001: Proceedings of the 10th World Congress on Medical Informatics* (p. 1544). Amsterdam, The Netherlands: IOS Press.

Saba, V. K., & Irwin, R. G. (2001). An electronic system for home care protocols. In S. Bakken (Ed.), *Proceedings of the AMIA 2005 Annual Symposium* (p. 1013). Philadelphia, PA: Hanley & Belfus, Inc.

2000

Bakken, S., Campbell, K. E., Comino, J. J., Huff, S. M., & Hammond, W. E. (2000). Toward vocabulary domain specifications for health level 7-coded data elements. *Journal of the American Medical Informatics Association, 7,* 333–342.

Bakken, S., Cashen, M. S., Mendonca, E. A., O'Brien, A., & Zieniewicz, J. (2000). Representing nursing activities within a concept-oriented terminological system: Evaluation of a type definition. *Journal of the American Medical Informatics Association, 7,* 81–89.

Bakken, S., Cimino, J. J., Haskell, R., et al. (2000). Evaluation of clinical LOINC (logical observation identifiers, names, and codes). *Journal of the American Medical Informatics Association, 7,* 529–538.

Bakken, S., Parker, J., Konicek, D., & Campbell, K. (2000). An evaluation of ICNP intervention axes as terminology model components. In J. M. Overhage (Ed.), *Proceedings of the AMIA 2000 Annual Symposium* (pp. 42–46). Nashville, TN: Hanley & Belfus.

Bakken, S., Wage, G., Bain, C., Cashen, M. S., Sklar, B., & Kelber, C. (2000). Standardized terminology requirements for nurse practitioner documentation of clinical findings. In V. K. Saba, R. Carr, W. Sermeus, & P. Rocha (Eds.), *7th International Congress: Nursing informatics one step beyond: The evolution of technology and nursing* (pp. 177–182). Auckland, New Zealand: Adis International Ltd.

Bakken, S., Button, P., Konicek, D., et al. (2000). Standardized terminologies for nursing concepts: Collaborative activities in the United States. In *7th International Congress of Nursing Informatics: Post-congress workshop* (pp. 21–32). Rotorua, New Zealand, May 3–6, 2000. Auckland, New Zealand: Premier Print.

Saba, V. K., & Irwin, R. G. (2000). An electronic tracking system for home care protocols. In V. K. Saba, R. Carr, W. Sermeus, & P. Rocha (Eds.), *One step beyond: The evolution of technology and nursing: Proceeding of the 7th Nursing Informatics Congress* (p. 779). Auckland, New Zealand: Adis International.

Strachan, H., Hoy, D., Moen, A., Park, H. A., Saba, V., & Skiba, D. (2000). Critical pathways and outcomes: Using evidence based practice in community and home health care. In *7th International Congress on Nursing Informatics: Post-congress workshop.* Rotorua, New Zealand, May 3–6, 2000. Auckland, New Zealand: Premier Print.

1999

Bakken, S., Button, P., Hardiker, N. R., Mead, C. N., Ozbolt, J. G., Warren, J. J. (1999). On the path to a reference terminology for nursing concepts. In C. G. Chute (Ed.), *IMIA Working Group: 6th Conference on Natural Language and Medical Concept Representation.* Phoenix, AZ: IOS Press.

Beyea, S. C. (1999). Standardized language: Making nursing practice count. *AORN Journal, 70,* 831–832, 834, 837, 838.

1998

Anderson, M. A., Pena, R. A., & Helms, L. B. (1998). Home care utilization by congestive heart failure patients: A pilot study. *Public Health Nursing, 15,* 126–162.

Button, P., Androwich, I., Hibben, L., et al. (1998). Challenges and issues related to implementation of nursing vocabularies in computer-based systems. *Journal of the American Medical Informatics Association, 5,* 332–334.

Hardiker, N. R., & Rector, A. L. (1998). Modeling nursing terminology using the GRAIL representation language. *Journal of the American Medical Informatics Association, 5,* 120–128.

Henry, S. H., Warren, J. J., Lange, L., & Button, P. (1998). A review of major nursing vocabularies and the extent to which they have the characteristics required for implementation in computer-based systems. *Journal of the American Medical Informatics Association, 5,* 321–328.

McCormick, K. A., & Jones, C. B. (1998, September). Is one taxonomy needed for health care vocabularies and classifications? *Online Journal of Issues in Nursing.* Retrieved from <http://www.nursingworld.org/ojin/tpc7/tpc7_2htm>.

Parlocha, P. K., & Henry, S. B. (1998). The usefulness of the Georgetown home health care classification system for coding patient problems and nursing interventions in psychiatric home care. *Computers in Nursing, 16,* 45–52.

Saba, V. K. (1998). A new paradigm for computer-based nursing information systems: Twenty care components. In V. K. Saba, D. P. Pocklington, & K. P. Miller (Eds.), *Nursing and computers: An anthology, 1987–1996* (pp. 29–32). New York: Springer.

Saba, V. K., & Sparks, S. M. (1998). Twenty care components: An educational strategy to teach nursing science. In B. Cesnik, A. T. Cray, & J. R. Scherrer (Eds.), *Medinfo '98: Ninth World Congress on Medical Informatics* (pp. 756–759). Amsterdam, The Netherlands: IOS Press.

Zielstorff, R. D. (1998). Characteristics of a good nursing nomenclature from an informatics perspective. *Online Journal of Issues in Nursing.* Retrieved from <http://www.nursingworld org/ojin/tpc7/tpc7_4htm>.

Zielstorff, R. D., Tronni, C., Basque, J., Griffin, L. R., & Welebob, E. M. (1998). Mapping nursing diagnosis nomenclatures for coordinated care. *Image: Journal of Nursing Scholarship, 30,* 369–373.

1997

Henry, S. H., & Mead, C. N. (1997). Nursing classifications systems; necessary but not sufficient for representing "what nurses do" for inclusion in computer-based patient record systems. *Journal of the American Medical Informatics Association, 4,* 222–232.

Henry, S. B., Morris, J. A., & Holzemer, W. L. (1997). Using structured text and templates to capture health status outcomes in the electronic health record. *Journal of Quality Improvement, 23,* 667–677.

Holzemer, W. L., Henry, S. B., Dawson, C., Sousa, K., Bain, C., & Hsieh, S.-F. (1997). An evaluation of the utility of the home health care classification for categorizing patient problems and nursing interventions from the hospital setting. In U. Gerdin, M. Tallberg, & P. Wainwright (Eds.), *NI'97: nursing informatics: The impact of nursing knowledge on health care informatics* (pp. 21–26). Stockholm, Sweden: IOS Press.

Saba, V. K. (1997). Georgetown University home care project: Home health care classification (HHCC) system. *Inventory of health care information standards pertaining to: The Health Insurance Portability and Accountability Act (HIPAA) of 1996* (P.L. 104-191). Washington, DC: American National Standards Institute-Healthcare Informatics Standards Board.

Saba, V. K. (1997) An innovative home health care classification system for continuity of care. In U. Gerdin, M. Tallberg, & P. Wainwright (Eds.), *Nursing informatics: The impact of nursing knowledge on health care informatics* (p. 607). Amsterdam: IOS Press.

Saba, V. K. (1997). An innovative home health care classification (HHCC) system. In *Classification of nursing diagnoses: Proceedings of the 12th Conference*, April 11–14, 1996 (pp. 13–15). NANDA. Pasadena, CA: Western Adventist Health Services (CINAHL).

Saba, V. K. (1997). Home health care classification (HHCC) system. In G. K. McFarland & E. A. McFarlane (Eds.), *Nursing diagnosis & intervention: Planning for patient care* (3rd ed., pp. 867–872). St. Louis: Mosby.

Saba, V. K. (1997). The home health care classification of nursing diagnoses and interventions. In M. D. Harris (Ed.), *Handbook of home health care administration* (2nd ed., pp. 215–219). Gaithersburg, MD: Aspen Publications.

Saba, V. K. (1997). Why the home health care classification is a recognized nomenclature. *Computers in Nursing, 15,* S69–S76.

Sparks, S. M. (1997). Noun phrases for nursing diagnoses. *Nursing Diagnosis, 8,* 49–54.

1996

Saba, V. K. (1996). Community health applications. In V. K. Saba & K. A. McCormick, (Eds.), *Essentials of computers for nurses* (2nd ed., pp. 429–484). New York: McGraw-Hill.

Saba, V. K. (1996). Appendix: Home health care classification: Nursing diagnoses and nursing interventions. In V. K. Saba & K. A. McCormick, *Essentials of computers for nurses* (2nd ed., pp. 619–635). New York: McGraw-Hill.

Saba, V. K., & Hollers, K. (1996). An innovative home health care classification system for managing managed care. In J. J. Cimino (Ed.), *Proceedings: 1996 AMIA Annual Fall Symposium* (p. 936). Philadelphia, PA: Hanley & Belfus, Inc.

1995

Anderson, B., Hannah, K., Besner, J., et al. (1995). Classification systems for health information: Nursing components, Part 1. *AARN Newsletter, 51,* 10–11.

Lang, N. M., Hudgins, C., Jacox, A., et al. (1995). Toward a national database for nursing practice. In *American Nurses Association nursing data systems: The emerging framework* (pp. 7–18). Washington, DC: ANA.

Lang, N. M., & Marek, K. D. (1995). Quality assurance: The foundation of professional care. *Journal of the New York State Nurses Association, 26,* 48–50.

Lazerowich, V. (1995). Development of a patient classification system for a home-based hospice program. *Journal of Community Health Nursing, 12,* 121–126.

Mackenzie, W., Hannah, K., Anderson, B., et al. (1995, March). Classification systems for health information: Nursing components, Part 11. *AARN Newsletter, 51,* 32–33.

Saba, V. K. (1995). A new paradigm for computer-based nursing information systems twenty care components. In R. A. Greenes, H. E. Peterson, & D. J. Protti (Eds.), *Medinfo*

'95: Proceedings of the 8th World Congress on Medical Informatics (pp. 1401–1406). Amsterdam, The Netherlands: North-Holland. [Reprinted in: Saba, V. K., Pocklington, D. B., & Miller, K. P. (1998). *Nursing and computers: An anthology* (pp. 29–32). New York: Springer Publishing.]

Saba, V. K. (1995). Home health care classification (HHCC). In R. A. Mortensen (Ed.), *Creating a European platform: Proceedings of the 1st European Conference on Nursing Diagnoses* (pp. 302–308). Copenhagen, Denmark: Danish Institute for Health and Nursing Research.

Saba, V. K. (1995). Home health care classifications (HHCCs): Nursing diagnoses and nursing interventions. In N. M. Lang (Ed.), *Nursing data systems: The emerging framework* (pp. 61–103). Washington, DC: American Nurses Association.

Zielstorff, R. D., Lang, N. M., Saba, V. K., McCormick, K. A., & Milholland, D. K. (1995). Toward a uniform language for nursing in the US: Work of the American Nurses Association steering committee on databases to support clinical practice. In R. A. Greenes, H. E. Peterson, & D. J. Protti (Eds.), *Medinfo '95: Proceedings of the 8th World Congress on Medical Informatics* (pp. 1362–1366). Amsterdam, The Netherlands: North-Holland. [Reprinted in: Saba, V. K., Pocklington, D. B., & Miller, K. P. (1998). *Nursing and computers: An anthology* (pp. 22–28). New York: Springer Publishing.]

1994

Henry, S. B., Holzemer, W. L., Reilly, C. A., & Campbell, K. E. (1994). Terms used by nurses to describe patient problems: Can SNOLED III represent nursing concepts in the patient record. *Journal of the American Medical Informatics Association, 1,* 61–74.

McCormick, K. A., Lang, N., Zielstorff, R., Milholland, D. K., Saba, V. K., & Jacox, A. (1994). Toward standard classification schemes for nursing languages: Recommendations of the American Nurses Association steering committee on databases to support clinical nursing practice. *Journal of the American Medical Informatics Association, 1,* 421–427.

Miller, J. M., & Bakken, S. (1994, Spring). Toward a common healthcare language. *Computertalk, 2,* 40–42.

Ozbolt, J., Fruchtnicht, J. N., & Hayden, J. R. (1994). Toward data standards for clinical nursing information. *Journal of the American Medical Informatics Association, 1,* 175–185).

Saba, V. K. (1994). A home health classification system. In S. J. Grobe & E. S. P. Pluyter-Wenting (Eds.), *Nursing informatics: An international overview for nursing in a technological era* (pp. 697–701). Amsterdam, The Netherlands: Elsevier.

Saba, V. K. (1994). Coding systems for nursing. In P. Waegeman (Ed.), *Toward an electronic patient record '94: 10th International Symposium on the Creation of Electronic Health Record System & 6th Global Congress on Patient Cards* (pp. 223–225). Newton, MA: Medical Records Institute.

Saba, V. K. (1994). *Home health care classification (HHCC) of nursing diagnoses and interventions, revised.* Washington, DC: Georgetown University.

Saba, V. K. (1994). Twenty nursing diagnosis home health care components. In R. M. Carroll-Johnson & M. Paquette (Eds.), *Classification of nursing diagnoses: Proceedings of the 10th Conference* (p. 301). Philadelphia, PA: J. B. Lippincott Co.

Saba, V. K., & Zuckerman, A. E. (1994). Home health care classification (HHCC) system. In J. G. Ozbolt (Ed.), *Transforming Information, Changing Health Care: Proceedings of the 18th Annual Symposium on Computer Applications in Medical Care* (p. 1046). Philadelphia, PA: Hanley & Belfus, Inc.

1993

Saba, V. K. (1993). Nursing diagnostic schemes. In Canadian Nurses Association (Ed.), *Proceedings: Nursing minimum data set conference. Alberta, December, Canada 1992* (pp. 54–63). Alberta, Canada: Canadian Nurses Association.

1992

Fuiper, M. (1992). (Dutch Translation). Diagnose en interventie. In L. Regeer (Ed.), *Verpleegkundige Diagnostiek in Nederland* (pp. 73–82). Amsterdam, The Netherlands: LEO Verpleegkundig Management.

Gabrieli, E. R. (1992). *6-3-1-10 Nursing terminology.* Buffalo, NY: Gabrieli Associates.

Milholland, D. K. (1992). Naming what we do: Nursing vocabularies. *Journal of AHIMA, 63,* 68–61.

Saba, V. K. (1992). A classification of home health care nursing diagnoses and interventions. *Caring, 11,* 50–57.

Saba, V. K. (1992). Home health care classification. *Caring, 11,* 58–60.

Saba, V. K. (1992). *Home health care classification (HHCC) of nursing diagnoses and interventions.* Washington, DC: Georgetown University.

Saba, V. K. (1992). The classification of home health care nursing diagnoses and interventions. In L. Regeer (Ed.), *Verpleegkundige Diagnostiek in Nederland* (pp. 62–82). Amsterdam, The Netherlands: LEO Verpleegkundig Management. (First Translation of HHCC Version 1.0 in Dutch by Marlou de Fuiper, RN, MsN, for Conference Proceedings.)

Saba, V. K., & Zuckerman, A. E. (1992). A new home health classification method. *Caring, 11,* 27–34.

Saba, V. K., & Zuckerman, A. E. (1992). A home health care classification system. In K. C. Lun, P. DeGoulet, T. E. Piemme, & O. Reinhoff (Eds.), *MEDINFO '92: Proceedings of the 7th World Congress on Medical Informatics* (pp. 344–348). Amsterdam, The Netherlands: North Holland.

1991

Saba, V. K. (1991). *Final report: Home care classification project.* Washington, DC: Author. (NTIS No. PB92-177013/AS)

Saba, V. K. (1991). Home health care classification system. In *Computers in health care: 2nd Annual Conference & Exhibits* (pp. 19–20). Washington, DC: Georgetown University.

Saba, V. K. (1991). The international classification of diseases (ICD): Classification of nursing diagnosis. In R. M. Carroll-Johnson (Ed.), *Classification of nursing diagnoses: Proceedings of the ninth conference* (pp. 14–18). New York: J. B. Lippincott Co.

Saba, V. K., O'Hare, A., Zuckerman, A. E., Boondas, J., Levine, E., & Oatway, D. M. (1991). A nursing intervention taxonomy for home health care. *Nursing and Health Care, 12,* 296–299.

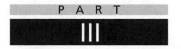

PART

III

TERMINOLOGY USES

12

A CLINICAL CARE CLASSIFICATION (CCC) COST METHOD

JEAN ARNOLD
VIRGINIA K. SABA

PURPOSE

The purpose of this chapter is to propose a method for determining the cost of nursing services using the Clinical Care Classification (CCC) system. The method uses three major indicators that document patient care in accord with the nursing process and is designed for the electronic health record (EHR). The CCC Cost Method (CCC-CM) uses a formula that employs relative value units (RVUs) to establish the financial value for nursing services similar to a method used by the federal government and private organization units.

BACKGROUND

Nursing is lagging behind the other health care disciplines in developing methods to cost out their services. Traditionally, hospital nursing departments calculate nursing personnel within the room rate, using the nurse-to-patient ratios and not the cost of their individualized patient services. Nursing departments do not function as cost centers, do not generate revenue, and do not collect or code nursing care like other hospital departments such as radiology, pharmacy, or laboratory. As a result, the cost of nursing care is not calculated and generally not included on a patient's hospital statement.

Patient Acuity Systems

In the past, patient acuity classification systems were developed to determine nurse staffing for nursing units based on the patients' care requirements but not for care costs. Nurse staffing was determined from time-based tasks that were scored to predict the hours of nursing care needed for a specific hospital unit. The nursing task list developed by hospitals and/or vendors varied not only by the number of tasks, but also by the calculated time allocated for each task. Since there was no national standardized list of nursing tasks, the acuity systems varied from hospital to hospital, and were subjective and unreliable, thus making it difficult to accurately cost out nursing care.

Halloran and colleagues (1987) developed a nursing diagnoses-based patient classification system in an attempt to relate nursing diagnoses to nursing services and cost. They calculated patient care based on the total time nurses spent daily treating patients with specific nursing diagnoses instead of by nursing tasks. They indicated that nurses treating nursing diagnoses of patients provided a more holistic approach to their care and that the time they spent each day treating patients with specific nursing diagnoses was the major factor needed for costing their services.

The American Nurses Association (ANA) also recommended a change from the patient acuity classification systems to a professional model that includes intensity of the patient units, care needs, context, and nurse expertise (ANA, 2005). The acuity classification task-time methods are generally incongruent with the decision-making processes employed by the nurses (Halloran, 1988). Nursing care is more than nursing tasks. It includes decision making and follows the standards of care demonstrated by the six steps of the nursing process (ANA, 1998). The nursing process is the theoretical model used by the CCC to cost out care.

Coded Terminologies

With the introduction of hospital/medical information systems, many of the medical classification systems, such as the International Classification of Diseases (ICD-10) (WHO, 1992), were already in existence and used to code medical diagnoses and surgical procedures. They served as the basis for physician claims for reimbursement. At that time, before the 1980s, the nursing profession did not have any recognized standardized classification systems. As a result, nursing care plans were not computerized, and nurses continued to document the care they gave as narrative nursing notes in the patients' paper charts.

Nursing Terminologies

In the 1990s, with the emergence of several recognized standardized nursing terminologies, the documentation of nursing care by computer became possible. Many nurses began to use nursing terminologies for research purposes; however, nursing care plans, outcome measures, and/or care costs were still not computerized or included in the EHR or the computer-based patient record

(CPR) systems. They were primarily excluded because computerized care plans were not cost-effective, nor were they required for claims data by the federal government or insurance companies.

Federal Initiatives

In 1996, with the enactment of the Health Insurance Portability and Accountability Act of 1996 (HIPAA), the federal government began to implement legislation focusing on health care measures needed to ensure patient safety and quality. The federal government implemented this aspect of the HIPAA legislation by mandating the use of electronic billing for the reimbursement of medical claims. In 2003, the National Committee for Vital and Health Statistics (NCVHS) convened a committee to select the concept-oriented code sets to implement the patient medical record information (PMRI), another part mandated by the HIPAA legislation.

The NCVHS committee conducted hearings as well as obtained analysis of existing terminologies in order to select and recommend to the Secretary of the Department of Health and Human Services (DHHS) the code sets for the PMRI addressing physician orders, surgical procedures, and other clinical services. Approximately 10 code sets were selected—including Systemized Nomenclature of Medical Clinical Terms (SNOMED CT)—and recommended for implementing the PMRI requirement. However, since several nursing terminologies, including the CCC system, were already integrated in the approved SNOMED CT, nursing terminologies were excluded from being accepted as separate code sets for the PMRI. As a result, nursing terminologies were still not mandated for the EHR systems. However, with the emerging focus on computerized physician order entry (CPOE) systems and evidenced-based practices, the need for data on the nursing care of patients emerged as critical to ensure that the physician orders were carried out and that their outcomes were measured.

Today, patient care data represent one of the largest gaps of data required by Centers for Medicare and Medicaid Services (CMS) on hospitalized patients. They include clinical services data, complexity of patient conditions, and the time and depth of services performed by professional nurses and allied health personnel. To ensure that safe and quality care are being performed, patient care data should be integrated into EHR systems; this can be accomplished by using a coded, standardized nursing terminology, such as the CCC system. Such a system is needed to obtain accurate outcomes and other measures that could determine care costs, as well as demonstrate the value of professional nursing practice.

Costing Methods

Relatively few methods have been developed that address the actual cost of nursing services. Nursing services continue to be considered part of the daily cost or room rate of hospital care. These authors are proposing a cost method that uses three major CCC indicators: (1) nursing diagnoses, (2) nursing intervention action types, and (3) nursing outcomes. It consists of a formula that uses RVUs for the nursing intervention action types variable. These authors are proposing this method as a possible approach for costing nursing services in hospitals and other health care facilities. According to Stone and colleagues (2004): "the name of the nursing intervention alone is not sufficient for its use in economic analyses; some method of estimating the resources associated with the intervention is necessary because time alone is an inadequate measure" (p. 107). These authors are recommending that the CCC system be used to determine care costs. Also, that the methodology (1) follow the nursing process; (2) focus on the nursing diagnoses, interventions action types, and outcomes; and (3) apply RVUs for the allocated nursing intervention action types provided by nurses' encounters with patients during an episode of care.

For the purpose of demonstrating the CCC-CM, these authors are highlighting a similar cost method used by ABC Coding Solutions–Alternative Link Inc. They use RVUs based on resource costs for their ABC Codes to produce a cost value for a service to a patient. The ABC Codes contain both RVUs and corresponding resource-based relative value scale (RBRVS) values used by the Centers for Medicare and Medicaid Services (CMS). CMS uses RBRVS as a standardized physician payment schedule for the assessments of the financial worth of their various health care interventions that also supports the fee schedules for conventional health care services (Molina, 2004).

The ABC costing method has been approved by the CMS on a trial basis for reimbursement of claims for services provided by non-physician providers who are eligible for physician payments. Although direct reimbursement for nursing care of patients does not occur at this time, the methodology is in place and nursing care costs can be determined.

Clinical Care Classification

The CCC system is being proposed as the terminology to determine nursing care costs for the CCC-CM. The CCC consists of two interrelated terminologies: CCC of Nursing Diagnoses and Outcomes and the CCC of Nursing Interventions—both of which are classified by 21 Care Components that provide a standardized framework. The CCC system is used to document, classify, and code clinical nursing services in all health care settings. The two terminologies use a coding scheme that links the six steps of the nursing process to each other as well as map to other coding systems, such as SNOMED CT. The coding structure for the CCC system consists of five alphanumeric characters that have been described in other chapters.

CLINICAL CARE CLASSIFICATION COSTING METHOD

The CCC Costing Method (CCC-CM) requires the CCC system's two interrelated terminologies to provide the inter-relationships and linkages between: nursing diagnoses, nursing interventions action types, and nursing outcomes, which are the three major CCC-CM indicators (Arnold & Saba, 2004). The purpose of the proposed CCC-CM is to determine the cost of the clinical nursing care services provided to treat a patient with a specific nursing (medical) diagnosis for an episode of care in any health care setting. The proposed CCC-CM, once applied, could also determine (or predict) the amount of nursing services needed by a patient as well as other measurable practices.

Three nursing indicators—**Diagnoses**, **Actions**, and **Outcomes**—are proposed as the three major indicators for the CCC-CM. The first indicator—Nursing **Diagnoses**—is derived from the signs and symptoms of the assessed patient problems and provides the starting point for the CCC-CM. The CCC of Nursing Diagnoses consists of 172 diagnostic concepts and has three qualifiers (improve, stabilize, or deteriorate) that represent 546 Nursing Outcomes. The second indicator—**Actions**—is selected for the nursing interventions to treat the delineated nursing diagnoses. The CCC of Nursing Interventions consists of 198 concepts with four qualifiers (assess, care, teach, or manage) that represent 792 unique Nursing Intervention Action types. The Action Types form the basis for allocating the time used to carry out the nursing interventions.

The third indicator—**Outcomes**—provides evidence of the impact of the Nursing Intervention Action Types used to treat the delineated nursing diagnoses. The Outcomes evaluate and measure the actual resolutions of the nursing diagnoses. The Outcome indicators are first described in the present tense as expected outcomes (to improve, stabilize, or deteriorate) when the assessed nursing diagnoses are first identified. When the specific nursing diagnoses are resolved, the actual outcomes are described in the past tense as improved, stabilized, or deteriorated. The Outcomes provide the evidence that the Nursing Interventions Action Types did impact on the assessed patient's nursing diagnoses.

The CCC-CM requires the linkage between nursing diagnoses, nursing interventions, and nursing outcomes. One **cannot select** a nursing intervention without **linking** it to a nursing diagnosis and one **cannot calculate** the care costs until the outcomes have been evaluated. The definition of a nursing intervention describes this interrelationship.

> *A nursing intervention is a single nursing action which is a treatment, procedure or activity, designed to achieve a nursing diagnosis outcome for which the nurse is held accountable* (Saba, 2005).

The CCC-CM follows the nursing process for documenting patient care for an episode of care before the care costs can be calculated.

Nursing Process

This nursing process is used to link together the nursing diagnoses, nursing intervention action types, and nursing outcomes identified for a patient encounter. The process starts by evaluating the **assessed signs and symptoms** needed to determine the **nursing diagnoses,** which are selected from the CCC of Nursing Diagnoses. Then the nurse determines one **expected outcome** from the three possible qualifiers (improve, stabilize, or deteriorate) for each delineated nursing diagnosis. The nurse next selects the **nursing interventions** or services from the

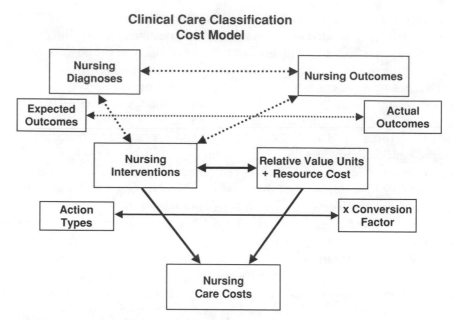

FIGURE 12.1. Clinical Care Classification Cost Model.

CCC of Nursing Interventions to treat the nursing diagnoses. Each specified nursing intervention also requires that one **action type** from the four possible qualifiers (assess, care, teach, and manage) is documented for each intervention. Upon completion of the patient care process, one **actual outcome** from the three possible qualifiers (improved, stabilized, deteriorated) is selected to determine and evaluate the delineated nursing diagnosis.

CLINICAL CARE CLASSIFICATION COST METHOD MODEL

The CCC-CM Model in Figure 12.1 illustrates the relationships among the CCC system terminologies and the cardinal elements of the costing method. The three CCC nursing indicators: (1) nursing diagnoses, (2) nursing interventions action types (four qualifiers), and (3) nursing outcomes (three expected or actual qualifiers) are represented with dotted lines. The RVU cost factors—nursing intervention action types, resource cost, and conversion factor—are connected by solid lines that are bi-directional, thus indicating that there is continual flow among them.

The CCC-CM uses RVU cost values based on nursing intervention action types, resource costs, and a conversion factor. The RVU is based on the nursing intervention action types time, and frequency for each nurse–patient encounter. Resource costs include the hourly wage of the nurses, length of encounter, supplies used for patient care, and overhead related to the physical setting where patient care takes place. The conversion factor is a dollar amount, which is

EXHIBIT 12.1. CLINICAL CARE CLASSFICATION COST METHOD STEPS

Nursing Diagnoses:

- Evaluate assessed signs and symptoms.
- Determine nursing diagnoses.
- Identify nursing services needed to treat nursing diagnoses.

Outcomes:

- Determine an expected outcome for each nursing diagnosis.

Actions:

- Select nursing interventions needed to treat nursing diagnoses.
- Determine an action type for each nursing intervention.
- Determine allocated time for each nursing action type.
- Determine relative value unit (RVU) for each nursing action type.

Outcomes:

- Delineate actual outcome for each nursing diagnosis.

Costs:

- Total specified nursing diagnoses.
- Total nursing interventions.
- Total action types for each nursing intervention.
- Total action types time allocated for each nursing intervention.
- Calculate frequency of total action types.
- Determine **resource cost** for nursing intervention actions types, including type of nursing personnel, overhead, equipment, and supplies.
- Determine **conversion factor** for the interventions actions types (regional differences).
- Calculate nursing care cost by using the formula: **relative value unit** for each nursing intervention action type plus their frequency and allocated time, which is then added to **resource cost** and multiplied by the regional **conversion factor**.

based on regional differences in the U.S. geographical areas (e.g., the Northeast versus the West). The conversion factor is updated annually by the federal government. Each nurse–patient encounter is calculated by its RVUs plus resource cost and multiplied by the regional conversion factor. The steps for determining nursing care costs are outlined in Exhibit 12.1.

CCC-CM Formula

The cardinal indicators of the CCC-CM are the **Nursing Diagnoses**, Intervention **Action Types**, and **Outcomes**. The cost factors include the identification of the **RVUs**, **resource cost**, and the **conversion factor**. The formula for determining cost is demonstrated and discussed further with the CCC-CM examples based on ABC Codes.

The CCC-CM requires the nurse to evaluate the assessed signs and symptoms for a patient to determine the nursing diagnoses using the CCC of Nursing Diagnoses. Next, the nurse identifies the nursing interventions/services needed to treat the nursing diagnoses. Then, the nurse needs to determine an expected outcome qualifier for each delineated nursing diagnosis. This is followed by the selection of the nursing interventions, including an action type qualifier for each, that are needed to achieve the expected outcomes.

For the demonstration of the CCC-CM, if the crosswalk between the CCC Nursing Intervention Action Type and the ABC Nursing Intervention can be made, then the ABC RVU can be used. This process can be used for only those nursing intervention action types adapted by the ABC codes, with their associated CCC nursing diagnoses that have been identified for the patient encounter. At this time each CCC of Nursing Intervention Action Type does not have an RVU, but each ABC Nursing Intervention does has a specific RVU. The cost for the nursing services is based on the total intervention action types, with their allocated time and frequency used to treat the nursing diagnoses. Note that any health care facility can calculate the cost for the CCC of Nursing Intervention Action Types by developing their own RVU values as outlined in Exhibit 12.1 or, as described above, can select an RVU, if available, from the *ABC Coding Manual* (ABC Coding Solutions, 2006).

The CCC-CM uses RVU values, resource cost, and a conversion factor. The RVU establishes the financial worth of health care intervention action types based on a variety of factors associated with the delivered nursing care: time, skill, risk to patient, risk to practitioner, and severity of the health condition. The resource cost is determined because it varies with the setting where the nurse treats the patient. The nurse's salary is a major factor that is determined by education and experience. The conversion factor reflects health care practice costs in a particular office, group practice, health care institution, or region. The conversion factor takes into account cost-drivers, including current fees, prevailing area rates, and overhead cost such as malpractice insurance, rent, salaries, and the cost of doing business (Molina, 2004).

Remember in the examples the time requirement for providing services is included in the RVUs found in the ABC Codes, which is 15 minutes for each encounter. The time requirement for teaching is usually longer; or two RVUs (30 minutes). (See Exhibit 12.2, Tables 12.1–12.3).

Example Case Studies

EXHIBIT 12.2. EXAMPLE: MRS. M. CASE STUDY

This case study provides the basis for nursing diagnoses, outcomes, and interventions in the following tables. Mrs. M. is a 90-year-old White female who is 5'6" tall and weighs 100 lbs. She ambulates without assistive devices, but has some difficulty with balance. During the encounter, Mrs. M. declines the suggestion to use a cane. "I don't need a cane. I need help with my medications." The nurse also determined that Mrs. M. does not eat properly. Note: Mrs. M. resides in the southwestern region of the United States.

A nurse assessed the patient and identified three nursing diagnoses:

- Activity Intolerance—A01.1
- Body Nutrition Deficit—J24.1
- Medication Risk—H21

TABLE 12.1. EXAMPLE FOR CCC OF NURSING DIAGNOSIS—ACTIVITY INTOLERANCE—A01.1

Expected Outcome:	To Improve Activity Intolerance—A01.1.1			
Actual Outcome:	Activity Intolerance Improved—A01.1.1			
	Evidence:	Able to conserve energy		
		Walking without assistance		

CCC of Nursing Interventions	CCC Code[a]	ABC Code[a]	RVU[a,b]	RVU Plus Time × Conversion Factor
Energy Conservation Assessment (Assess)	A01.2.1	NAAPQ	.55 Allocated time = 15 minutes	.55
Energy Conservation (Perform)	A01.2.2	NAAPR	.68 Allocated time = 15 minutes	.68
Energy Conservation Training (Teach)	A01.2.3	NAALG	.33 × 2 Allocated time = 30 minutes	.66
Total			1.56	1.89 × $25.00 = $47.25

[a]ABC Code, Complete Complementary Alternative Medical Billing and Coding Reference; CCC, Clinical Care Classification; RVU, relative value unit.
[b]Relative Value Unit and Conversion Factor are hypothetical.

Each RVU plus allocated time is multiplied by the conversion factor of $25.00. The nursing diagnosis **Activity Intolerance** has three intervention actions with RVUs: (1) **assessing** energy conservation (.55), (2) **performing** energy conservation (.68), and (3) **teaching** energy conservation (.33). A 15-minute time interval is allocated for **assessing** energy conservation, a 15-minute time interval is allocated for **performing** energy conservation, and a 30-minute time interval (or two RVUs) is allocated for the **teaching** energy conservation for a total of 1 hour. The total for the four RVUs is 1.56 and multiplied for the

TABLE 12.2. EXAMPLE FOR CCC OF NURSING DIAGNOSIS—BODY NUTRITION DEFICIT—J24.1

Expected Outcome:	To Improve Body Nutrition Deficit—J24.1.1			
Actual Outcome:	Body Nutrition Deficit Improved—J24.1.1			
	Evidence:	Weight under control		
		Understands proper nutrition		

CCC of Nursing Interventions	CCC Code[a]	ABC Code[a]	RVU[a,b]	RVU Plus Time × Conversion Factor
Weight Control Assessment (**Assess**)	J67.0.1	BFBAI	.44 Allocated time = 15 minutes	.44
Weight Control (**Perform**)	J67.0.2	BFBAI	.53 Allocated time = 15 minutes	.53
Nutrition Care Instruction (**Teach**)	J29.0.3	BFAAG	.65 × 2 Allocated time = 30 minutes	1.3
Total	3		1.62	2.27 × $25.00 = $56.75

[a]ABC Code, Complete Complementary Alternative Medical Billing and Coding Reference; CCC, Clinical Care Classification; RVU, relative value unit.
[b]Relative Value Unit and Conversion Factor are hypothetical.

TABLE 12.3. EXAMPLE FOR CCC OF NURSING DIAGNOSIS—MEDICATION RISK—H21

Expected Outcome:	To improve Medication Risk—H21.0.1
Actual Outcome:	Medication Risk improved—H21.0.1
	Evidence: Able to pre-fill medications
	Able to give own medications
	Able to verbalize medication side effects

CCC of Nursing Interventions	CCC Code[a]	ABC Code[a]	RVU[a,b]	RVU Plus Time × Conversion Factor
Medication Pre-fill Preparation (**Perform**)	H24.2.2	NAATC	.39 Allocated time = 15 minutes	.39
Medication Treatment Teaching (**Teach**)	H24.4.3	NBAAG	.48 Allocated time = 30 minutes	.48 × 2 = .96
Medication Side Effects Teaching (**Teach**)	H24.3.3	NAATF	.28 Allocated time = 30 minutes	.28 × 2 = .56
Total Cost			1.15	1.91 × $25.00 = $47.75

[a]ABC Code, Complete Complementary Alternative Medical Billing and Coding Reference; CCC, Clinical Care Classification; RVU, relative value unit.
[b]Relative Value Unit and Conversion Factor are hypothetical.

conversion factor of $25.00, resulting in a total of $47.25 for this encounter. The conversion factor for the given region is also considered. Hypothetically the conversion factor for Mid-West, USA is $25.00.

Each RVU plus allocated time is multiplied by the conversion factor of $25.00. The nursing diagnosis **Body Nutrition Deficit** has three intervention actions with RVUs: (1) **assessing** weight control (.44), (2) **performing** weight control (.53), and (3) **teaching** individual nutrition care counseling (.65). A 15-minute time interval is allocated for **assessing** weight control, a 15-minute time interval is allocated for **performing** weight control, and a 30-minute time interval (or two RVUs) is allocated for **teaching** nutrition care instruction for a total of 1 hour. The total for the four RVUs is 2.27 and is multiplied for the Conversion Factor of $25.00, resulting in a total of $56.75 for this encounter.

Each RVU plus resource cost is multiplied by the conversion factor of $25.00. The nursing diagnosis **Medication Risk** has three nursing actions with RVUs: (1) **performing** medication pre-fill (.39), (2) **teaching** medication treatments (.48), and (3) **teaching** medication side effects (.28). A 15-minute time interval is allocated for **performing** the medication pre-fill, a 30-minute time interval is allocated for **teaching** medication treatments, and a 30-minute time interval is allocated for **teaching** medication side effects of Mrs. M.'s medications. The total RVUs of 1.91 multiplied by the South West conversion factor of $25.00 results in a total cost of $47.75 for this 1 hour and 15-minute encounter.

CONCLUSION

These examples demonstrate the crosswalk mapping between the CCC of Nursing Interventions Action Types codes and the ABC Nursing Intervention codes.

The RVUs for the nursing interventions Action Types are summed up and multiplied by the regional conversion factor, resulting in the actual nursing care cost for a nurse–patient encounter. If a user prefers to use their own method to develop the RVU, then one can use the CCC-CM formula and assign their own RVUs. One can also use the ABC codes if it has an RVU for a specific nursing intervention action type.

The examples also demonstrate that costs for nursing services using the CCC system can be calculated. Why use nursing terminology for reimbursement? It is more descriptive of nursing services than medical Current Procedure Terminology (CPT) (American Medical Association, 2003). The CPT provides codes and fees for primarily medical procedures that nurse practitioners have used for reimbursement even though it does not incorporate specific nursing interventions or services as depicted in the CCC of Nursing Interventions.

The CCC-CM formula offers nursing the means for costing nursing services as a separate budget item. The time has come for the value of professional nursing to be visible in the cost of health care by all of the regulators of health care services.

REFERENCES

ABC Coding Solutions—Alternative Link Inc. (2006). *ABC coding manual: For integrative healthcare.* Albuquerque, NM: ABC Coding Solutions—Alternative Link Inc.

American Medical Association. (2003). *Current procedure terminology (CPT).* Chicago, IL: AMA.

American Nurses Association. (2005). *Principles for nurse staffing.* Retrieved May 4, 2005, from <http://www.nursingworld.org/readroom/stffprnc.htm.>

American Nurses Association. (1998). *Standards of clinical nursing practice.* Washington, DC: ANA.

Arnold, J. M., & Saba, V. K. (2004). A clinical care costing method. In M. Fieschi (Ed.), *MEDINFO 2004 Proceedings* (pp. 1371–1373). The Netherlands: IOS Press.

Halloran, E. J. (1988). Conceptual considerations, decision criteria, and guidelines for development of the nursing minimum data set from an administrative perspective. In H. H. Werley & N. M. Lang (Eds.), *Identification of the nursing minimum data set.* New York: Springer Publishing.

Halloran, E. J., Paterson, C., & Kiley, M. (1987). Case mix: Matching patient need with nursing resources. *Nursing Management, 18,* 27–42.

Molina, S. (2004). A new opportunity to capture CNS contributions to U.S. Health. *Clinical Nurse Specialist, 18,* 238–245.

Saba, V. K. (2005). *Clinical care classification (CCC) of nursing interventions.* Retrieved December 15, 2005, from <http://www.sabacare.com.>

Stone, P. W., Lee, N. J., Giannini, M., & Bakken, S. (2004). Economic evaluations and usefulness of standardized nursing terminologies. *International Journal of Nursing Terminologies and Classifications, 15,* 101–113.

World Health Organization. (1992). *ICD-10: International statistical classification of diseases and related health problems: Tenth Revision: Volume 1.* Geneva, Switzerland: WHO.

DOCUMENTATION STRATEGIES

If we cannot name it, we cannot control it, finance it, teach it, research it, or put it into public policy.

Clark & Lang (1992)

GETTING STARTED

This chapter provides **getting started** strategies for how to document and code plans of care using the Clinical Care Classification (CCC) system for electronic health record (EHR) systems. This chapter provides background information as well as why documented plans of care are required. It also provides the CCC system model as the road map for the electronic documenting of patient care using the nursing process as its theoretical framework. In this chapter, the basic activities of a system life cycle are outlined for configuring a nursing documentation application for an EHR system. Additionally, the format for different electronic plans of care using CCC is described, including examples.

ELECTRONIC PLANS OF CARE

Electronic plans of care are being configured using different formats and developmental strategies, depending on their purposes, objectives, and/or uses, as well as their clinical content that can be derived from many different sources. Thus, the coding strategies for the plans of care **differ**. This chapter highlights three different electronic plans of care: (1) **standardized**, (2) **individualized**, or (3) **interactive**. These plans will be described according to their format, structure, developmental strategy, and source of content. The reader will also learn how CCC is used to code them.

Standardized Plan of Care

The first strategy is a **standardized** plan of care and is pre-defined for a specific disease or medical condition. This plan of care consists of a pre-defined set of time-sequenced interventions and action types for their respective nursing diagnoses. The plan is usually coded manually using the CCC system and then uploaded into the EHR system. The plan is structured as a clinical pathway or as any other set format. The content is pre-determined and generally obtained from the health care facility's printed plans of care or textbooks, clinical guidelines, and/or literature.

Individualized Plan of Care

The second strategy is an **individualized** plan of care, entered real-time for a specific patient with a specific medical condition. The plan of care is configured by the nurse following the traditional plan of care format and is based on nursing knowledge of clinical practices. It complements the medical therapeutic regimen. The CCC codes are either added manually for uploading into the EHR system or electronically from the system's vocabulary manager or data dictionary, which contains the CCC system.

Interactive Plan of Care

The last strategy is an **interactive** plan of care with online branching logic, allowing for individualized menu-driven options, and adapted for a patient's condition. This type plan of care is designed and pre-coded manually using the CCC system for specific nursing diagnoses and/or medical conditions. The plans of care are compiled as a **Set** for integration into an EHR system. The design of the branching logic content requires nursing knowledge of clinical practices, as well as system design strategies. Once configured, the integrated application can also be linked to an executable knowledgebase, evidenced-based guidelines, and/or nursing literature.

NURSING FOCUS

With the introduction of information technology (IT) systems in hospitals, the revenue-generating departments—such as pharmacy, radiology, or the laboratory—were the first clinical departments to be computerized. The nursing departments, on the other hand, were neglected even though they generally had printed manuals with policies, plans of care, and/or clinical pathways that guided the documentation of patient care in their facilities. The plans of care were manual, generally home grown, specific to a nursing department, and varied from one facility to another. As a result, when management evaluated EHR systems for the facility, the nursing personnel typically were not included because they were too busy, not interested, or not knowledgeable about the benefits of computerized nursing applications.

CCC System Solution

The original Home Health Care Classification (HHCC) System Version 1.0 has been implemented by vendors of EHR systems in several home health agencies for documenting patient care. More recently, the revised and renamed CCC system Version 2.0 is being integrated in several of today's EHR systems to document plans of care for hospitals and other health care facilities. This has occurred because the federal government is beginning to focus its attention on requiring hospitals and other health care facilities to provide evidence of patient safety, quality, and outcome measures.

To address the new federal government requirements, vendors of EHR systems have started to offer different electronic documentation and/or pre-coded plans of care using the CCC system for nurses and allied health personnel. Also, the emerging computerized physician order entry (CPOE) systems require evidence that the physician orders have been carried out, which can only be done with the documentation of patient care. Additionally, patient care clinicians and hospital nurses who are enhancing, updating, or implementing the EHR systems are demanding that their services be captured, coded, and integrated in the systems so that they can evaluate their practices and demonstrate the value of nursing. Thus, many hospitals are requiring vendors to integrate their plans of care documentation as an application in their EHR systems. Some hospitals are requesting that the EHR vendors provide **starter sets** of integrated plans of care, others provide standardized plans of care, and still others the integration of the CCC terminologies into their vocabulary managers or data dictionaries for users to create their own plans using this standardized nursing terminology.

Essence of Care

The dilemmas for the configuration of a patient care documentation application are: What should the focus be, how much detail should be provided, and how responsive should the vendor be to make the application both useful and "easy" for a user of an EHR system to use? One strategy is to document and code only the **essence of care**, which primarily refers to the treatment of the patient's presenting problem; that is, to identify the nursing diagnoses based on the evaluation of the assessed signs and symptoms, followed by the selection of nursing intervention and actions needed to treat the patient. This process also requires documenting the outcomes of the care process. This strategy excludes **reminders** of what to look for, nice to know data, or other unrelated information.

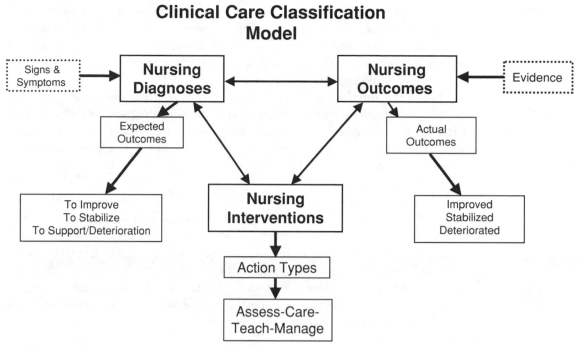

FIGURE 13.1. Clinical Care Classification Model.

Such reminders could be placed in a procedure manual that can be retrieved on demand as an electronic resource. In other words, the **essence of care** is documenting and coding the reason that a patient needs nursing care.

CLINICAL CARE CLASSIFICATION MODEL

The CCC system provides a new approach for organizing and capturing the plans of care data in the EHR and can be used to guide the documentation design. The CCC model shown in Figure 13.1 depicts the documenting of patient care performed by nursing and allied health providers in health care settings as an interactive, interrelated, continuous feedback nursing process. The model illustrates the interrelationship between the CCC of Nursing Diagnoses and Outcomes and the CCC of Nursing Interventions and Actions. The arrows in the model are bi-directional, indicating that there is continual flow, as well as feedback among these three major nursing variables. It also depicts the six steps of the nursing process.

Example

An example of the CCC system model to document patient care following the six steps of the nursing process starts with the **assessed sign and symptom**, such as *difficulty breathing*, which leads to the selection of the **nursing diagnosis** *respiration alteration*, and is the starting point of the care process.

An **expected outcome** is next determined *to improve respiration alteration* and has to be identified before a nursing intervention is selected and performed. The expected outcome is represented by using one of the three qualifiers as the reason or objective for the care, and is stated in present-tense terms to improve, to stabilize, or to support deterioration.

Next, the **nursing intervention** is selected to treat the nursing diagnosis, such as *breathing exercises*. **Note that a nursing diagnosis can be treated with more than one intervention.** Each nursing intervention, however, requires the selection of one of four action type qualifiers: (1) assess/monitor, (2) care/perform direct care, (3) teach/instruct, or (4) manage/refer, such as *teach breathing exercises*.

Once the objective is met or deemed as not able to be met for the nursing diagnosis *respiration alteration*, the **actual outcome** is then documented for the nursing diagnosis as *respiration alteration improved*. The actual outcome is described in the past tense to indicate the results of the nursing interventions/actions. The **evidence** for the actual outcome is the resolution or non-resolution of the assessed sign and/or symptom *difficulty breathing* and nursing diagnosis being treated by the two nursing interventions and action types—*perform breathing exercises* and *teach breathing exercises*.

CARE PLANNING NEEDS

To **get started** using the CCC system, the nursing members of the plan of care team need to have sound nursing knowledge and an understanding of the principles of nursing practice. The team members also need to have an understanding of the principles of data, data structures, and databases, and how and why a standardized terminology is needed to code the data. This means that they should have an understanding of: how data are organized in a database, processed, and retrieved; how and why data are coded; and why CCC, a standardized coded terminology, should be used for the documenting of patient care.

The CCC terminologies consist of atomic (data) concepts—each having a unique meaning—making it possible to code and process plans of care electronically. The CCC (data) concepts can be manipulated and processed by computer for multiple purposes (i.e., **data are entered once for use multiple times**). The CCC can also be analyzed in "use cases," which depict the sequence of activities and the flow of data from input to output, including how the data are coded, classified, processed, stored, and retrieved.

LIFE CYCLE OF A SYSTEM

The plan of care team should also understand the principles of the system life cycle and the impact these principles have on the configuration of an application for an EHR system. The system life cycle provides the outline for the sequence of activities needed to describe to the nurse executive of a hospital, health care facility or EHR vendor, or an individual clinician (the steps required to meet the outlined objectives). The system life cycle phases have been described in the literature for designing, implementing, or upgrading a nursing documentation system. The major phases focus on: System Planning, Analysis, Design, Development, Implementation, and Evaluation (Douglas & Celli, 2006). The phases of the system life cycle outline the major activities that should be addressed in configuring a documentation application and provide a guide on how to proceed. The activities are seamless and listed below with italicized examples.

Planning Phase

Regardless of the focus of type of plan of care or documentation application being configured, someone in authority has to approve the project. In general, it is the nurse executive of a hospital, health care facility or EHR vendor, or an individual clinician in a freestanding facility. Regardless of the setting, a nursing informatics expert should take the lead and assist in directing the **planning** of the project. This project leader should develop a business plan that identifies the purpose, objective, and scope of the application using the CCC. The plan should include: how the endproduct will look, how will it be used, who will use it, and what are the benefits derived from it. The project leader should be responsible for the configuration of a documentation plan of care application for an EHR system using the CCC system and should consider the following major activities:

- Determine the purpose and objectives:
  —*Use CCC terminology to code and document patient care.*
- Identify the specific format for the plans of care application:
  —*Select the form and/or type of plan of care from the three possible approaches: (1) Standardized, (2) Individualized, or (3) Interactive.*
- Obtain administrative and staff support, funds, and working committee:
  —*Convene a formal group of nurses and IT personnel to work on system.*
  —*Develop a realistic budget for the life of the project.*
- Identify benefits of why CCC is selected:
  —*Consider "Why CCC?" (found in Chapter 3).*

Analysis Phase

Once the initial business plan or project proposal has been approved, funds allocated, and staff involved, the next step is to conduct an **analysis** of the existing plan of care documentation system (manual or electronic) to determine what should be deleted, revised, and configured. The major analysis activities should include:

- Analyze the existing manual or electronic plans of care data:
  Focus on what content is collected, used, and what reports are generated.

- Track the work flow of existing plans of care:
  —*List the logical flow and sequence of patient care documents, forms, and/or computer screens from admission to discharge.*
- Evaluate how the existing plans of care are documented and if coded in what format:
  —*Identify the pros and cons.*

Design Phase

Use the analyzed information to **design** the scope, format, and/or prototype for the actual application. This is the creative phase and focuses on configuring the format of the plans of care application, as well as the scope of what essential data are needed. The major design phase activities should include:

- Design a model or framework following the nursing process:
  —*Use CCC model and framework and structure content in the manual.*
- Design the functional specifications and scope:
  —*Select the pre-determined plan of care format type to design: a clinical pathway for the **Standardized** Plan of Care, a structure for the **Individualized** Plan of Care, or the branching logic for an **Interactive** Plan of Care.*
- Determine content of the plans of care:
  —*Identify sources of content, such as facility care plans, nurses' notes, care planning manuals, textbooks, guidelines, or the literature.*
- Determine level of specificity:
  —*What level of specificity should be collected, coded, and/or documented. Remember to code only the **essence of care**.*
  —*Remember, the goal is "to code data only once for use many times."*
- Develop an example of plan of care for the pre-determined format:
  —*Identify proposed benefits of the pre-determined plan of care format.*

Development Phase

Once the design is completed, it is turned over to the **development** team to configure for the specific EHR system. The team not only creates the software, but also has to test and evaluate it with the users in the clinical test sites. The major activities should include:

- Review inputs and outputs:
  —*Review the screen formats for input and how it is processed for output.*
- Test and evaluate the scope of the software:
  —*Test, revise, and retest continuously until software is acceptable to the users and functioning as designed.*
- Train users:
  —*Once software is accepted, the users need to be trained on the system.*
  —*A user's manual should be developed.*

Implementation Phase

This phase requires that the software be **implemented** in the hospital or health care facility and that it should be organized and described. The project leader should provide the users with technical and professional support when the application goes **live**. The implementation phase should be done at a time when the hospital census is low and the staff has time to learn. These activities should include:

- Identify ongoing training needs:
  —*Develop manuals and initiate online help (help desk).*
  —*Conduct on-the-job training.*
- Support users:
  —*Provide technical support until the staff is able to use the software with ease.*
- Establish maintenance procedures and policies, including storage considerations:
  —*The procedures and polices should be in writing and updated routinely.*

Evaluation Phase

The **evaluation** phase is the last phase to be conducted and is usually conducted in two stages. Evaluation measures should also be analyzed once the system goes **live** to ensure it is functioning as planned and configured. The users need online, real-time assistance from those implementing the application in order to get problems corrected as they occur. This is an ongoing process until all the **bugs** are resolved.

The second stage occurs after the application has been running for at least 6 months. That is time when the true effects of the plans of care application in an EHR system can be determined. Only with a span of time can the project leader determine how the application benefits patient care and/or staff, and other nursing and hospital users. This also is the time when a research study should be conducted to identify the impact of the application on patient care. The major activities should focus on:

- Establish an error reporting process:
  —*Set up a real-time procedure for resolving errors and problems.*
- Test utility of plans of care:
  —*Review and evaluate output and other reports.*
- Determine satisfaction of users with software:
  —*Administer a user satisfaction questionnaire to measure the value of the software application.*
- Conduct research before and after implementation of the project:
  —*Conduct a research study to determine the value/impact of the application.*

Major Points

Some other major points that also should be considered by the project leader focus on several general concerns. They include:

- What degree of specificity and/or level of care should be coded versus what information can be recorded as narrative text?

  —*Remember that more **specificity** requires more software programming that may increase the resources required.*

- What data need to be collected, stored, analyzed, and retrieved for decision making?

  —*Remember **nice to know** data can be collected but may not have to be coded.*

- Whether reminders of diseases or medical conditions should be integrated and coded in the software?

  —*Remember, **reminders** are educational and can be provided in an electronic policy manual that can be easily accessed.*

- Whether physician-to-nurse **orders** have to be integrated and coded in the nursing plan of care application?

  —*Remember the physician-to-nurse orders are generally in the order entry dictionary of the EHR system.*

- What sources of **content** should be selected?

  —*Content can be selected from several sources, such as: existing nursing notes or plans of care, adapting a standardized plan of care, or configuring the plans of care from evidence-based literature.*

In summary, the plan of care application proposed in this manual should be configured to document and code the actual **essence of care** provided by nurses and allied health personnel. The system life-cycle phases provide a guide for configuring the documentation or plans of care application for an EHR system using the CCC. The application configuration should be directed by a knowledgeable nurse informatics expert.

PLANS OF CARE EXAMPLES

Examples of the three different types of plans of care are presented that address the different strategies for configuring an application using the CCC for an EHR system.

Standardized Plan of Care

The first set of examples present three case studies as **standardized** plans of care represented as clinical pathways. They consist of time-sequenced interventions with their respective nursing diagnoses. The content for each of the examples focuses on a disease condition that is selected by the clinician and coded manually using the CCC. The nursing interventions are documented as three discrete encounters for each of the assessed nursing diagnoses. The object is to demonstrate the time sequences for the clinical pathway. Once the expected outcome for each nursing diagnosis is **met**, its respective interventions are discontinued and the pathway ends. Examples include:

- Exhibit 13.1: Pneumonia Plan of Care
- Exhibit 13.2: Deep Venous Thrombosis (DVT) Plan of Care
- Exhibit 13.3: Fractured Hip Plan of Care

EXHIBIT 13.1. STANDARDIZED PLAN OF CARE EXAMPLE: PNEUMONIA

Care Component/ Nursing Diagnosis Signs & Symptoms	Care Component/ Nursing Diagnosis Expected Outcome	Encounter/Day 1 Nursing Interventions Action Types	Encounter/Day 2 Nursing Interventions Action Types	Encounter/Day 3 Nursing Interventions Action Types	Care Component/ Nursing Diagnosis Actual Outcome
Q Sensory	Q Sensory	Q Sensory			Q Sensory
					Q45.1.1 Acute Pain Alteration **Improved/Goal Met**
Q45.1 Acute Pain Alteration Pain when coughing or deep breathing	Q45.1.1 To Improve Acute Pain	**Q47.1.1 Assess Acute Pain Control** *Determine location and intensity of pain	>>>>>>>>>>>	>>>>>>>>>>>	*No pain when coughing
		Q47.1.3 Teach Acute Pain Control *Splint with pillow when coughing	>>>>>>>>>>>	>>>>>>>>>>>	*Does not need pain medication
		H24.4.2 Perform Medication Treatment *Give pain medication prn	>>>>>>>>>>>	>>>>>>>>>>>	
L Respiratory	L Respiratory				L Respiratory
L26.2 Breathing Pattern Impairment Shortness of breath when walking more than 20 feet	L26.2.2 To Stabilize Breathing Pattern Impairment	**L35.0.2 Perform Oxygen Therapy Care** *Administer oxygen – 10 liters	>>>>>>>>>>>	>>>>>>>>>>>	L26.2.2 Breathing Pattern Impairment **Stabilized/ Goal Met**
		L36.1.3 Teach Breathing Exercises *Instruct pursed lip breathing	>>>>>>>>>>>	>>>>>>>>>>>	*Does not need oxygen
		H24.4.2 Perform Medication Treatment *Give dose of mist inhalant qid	>>>>>>>>>>>	>>>>>>>>>>>	*Able to walk more than 20 feet without shortness of breath
		H24.4.3 Teach Medication Treatment *Instruct use of mist inhaler	>>>>>>>>>>>	Outcome Achieved	*Able to breathe with lips pursed *Able to use mist inhaler
K. Physical Regulation	K. Physical Regulation				K. Physical Regulation
K25.2 Hyperthermia *Has Temperature (102°F)	K25.2.1 To Improve (Lower) Temperature	**H23.0.2 Perform Injection Administration** *Give IM Injection of antibiotic	>>>>>>>>>>>	>>>>>>>>>>>	K25.2.1 Hyperthermia **Improved.** Temperature Normal

VKS/ 2004 Rev 2005/2006

EXHIBIT 13.2. STANDARDIZED PLAN OF CARE EXAMPLE: DEEP VENOUS THROMBOSIS

Care Component/ Nursing Diagnosis Signs & Symptoms	Care Component/ Nursing Diagnosis Expected Outcome	Encounter/Day 1 Nursing Interventions/ Action Types for	Encounter/Day 2 Nursing Interventions/ Action Types for	Encounter/Day 3 Nursing Interventions/ Action Types for	Care Component/ Nursing Diagnosis Actual Outcome
S-Tissue Perfusion	S-Tissue Perfusion	S-Tissue Perfusion			S-Tissue Perfusion
S48 Tissue Perfusion Alteration *Edema of left leg calf	S48.0.1 To Improve Tissue Perfusion	S69.0.2 Perform Edema Control *Elevate left leg on two pillows	>>>>>>>>>	>>>>>>>>>	S48.0.1 Tissue Perfusion Improved *Minimal edema in left leg
*Skin redness & tenderness in left leg calf		S69.0.2 Perform Edema Control *Measure lower left leg & calf measurement q4 hrs	>>>>>>>>	>>>>>>>>	*Minimal skin redness & tenderness in left leg *Left leg measurements within normal limits
		S69.0.1 Assess Edema Control *Observe skin redness	>>>>>>>	>>>>>>>	*Blood specimen in normal limits
		H24.4.2 Perform Medication Treatment *Give blood thinning drug daily	>>>>>>>	>>>>>>>	
		K32.1.4 Manage Blood Specimen Care *Have lab take blood daily		>>>>>>>	
Q Sensory	Q Sensory	Q Sensory			Q Sensory
Q45.1 Acute Pain *Pain when moving & touching left leg	Q45.1.1 To Improve Acute Pain	Q47.1.2 Perform Acute Pain Control *Use Pain Scale measure severity	>>>>>>>>>	Outcome Achieve Pain Scale not used	Q45.1.1 Acute Pain Improved *No left leg pain
		H24.4.2 Perform Medication Treatment Give analgesics prn for pain	>>>>>>>>>	Outcome achieved: Pain scale within normal limits	
A-Activity	A-Activity	A-Activity			A-Activity
A01.6 Sleep Pattern Disturbance *Unable to sleep	A01.6.2 To Stabilize Sleep Pattern Disturbance	A04.0.3 Teach Sleep Pattern Control *Request analgesics prn when unable to sleep	>>>>>>>>>	*Outcome achieved: Able to sleep	A01.6.2 Sleep Pattern Disturbance Stabilized *Able to sleep

EXHIBIT 13.3. STANDARDIZED PLAN OF CARE EXAMPLE: FRACTURED HIP

Care Component/ Nursing Diagnosis Signs & Symptoms	Care Component/ Nursing Diagnosis Expected Outcome	Encounter/Day 1 Nursing Interventions/ Action Types for	Encounter/Day 2 Nursing Interventions/ Action Types for	Encounter/Day 3 Nursing Interventions/ Action Types for	Care Component/ Nursing Diagnosis Actual Outcome
H-Skin Integrity H46.4 Skin Incision	H-Skin Integrity H46.4.1 To Improve Skin Incision	H-Skin Integrity R55.2.2 – Perform Dressing Change R55.0.2 – Assess Wound Care	>>>>>>>>>>> >>>>>>>>>>>	>>>>>>>>>>> >>>>>>>>>>>	H-Skin Integrity H46.4.1 Skin Integrity Improved *No wound drainage *Wound health
S-Tissue Perfusion S48 Tissue Perfusion Alteration *Edema of left leg calf	S-Tissue Perfusion S48.0.1 To Improve Tissue Perfusion	S-Tissue Perfusion S69.0.2 Perform Edema Control *Elevate right leg on two pillows S69.0.2 Assess Edema Control *Monitor right leg edema	>>>>>>>>>>> >>>>>>>>>>>	>>>>>>>>>>> >>>>>>>>>>>	S-Tissue Perfusion S48.0.1 Tissue Perfusion Improved *Minimal edema in right leg
Q Sensory Q45.1 Acute Pain *Surgical pain in right leg	Q Sensory Q 45.1.1 To Improve Acute Pain	Q Sensory H24.4.2 Perform Medication Treatment *Give pain medication as needed	>>>>>>>>>>>	>>>>>>>>>>>	Q Sensory Q45.1.1 Acute Pain Improved *No pain in right leg
A-Activity A01.5 Physical Mobility Impairment *On bed rest *Has to use wheelchair or crutches	A-Activity A01.5.2 To Stabilize Physical Mobility Impairment	A-Activity A61.0.1 Assess Bedbound Care *Monitor bed rest A02.2.3 Teach Immobilizer Care *Instruct use of crutches	>>>>>>>>>>> >>>>>>>>>>>	>>>>>>>>>>> >>>>>>>>>>>	A-Activity A01.5.2 Physical Mobility Stabilized *Able to use wheelchair *Able to use crutches

Individualized Plan of Care

The second set of examples consists of three case studies with their **individualized** plans of care. Each provides a step-by-step overview of how a nurse configures the plan in real time, for a specific patient with a specific medical condition, and codes it using the CCC system. Note that the nurse uses his/her nursing knowledge of clinical nursing practices to determine the nursing orders to complement the medical orders for the specific case.

Each of the three case study examples lists the **nursing diagnoses** from the assessed signs and symptoms and the rationale for hospitalization. The treatable **nursing diagnoses** are listed by their respective care components and **expected outcomes** using one of the three outcome qualifiers. The **nursing orders** are then determined to treat the nursing diagnoses, listed, and documented as **nursing interventions** each with one of the four action types. Once the expected outcome for each nursing diagnosis has been met or not met, the actual outcome is documented also using one of the three outcome qualifiers. The treated signs and symptoms serve as the **evidence** for the actual outcome of the care process. They include:

- Exhibit 13.4: Pneumonia Plan of Care
- Exhibit 13.5: Deep Venous Thrombosis (DVT) Plan of Care
- Exhibit 13.6: Fractured Hip Plan of Care

Interactive Plans of Care

The last set of examples are the plans of care based on nursing diagnoses or medical conditions with the branching logic, including electronic, menu-driven options for a nurse user to select in order to individualize the plan of care. Once completed, the plans of care are compiled as a **set** for the application that is provided to a vendor to integrate in an EHR system.

Note that the plans of care will be extremely long and detailed in order to allow for the possible pre-determined branching logic options that are pre-coded using the CCC system. The content is generally derived from the literature, textbooks, or any other resource selected by the nursing informatics project leader. This interactive strategy allows for the electronic plans of care application to be flexible and adaptable for the nurse and allied health personnel users. The three examples are based on nursing diagnoses, providing only one branching logic format. They include:

- Exhibit 13.7: Sleep Deprivation Disturbance Plan of Care
- Exhibit 13.8: Physical Mobility Impairment Plan of Care
- Exhibit 13.9. Breathing Pattern Impairment Plan of Care

EXHIBIT 13.4. INDIVIDUALIZED PLAN OF CARE EXAMPLE: PNEUMONIA

Case Study
Mr. Jones, age 70, was admitted to a unit complaining of acute pain when coughing and/or deep breathing. He has shortness of breath when he walks more than 20 feet. Mr. Jones's physician diagnosed his patient as having pneumonia and ordered oxygen therapy, antibiotic injection, pain medication, and inhalant mist.

Signs & Symptoms
- Acute pain on coughing
- Shortness of breath when walking more than 20 feet
- Temperature of 102°F

Medical Diagnosis
Pneumonia

Care Components/Nursing Diagnoses (Assessment/Diagnosis)
- **Sensory Component—Q**
  Nursing Diagnosis: Acute Pain Alteration – Q45.1
- **Respiratory Component—L**
  Nursing Diagnosis: Breathing Pattern Impairment – L26.2
- **Physical Regulation Component—K**
  Nursing Diagnosis: Hyperthermia – K25.2

Expected Outcomes/Goals of Care (Outcome Identification)
- To Improve Acute Pain – Q45.1.1
- To Stabilize Breathing Pattern Impairment – L26.2.2
- To Improve Hyperthermia – K.25.2.1

Nursing Orders Determined	Interventions and Action Types (Planning and Implementation)
Determine intensity of pain	*Assess*—Acute Pain Control – Q47.1.1
Administer oxygen therapy	*Perform*—Oxygen Therapy Care – L35.0.2
Instruct how to splint for coughing	*Teach*—Acute Pain Control – Q47.1.3
Give IM antibiotic injection–qid	*Perform*—Injection Administration – H23.0.2
Give dose of mist inhalant–qid	*Perform*—Medication Treatment – H24.4.2
Give pain medication–prn	*Perform*—Medication Treatment – H24.4.2
Instruct re-breathing exercises–qid	*Teach*—Breathing Exercises – L36.1.3
Instruct re-mist inhalant–qid	*Teach*—Medication Treatment – H24.4.3

Actual Outcomes/Goals Met (Evaluation)—(Care Components/Nursing Diagnoses)
- **Sensory Component—Q**
  Nursing Diagnosis: Acute Pain Improved – Q45.1.1
    Evidence = no pain when coughing
- **Respiratory Component—L**
  Nursing Diagnosis: Breathing Pattern Impairment Stabilized – L26.2.2
    Evidence = Able to walk more than 20 feet without shortness of breath
- **Physical Regulation Component—K**
  Nursing Diagnosis: Hyperthermia Improved – K25.2.1

VKS 2005/2006

EXHIBIT 13.5. INDIVIDUALIZED PLAN OF CARE EXAMPLE: DEEP VENOUS THROMBOSIS

Case Study

Mrs. Jones, age 69, has just returned home from a long trip overseas after a 20-hour flight. She is admitted to the hospital complaining of swelling of her left leg, ++pain in the calf when walking or touching the back of the leg. There is a red streak in the area of the calf, and it is hot and tender to the touch. She is having trouble sleeping because of the pain. She has been diagnosed as having deep venous thrombosis (DVT). Her physician has ordered the left leg to be elevated, medication to prevent clotting of the blood and tested daily, and medication prn for pain and sleeplessness.

Signs & Symptoms

- Edema of left leg
- Skin redness/tenderness in left leg
- Pain in left leg
- Trouble sleeping

Medical Diagnosis

Deep venous thrombosis (DVT) of the left leg

Care Components/Nursing Diagnoses (Assessment/Diagnosis)

- **Tissue Perfusion Component—S**
  Nursing Diagnosis: Tissue Perfusion Alteration – S48
- **Sensory Component—Q**
  Nursing Diagnosis: Acute pain – Q45.1
- **Activity Component—A**
  Nursing Diagnosis: Sleep pattern disturbance – A01.6

Expected Outcomes/Goals of Care (Outcome Identification)

- To Improve Nursing Diagnosis—Tissue Perfusion Alteration – S48.0.1
- To Improve—Nursing Diagnosis – Acute Pain – Q45.1.1
- To Stabilize—Nursing Diagnosis – Sleep Pattern Disturbance – A01.6.2

Nursing Orders	Interventions and Actions Types (Planning and Implementation)
Elevate edematous left leg on two pillows	*Perform*—Edema Control – S69.0.2
Measure lower leg and calf q4hrs	*Perform*—Edema Control – S69.0.2
Monitor left leg skin redness	*Assess*—Edema Control – S69.0.1
Give blood thinning drug daily	*Perform*—Medication Treatment – H24.4.2
Contact lab to take blood daily	*Manage*—Blood Specimen Care – K32.1.4
Measure pain severity using pain scale	*Perform*—Acute Pain Control – Q47.1.2
Give prn analgesics for leg pain	*Perform*—Medication Treatment – H24.4.2
Instruct on prn analgesics for sleeplessness	*Teach*—Sleep Pattern Control – A04.0.3

Actual Outcomes/Goals Met (Evaluation)—(Care Components/Nursing Diagnoses)

- **Tissue Perfusion Component—S**
  Nursing Diagnosis: Tissue Perfusion Alteration Improved – S48.0.1
  - Evidence = Skin Redness Minimal
  - Evidence = Left Leg Measurements within Normal Range
  - Evidence = Left Leg Edema Minimal
- **Sensory Component—Q**
  Nursing Diagnosis: Acute Pain Improved – Q45.1.1
  - Evidence = Acute Pain Gone
  - Evidence = Pain Scale within Normal Limits
- **Activity Component—A**
  Nursing Diagnosis: Sleep Pattern Disturbance Stabilized – A01.6.2
  - Evidence = Able to Sleep at Night

EXHIBIT 13.6. INDIVIDUALIZED PLAN OF CARE EXAMPLE: FRACTURED HIP

Case Study
Ms. Ivy, age 50, is hospitalized on the surgical orthopedic unit with a fractured hip of her right leg, which she received while playing tennis. Her surgeon operated to set the femur, and inserted several pins and a metal rod. The surgeon wrote orders to change her surgical wound dressing daily, give medication prn for pain, elevate right leg on two pillows, watch for leg edema, assign to bed rest or to be out of bed in a wheelchair only, have a normal diet, and be taught how to use crutches without any weight bearing on the right leg.

Signs & Symptoms
- Surgical wound in right leg
- Edema of right leg
- Surgical pain
- Activity restrictions

Medical Diagnosis
Fractured hip of right leg

Care Components/Nursing Diagnoses (Assessment/Diagnosis)
- **Skin Integrity Component—R**
  Nursing Diagnosis: Skin Incision – R46.4
- **Tissue Perfusion Component—S**
  Nursing Diagnosis: Tissue Perfusion Alteration – S48
- **Sensory Component—Q**
  Nursing Diagnosis: Acute pain – Q45.1
- **Activity Component—A**
  Nursing Diagnosis: Sleep pattern disturbance – A01.6

Expected Outcomes/Goals of Care (Outcome Identification)
- To Improve—Nursing Diagnosis: Skin Incision – R46.4.<u>1</u>
- To Improve—Nursing Diagnosis: Tissue Perfusion Alteration – S48.0.<u>1</u>
- To Improve—Nursing Diagnosis: Acute Pain – Q45.1.<u>1</u>
- To Stabilize—Nursing Diagnosis: Physical Mobility Impairment – A01.5.<u>2</u>

Nursing Orders	Interventions and Actions Types (Planning and Implementation)
Change wound dressing	*Perform*—Dressing Change – R55.2.2
Monitor wound drainage	*Perform*—Wound Care – R55.0.2
Elevate right leg on two pillows	*Perform*—Edema Control – S69.0.2
Monitor right leg swelling	*Assess*—Edema Control – S69.0.1
Give prn analgesics for right leg pain	*Perform*—Medication Treatment – H24.4.2
Monitor bed rest	*Assess*—Bedbound Care – A61.0.1
Instruct crutch walking	*Teach*—Immobilizer Care – A02.2.3

Actual Outcomes/Goals Met (Evaluation)—(Care Components/Nursing Diagnoses)
- **Skin Integrity Component—R**
  Nursing Diagnosis: Skin Incision Improved – R46.4.<u>1</u>
  - Evidence = No Wound Drainage
  - Evidence = Wound Healed
- **Tissue Perfusion Component—S**
  Nursing Diagnosis: Tissue Perfusion Alteration Improved – S48.0.<u>1</u>
  - Evidence = Left Leg Edema Minimal
- **Sensory Component—Q**
  Nursing Diagnosis: Acute Pain Improved – Q45.1.<u>1</u>
  - Evidence = Acute Pain Gone
  - Evidence = No Pain Medication Needed
- **Activity Component—A**
  Nursing Diagnosis: Physical Mobility Impairment Stabilized – A 01.5.<u>2</u>
  - Evidence = Able to Use Wheelchair
  - Evidence = Able to Walk with Crutches and Right Leg Not Touching Ground

EXHIBIT 13.7. INTERACTIVE PLAN OF CARE EXAMPLE—NURSING DIAGNOSES: SLEEP DEPRIVATION DISTURBANCE

Patient Problem Textbook Content	CCC of Nursing Diagnosis	CCC Code
Sleep Pattern Disturbance	Sleep Pattern Disturbance (Activity Component)	A01.6

Goal/Outcome	Expected Outcome	
■ Patient shows no physical sign indicative of sleep deprivation	■ Sleep Pattern Disturbance	
	Improve	A01.6.1
	Stabilize	A01.6.2
	Deteriorate	A01.6.3

Intervention/Process	Intervention/Action Types	
■ Educate patient in relaxation technique such as imagery	■ Sleep Pattern Control	
	Assess/Monitor	A04.0.1
	Care/Perform	A04.0.2
	Teach/Instruct	A04.0.3
	Manage/Refer	A04.0.4

	Actual Outcomes	
	■ Sleep Pattern Disturbance	
	Improved	A01.6.1
	Stabilized	A01.6.2
	Deteriorated	A01.6.3

VKS & ST/2006

DISCUSSION

These three sets of examples of plans of care depict different formats and strategies for nurses and allied health personnel to document their care. Each format demonstrates how the CCC terminologies can be used to document and code patient care based on the six steps of the nursing process (ANA, 1998). The first set of examples demonstrates how **standardized** plans of care are designed for specific disease conditions and how they can be structured as clinical pathways. The second set of examples demonstrates how **individualized** plans of care are structured for real-time configuration by clinicians for specific patients with specific medical conditions. The last set of examples demonstrates how **interactive** plans of care for nursing diagnoses and/or medical conditions are configured and compiled as a **set** for integration into the EHR system. It gives an example of how the branching logic options are designed, as well as how the content is determined.

Each example, regardless of format, depicts the **essence of care** by tracking and coding the documentation of the care process from admission to discharge. The plans of care demonstrate the relationship between the two CCC

EXHIBIT 13.8. INTERACTIVE PLAN OF CARE EXAMPLE—NURSING DIAGNOSES: PHYSICAL MOBILITY IMPAIRMENT

Patient Problem Textbook Content	CCC of Nursing Diagnosis	CCC Code
Mobility Impairment	Physical Mobility Impairment (Activity Component)	A01.5

Goal/Outcome	Expected Outcome	
■ Patient achieves highest level of mobility	■ Physical Mobility Impairment	
	Improve	A01.5.1
	Stabilize	A01.5.2
	Deteriorate	A01.5.3

Intervention/Process	Intervention/Action Types	
■ Provide range-of-motion exercises to joints	■ Immobilizer Care	
	Assess/Monitor	A02.2.1
	Care/Perform	A02.2.2
	Teach/Instruct	A02.2.3
	Manage/Refer	A02.2.4

	Actual Outcomes	
	■ Physical Mobility Impairment	
	Improved	A01.5.1
	Stabilized	A01.5.2
	Deteriorated	A01.5.3

VKS & ST/2006

terminologies and when integrated into an EHR system how it will be able to map to other systems. The CCC system is integrated with SNOMED CT (Systematized Nomenclature of Medical Clinical Terms) and is registered by HL7 (Health Level 7) standard as an approved terminology making communication and interoperability between other EHR systems possible.

WORKING TABLE

The last section in this chapter contains Table 13.1. It is a working table specially prepared to be a comprehensive resource for selecting the appropriate CCC concepts. This tool presents the CCC of Nursing Diagnoses side by side with the CCC of Nursing of Interventions for each of the 21 Care Components to help visualize the relationships between them. The individualized Nursing Diagnoses Outcomes and its three qualifiers and the Nursing Interventions Action types and its four qualifiers are presented at the top of each page. This table facilitates the building of a **standardized** clinical pathway, **individualized** patient-specific, or

EXHIBIT 13.9. INTERACTIVE PLAN OF CARE EXAMPLE—NURSING DIAGNOSES: BREATHING PATTERN IMPAIRMENT

Patient Problem Textbook Content	CCC of Nursing Diagnosis	CCC Code
Breathing Pattern Ineffective	Breathing Pattern Impairment (Respiratory Component)	L26.2
Goal/Outcome	**Expected Outcome**	
■ Patient reports feeling comfortable when breathing.	■ Breathing Pattern Impairment Improve Stabilize Deteriorate	L26.2.1 L26.2.2 L26.2.3
Intervention/Process	**Intervention / Action Types**	
■ Assist patient to comfortable position.	■ Breathing Exercises Assess/Monitor Care/Perform Teach/Instruct Manage/Refer	L36.1.1 L36.1.2 L36.1.3 L36.1.4
	Actual Outcomes	
	■ Physical Mobility Impairment Improved Stabilized Deteriorated	L26.2.1 L26.2.2 L26.2.3

VKS & ST/2006

an **interactive** plan of care while keeping the CCC codes accurate, thus making it a useful tool.

The table presents the codes for the three nursing diagnosis qualifiers for expected and/or actual outcomes that use a decimal point and code number (.1, .2, or .3), and the four action types for the nursing interventions that use a decimal point and the code number (.1, .2, .3, or .4), to help keep the codes accurate. Additionally, by including a column for the 21 Care Components, it can serve as an index to locate the nursing diagnosis or nursing intervention concepts more easily, as well as index the charting screens. **Note** that the 21 Care Components could also be used to design the admission assessment structure instead of using other approaches, such as body systems.

In summary, the Working Table and the plans of care examples, regardless of format, provide useful tools for the project team configuring the coding and documentation of the plans of care application for an EHR system. These tools will assist the nursing informatics project leader to make nurses accountable for their actions and demonstrate the value of nursing.

TABLE 13.1. CLINICAL CARE CLASSIFICATION WORKING TABLE—NURSING DIAGNOSES AND NURSING INTERVENTIONS, WITH DEFINITIONS, BY CARE COMPONENTS

Care Components	Nursing Diagnoses & Definitions	Nursing Interventions & Definitions
Coding structure consists of 5 Alphanumeric digits 1st – A to U – CCCs 2nd /3rd – Major Category 4th – SubCategory 5th – Qualifier	3 Qualifiers: 5th Digit Code **Expected Outcomes ——— Actual Outcomes** To Improve (.1)　　or　　Improved (.1) To Stabilize (.2)　　or　　Stabilized (.2) To Support Deterioration (.3)　　or　　Deteriorated (.3) Example: *Activity Alteration, Improved – A01.0.1*	4 Qualifiers: 5th Digit Code **Action Type & Intervention** Assess or Monitor – (.1) Care or Perform – (.2) Teach or Instruct – (.3) Manage or Refer – (.4) Example: *Perform Activity Care – A01.0.2*
A. – ACTIVITY COMPONENT: *Cluster of elements that involve the use of energy in carrying out musculoskeletal and bodily actions.*	**Activity Alteration – A01** *Change in or modification of energy used by the body.* 　**Activity Intolerance – A01.1** 　*Incapacity to carry out physiological or psychological daily activities.* 　**Activity Intolerance Risk – A01.2** 　*Increased chance of incapacity to carry out physiological or psychological daily activities.* 　**Diversional Activity Deficit – A01.3** 　*Lack of interest or engagement in leisure activities.* 　**Fatigue – A01.4** 　*Exhaustion that interferes with physical and mental activities.* 　**Physical Mobility Impairment – A01.5** 　*Diminished ability to perform independent movement.* 　**Sleep Pattern Disturbance – A01.6** 　*Imbalance in the normal sleep/wake cycle.* 　**Sleep Deprivation – A01.7** 　*Lack of the normal sleep/wake cycle.* **Musculoskeletal Alteration – A02** *Change in or modification of the muscles, bones, or support structures.*	**Activity Care – A01** *Activities performed to carry out physiological or psychological daily activities.* 　**Energy Conservation – A01.2** 　*Actions performed to preserve energy.* **Fracture Care – A02** *Actions performed to control broken bones.* 　**Cast Care – A02.1** 　*Actions performed to control a rigid dressing.* 　**Immobilizer Care – A02.2** 　*Actions performed to control a splint, cast, or prescribed bed rest.* **Mobility Therapy – A03** *Actions performed to advise and instruct on mobility deficits.* 　**Ambulation Therapy – A03.1** 　*Actions performed to promote walking.* 　**Assistive Device Therapy – A03.2** 　*Actions performed to support the use of products to aid in caring for oneself.* 　**Transfer Care – A03.3** 　*Actions performed to assist in moving from one place to another.* **Sleep Pattern Control – A04** *Actions performed to support the sleep and wake cycles.* **Musculosketal Care – A05** *Actions performed to restore physical functioning.* 　**Range of Motion – A05.1** 　*Actions performed to provide the active and passive exercises to maintain joint function.* 　**Rehabilitation Exercise – A05.2** 　*Actions performed to promote physical functioning.* **Bedbound Care – A61** *Actions performed to support an individual confined to bed.* 　**Positioning Therapy – A61.1** 　*Process to support changes in body positioning.*

(Continued)

TABLE 13.1. CLINICAL CARE CLASSIFICATION WORKING TABLE—NURSING DIAGNOSES AND NURSING INTERVENTIONS, WITH DEFINITIONS, BY CARE COMPONENTS (CONTINUED)

Care Components	Nursing Diagnoses & Definitions	Nursing Interventions & Definitions
Coding structure consists of 5 Alphanumeric digits 1st – A to U – CCCs 2nd /3rd – Major Category 4th – SubCategory 5th – Qualifier	3 Qualifiers: 5th Digit Code **Expected Outcomes ⎯⎯ Actual Outcomes** To Improve (.1) or Improved (.1) To Stabilize (.2) or Stabilized (.2) To Support Deterioration (.3) or Deteriorated (.3) Example: *Activity Alteration, Improved – A01.0.1*	4 Qualifiers: 5th Digit Code **Action Type & Intervention** Assess or Monitor – (.1) Care or Perform – (.2) Teach or Instruct – (.3) Manage or Refer – (.4) Example: *Perform Activity Care – A01.0.2*
B. – BOWEL/GASTRIC COMPONENT: *Cluster of elements that involve the gastrointestinal system.*	**Bowel Elimination Alteration – B03** *Change in or modification of the gastrointestinal system.* **Bowel Incontinence – B03.1** *Involuntary defecation.* **Colonic Constipation – B03.2** *Infrequent or difficult passage of hard, dry feces.* **Diarrhea – B03.3** *Abnormal frequency and fluidity of feces.* **Fecal Impaction – B03.4** *Feces wedged in intestines.* **Perceived Constipation – B03.5** *Belief and treatment of infrequent or difficult passage of feces without cause.* **Unspecified Constipation B03.6** *Other forms of abnormal feces or difficult passage of feces.* **Gastrointestinal Alteration – B04** *Change in or modification of the stomach or intestines.* **Nausea – B51** *Distaste for food/fluids and an urge to vomit.*	**Bowel Care – B06** *Actions performed to control and restore the functioning of the bowel.* **Bowel Training – B06.1** *Actions performed to provide instruction on bowel elimination conditions.* **Disimpaction – B06.2** *Actions performed to manually remove feces.* **Enema – B06.3** *Actions performed to administer fluid rectally.* **Diarrhea Care – B06.4** *Actions performed to control the abnormal frequency and fluidity of feces.* **Ostomy Care – B07** *Actions performed to control the artificial opening that removes waste products.* **Ostomy Irrigation – B07.1** *Actions performed to flush or wash out an ostomy.* **Gastric Care – B62** *Actions performed to control changes in the stomach and intestines.* **Nausea Care – B62.1** *Actions performed to control the distaste for food and desire to vomit.*
C. – CARDIAC COMPONENT: *Cluster of elements that involve the heart and blood vessels.*	**Cardiac Output Alteration – C05** *Change in or modification of the pumping action of the heart.* **Cardiovascular Alteration – C06** *Change in or modification of the heart or blood vessels.* **Blood Pressure Alteration – C06.1** *Change in or modification of the systolic or diastolic pressure.*	**Cardiac Care – C08** *Actions performed to control changes in the heart or blood vessels.* **Cardiac Rehabilitation – C08.1** *Actions performed to restore cardiac health.* **Pacemaker Care – C09** *Actions performed to control the use of an electronic device that provides a normal heartbeat.*

(Continued)

TABLE 13.1. (CONTINUED)

Care Components	Nursing Diagnoses & Definitions	Nursing Interventions & Definitions
D. – COGNITIVE COMPONENT: *Cluster of elements involving the mental and cerebral processes.*	**Cerebral Alteration – D07** *Change in or modification of thought processes or mentation.* **Confusion – D07.1** *State of being disoriented (mixed-up).* **Knowledge Deficit – D08** *Lack of information, understanding, or comprehension.* **Knowledge Deficit of Diagnostic Test – D08.1** *Lack of information on test(s) to identify disease or assess health condition.* **Knowledge Deficit Dietary Regimen – D08.2** *Lack of information on the prescribed food or fluid intake.* **Knowledge Deficit of Disease Process – D08.3** *Lack of information on the morbidity, course, or treatment of the health condition.* **Knowledge Deficit of Fluid Volume – D08.4** *Lack of information on fluid volume intake requirements.* **Knowledge Deficit of Medication Regimen – D08.5** *Lack of information on prescribed regulated course of medicinal substances.* **Knowledge Deficit of Safety Precautions – D08.6** *Lack of information on measures to prevent injury, danger, or loss.* **Knowledge Deficit of Therapeutic Regimen – D08.7** *Lack of information on regulated course of treating disease.* **Thought Process Alteration – D09** *Change in or modification of cognitive processes.* **Memory Impairment – D09.1** *Diminished or inability to recall past events.*	**Behavior Care – D10** *Actions performed to support observable responses to internal and external stimuli.* **Reality Orientation – D11** *Actions performed to promote the ability to locate oneself in an environment.* **Wandering Control – D63** *Actions performed to control abnormal movability.* **Memory Loss Care –D64** *Actions performed to control a person's inability to recall ideas and/or events.*
E. – COPING COMPONENT: *Cluster of elements that involve the ability to deal with responsibilities, problems, or difficulties.*	**Dying Process – E10** *Physical and behavioral responses associated with death.* **Community Coping Impairment – E52** *Inadequate community response to problems or difficulties.* **Family Coping Impairment – E11** *Inadequate family response to problems or difficulties.* **Compromised Family Coping – E11.1** *Inability of family to function optimally.* **Disabled Family Coping – E11.2** *Dysfunctional ability of family to function.* **Individual Coping Impairment – E12** *Inadequate personal response to problems or difficulties.*	**Counseling Service – E12** *Actions performed to provide advice or instruction to help another.* **Coping Support – E12.1** *Actions performed to sustain a person dealing with responsibilities, problems, or difficulties.* **Stress Control – E12.2** *Actions performed to support the physiological response of the body to a stimulus.* **Crisis Therapy – E12.3** *Actions performed to sustain a person dealing with a condition, event, or radical change in status.*

(Continued)

TABLE 13.1. CLINICAL CARE CLASSIFICATION WORKING TABLE—NURSING DIAGNOSES AND NURSING INTERVENTIONS, WITH DEFINITIONS, BY CARE COMPONENTS (CONTINUED)

Care Components	Nursing Diagnoses & Definitions	Nursing Interventions & Definitions
Coding structure consists of 5 Alphanumeric digits 1st – A to U – CCCs 2nd /3rd – Major Category 4th – SubCategory 5th – Qualifier	3 Qualifiers: 5th Digit Code **Expected Outcomes —— Actual Outcomes** To Improve (.1) or Improved (.1) To Stabilize (.2) or Stabilized (.2) To Support Deterioration (.3) or Deteriorated (.3) Example: *Activity Alteration, Improved – A01.0.1*	4 Qualifiers: 5th Digit Code **Action Type & Intervention** Assess or Monitor – (.1) Care or Perform – (.2) Teach or Instruct – (.3) Manage or Refer – (.4) Example: *Perform Activity Care – A01.0.2*
E. – COPING COMPONENT: *Cluster of elements that involve the ability to deal with responsibilities, problems, or difficulties.* **(cont.)**	**Adjustment Impairment – E12.1** *Inadequate adjustment to condition or change in health status.* **Decisional Conflict – E12.2** *Struggle related to determining a course of action.* **Defensive Coping – E12.3** *Self-protective strategies to guard against threats to self.* **Denial – E12.4** *Attempt to reduce anxiety by refusal to accept thoughts, feelings, or facts.* **Post-trauma Response – E13** *Sustained behavior related to a traumatic event.* **Rape Trauma Syndrome – E13.1** *Group of symptoms related to a forced sexual act.* **Spiritual State Alteration – E14** *Change in or modification of the spirit or soul.* **Spiritual Distress – E14.1** *Anguish related to the spirit or soul.* **Grieving – E53** *Feeling of great sorrow.* **Anticipatory Grieving E53.1** *Feeling great sorrow before the event or loss.* **Dysfunctional Grieving – E53.2** *Prolonged feeling of great sorrow.*	**Emotional Support – E13** *Actions performed to maintain a positive affective state.* **Spiritual Comfort – E13.1** *Actions performed to console, restore, or promote spiritual health.* **Terminal Care – E14** *Actions performed in the period surrounding death.* **Bereavement Support – E14.1** *Actions performed to provide comfort to the family/friends of the person who died.* **Dying/Death Measures – E14.2** *Actions performed to support the dying process.* **Funeral Arrangements – E14.3** *Actions performed to direct the preparatory for burial.*
F . – FLUID VOLUME COMPONENT: *Cluster of elements that involve liquid consumption.*	**Fluid Volume Alteration – F15** *Change in or modification of bodily fluid.* **Fluid Volume Deficit – F15.1** *Dehydration* **Fluid Volume Deficit Risk – F15.2** *Increased chance of dehydration* **Fluid Volume Excess – F15.3** *Fluid retention, overload, or edema.* **Fluid Volume Excess Risk – F15.4** *Increased chance of fluid retention, overload, or edema.*	**Fluid Therapy – F15.0** *Actions performed to provide liquid volume intake.* **Hydration Control – F15.1** *Actions performed to control the state of fluid balance.* **Intake/Output – F15.2** *Actions performed to measure the amount of fluid/flood and excretion of waste.* **Infusion Care – F16** *Actions performed to support solutions given through the vein.* **Intravenous Care – F16.1** *Actions performed to administer an infusion through a vein.* **Venous Catheter Care – F16.2** *Actions performed to control the use of infusion equipment.*

(Continued)

TABLE 13.1. (CONTINUED)

Care Components	Nursing Diagnoses & Definitions	Nursing Interventions & Definitions
G. – HEALTH BEHAVIOR COMPONENT: *Cluster of elements that involve actions to sustain, maintain, or regain health.*	**Health Maintenance Alteration – G17** *Change in or modification of ability to manage health related needs.* **Failure to Thrive – G17.1** *Inability to grow and develop normally.* **Health-Seeking Behavior Alteration – G18** *Change in or modification of actions needed to improve health state.* **Home Maintenance Alteration – G19** *Inability to sustain a safe, healthy environment.* **Noncompliance – G20** *Failure to follow therapeutic recommendations.* **Noncompliance of Diagnostic Test – G20.1** *Failure to follow therapeutic recommendations on tests to identify disease or assess health condition.* **Noncompliance of Dietary Regimen – G20.2** *Failure to follow the prescribed food or fluid intake.* **Noncompliance of Fluid Volume – G20.3** *Failure to follow fluid volume intake requirements.* **Noncompliance of Medication Regimen – G20.4** *Failure to follow prescribed regulated course of medicinal substances.* **Noncompliance of Safety Precautions – G20.5** *Failure to follow measures to prevent injury, danger, or loss.* **Noncompliance of Therapeutic Regimen – G20.6** *Failure to follow regulated course of treating disease or health condition.*	**Community Special Services – G17** *Actions performed to provide advice or information about special community services.* **Adult Day Center – G17.1** *Actions performed to direct the provision of a day program for adults in a specific location.* **Hospice – G17.2** *Actions performed to support the provision of offering and/or providing care for terminally ill persons.* **Meals-on-Wheels – G17.3** *Actions performed to direct the provision of community program of meals delivered to the home.* **Compliance Care – G18** *Actions performed to encourage conformity in therapeutic recommendations.* **Compliance with Diet – G18.1** *Actions performed to encourage conformity to food or fluid intake.* **Compliance with Fluid Volume – G18.2** *Actions performed to encourage conformity to therapeutic intake of liquids.* **Compliance with Medical Regimen – G18.3** *Actions performed to encourage conformity to physician's plan of care.* **Compliance with Medication Regimen – G18.4** *Actions performed to encourage conformity to follow prescribed course of medicinal substances.* **Compliance with Safety Precaution – G18.5** *Actions performed to encourage conformity with measures to protect self or others from injury, danger, or loss.* **Compliance with Therapeutic Regimen – G18.6** *Actions performed to encourage conformity with the health team's plan of care.* **Nursing Contact – G19** *Actions performed to communicate with another nurse.* **Bill of Rights – G19.1** *Statements related to entitlements during an episode of illness.*

(Continued)

TABLE 13.1. CLINICAL CARE CLASSIFICATION WORKING TABLE—NURSING DIAGNOSES AND NURSING INTERVENTIONS, WITH DEFINITIONS, BY CARE COMPONENTS (CONTINUED)

Care Components	Nursing Diagnoses & Definitions	Nursing Interventions & Definitions
Coding structure consists of 5 Alphanumeric digits 1st – A to U – CCCs 2nd /3rd – Major Category 4th – SubCategory 5th – Qualifier	3 Qualifiers: 5th Digit Code **Expected Outcomes —— Actual Outcomes** To Improve (.1) or Improved (.1) To Stabilize (.2) or Stabilized (.2) To Support Deterioration (.3) or Deteriorated (.3) Example: *Activity Alteration, Improved – A01.0.1*	4 Qualifiers: 5th Digit Code **Action Type & Intervention** Assess or Monitor – (.1) Care or Perform – (.2) Teach or Instruct – (.3) Manage or Refer – (.4) Example: *Perform Activity Care – A01.0.2*
G. – HEALTH BEHAVIOR COMPONENT: *Cluster of elements that involve actions to sustain, maintain, or regain health.* **(cont.)**		**Nursing Care Coordination – G19.2** *Actions performed to synthesize all plans of care by a nurse.* **Nursing Status Report – G19.3** *Actions performed to document patient condition by a nurse.* **Physician Contact – G20** *Actions performed to communicate with a physician.* **Medical Regimen Orders – G20.1** *Actions performed to support the physician's plan of treatment.* **Physician Status Report – G20.2** *Actions performed to document patient condition by a physician.* **Professional/Ancillary Services – G21** *Actions performed to support the duties performed by health team members.* **Health Aide Service – G21.1** *Actions performed to support care services by a health aide.* **Medical Social Worker Service – G21.2** *Actions performed to provide advice or instruction by a medical social worker.* **Nurse Specialist Service – G21.3** *Actions performed to provide advice or instruction by an advanced practice nurse or nurse practitioner.* **Occupational Therapist Service – G21.4** *Actions performed to provide advice or instruction by an occupational therapist.* **Physical Therapist Service – G21.5** *Actions performed to provide advice or instruction by a physical therapist.* **Speech Therapist Service – G21.6** *Actions performed to provide advice or instruction by a speech therapist.*

(Continued)

TABLE 13.1. (CONTINUED)

Care Components	Nursing Diagnoses & Definitions	Nursing Interventions & Definitions
H. – MEDICATION COMPONENT: *Cluster of elements that involve medicinal substances.*	**Medication Risk – H21** *Increased chance of negative response to medicinal substances* **Polypharmacy – H21.1** *Use of two or more drugs together.*	**Chemotherapy Care – H22** *Actions performed to control and monitor antineoplastic agents.* **Injection Administration – H23** *Actions performed to dispense a medication by a hypodermic.* **Insulin Injection – H23.1** *Actions performed to administer a hypodermic administration of insulin.* **Vitamin B12 Injection – H23.2** *Actions performed to administer a hypodermic administration of vitamin B12.* **Medication Care – H24** *Actions performed to direct the dispensing of prescribed drugs.* **Medication Actions – H24.1** *Actions performed to support and monitor the use of medicinal substances.* **Medication Prefill Preparation – H24.2** *Actions performed to ensure the continued supply of prescribed drugs.* **Medication Side Effects – H24.3** *Actions performed to control untoward reaction or conditions to prescribed drugs.* **Medication Treatment – H24.4** *Actions performed to administer drugs or remedies regardless of route.* **Radiation Therapy Care – H25** *Actions performed to control and monitor radiation therapy.*
I. – METABOLIC COMPONENT: *Cluster of elements that involve the endocrine and immunological processes.*	**Endocrine Alteration – I22** *Change in or modification of internal secretions or hormones.* **Immunologic Alteration – I23** *Change in or modification of the immune systems.* **Protection Alteration – I23.1** *Change in or modification of the ability to guard against internal or external threats to the body.*	**Allergic Reaction Care – I26.0** *Actions performed to reduce symptoms or precautions to reduce allergies.* **Diabetic Care – I27** *Actions performed to support the control of diabetic conditions.* **Immunological Care – I65** *Actions performed to protect against a particular disease.*
J. – NUTRITIONAL COMPONENT: *Cluster of elements that involve the intake of food and nutrients.*	**Nutrition Alteration – J24** *Change in or modification of food and nutrients.* **Body Nutrition Deficit – J24.1** *Less than adequate intake or absorption of food or nutrients.* **Body Nutrition Deficit Risk – J24.2** *Increased chance of less than adequate intake or absorption of food or nutrients.*	**Enteral Tube Care – J28** *Actions performed to control the use of an enteral drainage tube.* **Enteral Tube Insertion – J28.1** *Actions performed to support the placement of an enteral drainage tube.* **Enteral Tube Irrigation – J28.2** *Actions performed to flush or wash out an enteral tube.*

(Continued)

TABLE 13.1. CLINICAL CARE CLASSIFICATION WORKING TABLE—NURSING DIAGNOSES AND NURSING INTERVENTIONS, WITH DEFINITIONS, BY CARE COMPONENTS (CONTINUED)

Care Components	Nursing Diagnoses & Definitions	Nursing Interventions & Definitions
Coding structure consists of 5 Alphanumeric digits 1st – A to U – CCCs 2nd /3rd – Major Category 4th – SubCategory 5th – Qualifier	3 Qualifiers: 5th Digit Code **Expected Outcomes —— Actual Outcomes** To Improve (.1) or Improved (.1) To Stabilize (.2) or Stabilized (.2) To Support Deterioration (.3) or Deteriorated (.3) Example: *Activity Alteration, Improved – A01.0.1*	4 Qualifiers: 5th Digit Code **Action Type & Intervention** Assess or Monitor – (.1) Care or Perform – (.2) Teach or Instruct – (.3) Manage or Refer – (.4) Example: *Perform Activity Care – A01.0.2*
J. – NUTRITIONAL COMPONENT: *Cluster of elements that involve the intake of food and nutrients.* **(cont.)**	**Body Nutrition Excess – J24.3** *More than adequate intake or absorption of food or nutrients.* **Body Nutrition Excess Risk – J24.4** *Increased chance of more than adequate intake or absorption of food or nutrients* **Swallowing Impairment – J24.5** *Inability to move food from mouth to stomach.* **Infant Feeding Pattern Impairment – J54** *Imbalance in the normal feeding habits of an infant.* **Breast-feeding Impairment – J55** *Diminished ability to nourish infant at the breast.*	**Nutrition Care – J29** *Actions performed to support the intake of food and nutrients.* **Feeding Technique – J29.2** *Actions performed to provide special measures to provide nourishment.* **Regular Diet – J29.3** *Actions performed to support the ingestion of food and nutrients from established nutrition standards.* **Special Diet – J29.4** *Actions performed to support the ingestion of food and nutrients prescribed for a specific purpose.* **Enteral Feeding – J29.5** *Actions performed to provide nourishment through a gastrointestinal route.* **Parenteral Feeding – J29.6** *Actions performed to provide nourishment through intravenous or subcutaneous routes.* **Breast-feeding Support – J66** *Actions performed to provide nourishment of an infant at the breast.* **Weight Control – J67** *Actions performed to control obesity or debilitation.*
K. – PHYSICAL REGULATION COMPONENT: *Cluster of elements that involve bodily processes.*	**Physical Regulation Alteration – K25** *Change in or modification of somatic control.* **Autonomic Dysreflexia – K25.1** *Life-threatening inhibited sympathetic response to noxious stimuli in a person with a spinal cord injury at T7 or above.* **Hyperthermia – K25.2** *Abnormal high body temperature.* **Hypothermia – K25.3** *Abnormal low body temperature.* **Thermoregulation Impairment – K25.4** *Fluctuation of temperature between hypothermia and hyperthermia.* **Infection Risk – K25.5** *Increased chance of contamination with disease-producing germs.*	**Infection Control – K30** *Actions performed to contain a communicable disease.* **Universal Precautions – K30.1** *Practices to prevent the spread of infections and infectious diseases.* **Physical Health Care – K31** *Actions performed to support somatic problems.* **Health History – K31.1** *Actions performed to obtain information about past illness and health status.* **Health Promotion – K31.2** *Actions performed to encourage behaviors to enhance health state.*

TABLE 13.1. (CONTINUED)

Care Components	Nursing Diagnoses & Definitions	Nursing Interventions & Definitions
	Infection Unspecified – K25.6 *Unknown contamination with disease-producing germs.* **Intracranial Adaptive Capacity Impairment – K25.7** *Intracranial fluid volumes are compromised.*	**Physical Examination – K31.3** *Actions performed to observe somatic events.* **Clinical Measurements – K31.4** *Actions performed to conduct procedures to evaluate somatic events.* **Specimen Care – K32** *Actions performed to direct the collection and/or the examination of a bodily specimen.* **Blood Specimen Care – K32.1** *Actions performed to collect and/or examine a sample of blood.* **Stool Specimen Care – K32.2** *Actions performed to collect and/or examine a sample of feces.* **Urine Specimen Care – K32.3** *Actions performed to collect and/or examine a sample of urine.* **Sputum Specimen Care – K32.5** *Actions performed to collect and/or examine a sample of sputum.* **Vital Signs – K33** *Actions performed to measure temperature, respiration, pulse, and blood pressure.* **Blood Pressure – K33.1** *Actions performed to measure the diastolic and systolic pressure of the blood.* **Temperature – K33.2** *Actions performed to measure the body temperature.* **Pulse – K33.3** *Actions performed to measure rhythmical beats of the heart.* **Respiration – K33.4** *Actions performed to measure the function of breathing.*
L. – RESPIRATORY COMPONENT: *Cluster of elements that involve breathing and the pulmonary system.*	**Respiration Alteration – L26** *Change in or modification of carrying out responsibilities.* **Airway Clearance Impairment – L26.1** *Inability to clear secretions/obstructions in airway.* **Breathing Pattern Impairment – L26.2** *Inadequate inhalation or exhalation.* **Gas Exchange Impairment – L26.3** *Imbalance of oxygen and carbon dioxide transfer between lung and vascular system.* **Ventilatory Weaning Impairment – L56** *Inability to tolerate decreased levels of ventilator support.*	**Oxygen Therapy Care – L35** *Actions performed to support the administration of oxygen treatment.* **Pulmonary Care – L36** *Actions performed to support pulmonary hygiene.* **Breathing Exercises – L36.1** *Actions performed to provide therapy on respiratory or lung exertion.* **Chest Physiotherapy – L36.2** *Actions performed to provide exercises to provide postural drainage of lungs.* **Inhalation Therapy – L36.3** *Actions performed to support breathing treatments.*

(Continued)

TABLE 13.1. CLINICAL CARE CLASSIFICATION WORKING TABLE—NURSING DIAGNOSES AND NURSING INTERVENTIONS, WITH DEFINITIONS, BY CARE COMPONENTS (CONTINUED)

Care Components	Nursing Diagnoses & Definitions	Nursing Interventions & Definitions
Coding structure consists of 5 Alphanumeric digits 1st – A to U – CCCs 2nd /3rd – Major Category 4th – SubCategory 5th – Qualifier	3 Qualifiers: 5th Digit Code **Expected Outcomes ——— Actual Outcomes** To Improve (.1) or Improved (.1) To Stabilize (.2) or Stabilized (.2) To Support Deterioration (.3) or Deteriorated (.3) Example: *Activity Alteration, Improved – A01.0.1*	4 Qualifiers: 5th Digit Code **Action Type & Intervention** Assess or Monitor – (.1) Care or Perform – (.2) Teach or Instruct – (.3) Manage or Refer – (.4) Example: *Perform Activity Care – A01.0.2*

L. – RESPIRATORY COMPONENT: *Cluster of elements that involve breathing and the pulmonary system.* **(cont.)**		**Ventilator Care – L36.4** *Actions performed to control and monitor the use of a ventilator.* **Tracheostomy Care – L37** *Actions performed to support a tracheostomy.*
M. – ROLE RELATIONSHIP COMPONENT: *Cluster of elements involving interpersonal work, social, family, and sexual interactions.*	**Role Performance Alteration – M27** *Change in or modification of carrying out responsibilities.* 　**Parental Role Conflict – M27.1** 　*Struggle with parental position and responsibilities.* 　**Parenting Alteration – M27.2** 　*Change in or modification of nurturing figure's ability to promote growth.* 　**Sexual Dysfunction – M27.3** 　*Deleterious change in sex response.* 　**Caregiver Role Strain – M27.4** 　*Excessive tension of one who gives physical or emotional care and support to another person or patient.* **Communication Impairment – M28** *Diminished ability to exchange thoughts, opinions, or information.* 　**Verbal Impairment –M28.1** 　*Diminished ability to exchange thoughts, opinions, or information through speech.* **Family Processes Alteration – M29** *Change in or modification of usual functioning of a related group.* **Sexuality Patterns Alteration – M31** *Change in or modification of person's sexual response.* **Socialization Alteration – M32** 　*Change in or modification of personal identity.* 　**Social Interaction Alteration – M32.1** 　*Change in or modification of inadequate quantity or quality of personal relations.* 　**Social Isolation – M32.2** 　*State of aloneness, lack of interaction with others.* 　**Relocation Stress Syndrome – M32.3** 　*Excessive tension from moving to a new location.*	**Communication Care – M38** *Actions performed to exchange verbal information.* **Psychosocial Care – M39** *Actions performed to support the study of psychological and social factors.* 　**Home Situation Analysis – M39.1** 　*Actions performed to analyze the living environment.* 　**Interpersonal Dynamics Analysis – M39.2** 　*Actions performed to support the analysis of the driving forces in a relationship between people.* 　**Family Process Analysis – M39.3** 　*Actions performed to support the change and/or modification of a related group.* 　**Sexual Behavior Analysis – M39.4** 　*Actions performed to support the change and/or modification of a person's sexual response.* 　**Social Network Analysis – M39.5** 　*Actions performed to improve the quantity or quality of personal relationships.*

(Continued)

TABLE 13.1. (CONTINUED)

Care Components	Nursing Diagnoses & Definitions	Nursing Interventions & Definitions
N. – SAFETY COMPONENT: *Cluster of elements that involve prevention of injury, danger, loss, or abuse.*	**Injury Risk – N33** *Increased chance of danger or loss.* **Aspiration Risk – N33.1** *Increased chance of material into trachea-bronchial passages.* **Disuse Syndrome – N33.2** *Group of symptoms related to effects of immobility.* **Poisoning Risk – N33.3** *Exposure to or ingestion of dangerous products.* **Suffocation Risk – N33.4** *Increased chance of inadequate air for breathing.* **Trauma Risk – N33.5** *Increased chance of accidental tissue processes.* **Violence Risk – N34** *Increased chance of harming self or others.* **Suicide Risk – N34.1** *Increased chance of taking one's life intentionally.* **Self-Mutilation Risk – N34.2** *Increased chance of destroying a limb or essential part of the body.* **Perioperative Injury Risk – N57** *Increased chance of injury during the operative processes.* **Perioperative Positioning Injury – N57.1** *Damages from operative process positioning.* **Surgical Recovery Delay – N57.2** *Slow or delayed recovery from a surgical procedure.* **Substance Abuse – N58** *Excessive use of harmful bodily materials.* **Tobacco Abuse – N58.1** *Excessive use of tobacco products.* **Alcohol Abuse – N58.2** *Excessive use of distilled liquors.* **Drug Abuse – N58.3** *Excessive use of habit-forming medications.*	**Substance Abuse Control – N40** *Actions performed to control situations to avoid, detect, or minimize harm.* **Tobacco Abuse Control – N40.1** *Actions performed to avoid, minimize, or control the use of tobacco.* **Alcohol Abuse Control – N40.2** *Actions performed to avoid, minimize, or control the use of distilled liquors.* **Drug Abuse Control – N40.3** *Actions performed to avoid, minimize, or control the use of any habit-forming medication.* **Emergency Care – N41** *Actions performed to support a sudden or unexpected occurrence.* **Safety Precautions – N42** *Actions performed to advance measures to avoid, danger, or harm.* **Environmental Safety – N42.1** *Precautions recommended to prevent or reduce environmental injury.* **Equipment Safety – N42.2** *Precautions recommended to prevent or reduce equipment injury.* **Individual Safety – N42.3** *Precautions to reduce individual injury.* **Violence Control – N68** *Actions performed to control behaviors that may cause harm to oneself or others.*
O.– SELF-CARE COMPONENT: *Cluster of elements that involve the ability to carry out activities to maintain oneself.*	**Bathing/Hygiene Deficit – O35** *Impaired ability to cleanse oneself.* **Dressing/Grooming Deficit - O36** *Inability to clothe and groom oneself.* **Feeding Deficit – O37** *Impaired ability to feed oneself.* **Self-Care Deficit – O38** *Impaired ability to maintain oneself.* **Activities of Daily Living (ADLs) Alteration – O38.1** *Change in or modification of ability to maintain oneself.*	**Personal Care – O43** *Actions performed to care for oneself.* **Activities of Daily Living (ADLs) – O43.1** *Actions performed to support personal activities to maintain oneself.* **Instrumental Activities of Daily Living (IADLs) – 043.2** *Complex activities performed to support basic life skills.*

(Continued)

TABLE 13.1. CLINICAL CARE CLASSIFICATION WORKING TABLE—NURSING DIAGNOSES AND NURSING INTERVENTIONS, WITH DEFINITIONS, BY CARE COMPONENTS (CONTINUED)

Care Components	Nursing Diagnoses & Definitions	Nursing Interventions & Definitions
Coding structure consists of 5 Alphanumeric digits 1st – A to U – CCCs 2nd /3rd – Major Category 4th – SubCategory 5th – Qualifier	3 Qualifiers: 5th Digit Code **Expected Outcomes —— Actual Outcomes** To Improve (.1) or Improved (.1) To Stabilize (.2) or Stabilized (.2) To Support Deterioration (.3) or Deteriorated (.3) Example: *Activity Alteration, Improved – A01.0.1*	4 Qualifiers: 5th Digit Code **Action Type & Intervention** Assess or Monitor – (.1) Care or Perform – (.2) Teach or Instruct – (.3) Manage or Refer – (.4) Example: *Perform Activity Care – A01.0.2*
O. – SELF-CARE COMPONENT: *Cluster of elements that involve the ability to carry out activities to maintain oneself.* **(cont.)**	**Instrumental Activities of Daily Living (IADLs) Alteration – O38.2** *Change in or modification of more complex activities than those needed to maintain oneself.* **Toileting Deficit – O39** *Impaired ability to urinate or defecate for oneself.*	

P. – SELF-CONCEPT COMPONENT:
Cluster of elements that involve an individual's mental image of oneself.
	Anxiety – P40
	Feeling of distress or apprehension whose source is unknown.
	Fear – P41
	Feeling of dread or distress whose cause can be identified.
	Meaningfulness Alteration – P42
	Change in or modification of the ability to see the significance, purpose, or value in something.
	  Hopelessness – P42.1
	  Feeling of despair or futility and passive involvement.
	  Powerlessness – P42.2
	  Feeling of helplessness, or inability to act.
	Self-Concept Alteration – P43
	Change in or modification of ability to maintain one's image of self.
	  Body Image Disturbance – P43.1
	  Imbalance in the perception of the way one's body looks.
	  Personal Identity Disturbance – P43.2
	  Imbalance in the ability to distinguish between the self and the non-self.
	  Chronic Low Self-Esteem Disturbance – P43.3
	  Persistent negative evaluation of oneself.
	  Situational Self-Esteem Disturbance – P43.4
	  Negative evaluation of oneself in response to a loss or change.
		Mental Health Care – P45
		Actions taken to promote emotional well-being.
		  Mental Health History – P45.1
		  Actions performed to obtain information about past or present emotional well-being.
		  Mental Health Promotion – P45.2
		  Actions performed to encourage or further emotional well-being.
		  Mental Health Screening – P45.3
		  Actions performed to systematically examine the emotional well-being.
		  Mental Health Treatment – P45.4
		  Actions performed to support protocols used to treat emotional problems.

Q. – SENSORY COMPONENT:
Cluster of elements that involve the senses, including pain.
	Sensory Perceptual Alteration – Q44
	Change in or modification of the response to stimuli.
	  Auditory Alteration – Q44.1
	  Change in or modification of diminished ability to hear.
		Pain Control – Q47
		Actions performed to support responses to injury or damage.
		  Acute Pain Control – Q47.1
		  Actions performed to control physical suffering, hurting, or distress.

TABLE 13.1. (CONTINUED)

Care Components	Nursing Diagnoses & Definitions	Nursing Interventions & Definitions
	Gustatory Alteration – Q44.2 *Change in or modification of diminished ability to taste.* **Kinesthetic Alteration – Q44.3** *Change in or modification of diminished ability to move.* **Olfactory Alteration – Q44.4** *Change in or modification of diminished ability to smell.* **Tactile Alteration – Q44.5** *Change in or modification of diminished ability to feel.* **Unilateral Neglect – Q44.6** *Lack of awareness of one side of the body.* **Visual Alteration – Q44.7** *Change in or modification of diminished ability to see.* **Comfort Alteration – Q45** *Change in or modification of sensation that is distressing.* **Acute Pain – Q45.1** *Physical suffering or distress to hurt.* **Chronic Pain – Q45.2** *Pain that continues for longer than expected.* **Unspecified Pain – Q45.3** *Pain that is difficult to pinpoint.*	**Chronic Pain Control – Q47.2** *Actions performed to control physical suffering, hurting, or distress that continues longer than expected.* **Comfort Care – Q48** *Actions performed to enhance or improve well-being.* **Ear Care – Q49** *Actions performed to support ear problems.* **Hearing Aid Care – Q49.1** *Actions performed to control the use of a hearing aid.* **Wax Removal – Q49.2** *Actions performed to remove cerumen from ear.* **Eye Care – Q50** *Actions performed to support eye problems.* **Cataract Care – Q50.1** *Actions performed to control cataract conditions.* **Vision Care – Q50.2** *Actions performed to control vision problems.*
R. – SKIN INTEGRITY COMPONENT: *Cluster of elements that involve the mucous membrane, corneal, integumentary, or subcutaneous structures of the body.*	**Skin Integrity Alteration – R46** *Change in or modification of skin conditions.* **Oral Mucous Membranes Impairment – R46.1** *Diminished ability to maintain the tissues of the oral cavity.* **Skin Integrity Impairment – R46.2** *Decreased ability to maintain the integument.* **Skin Integrity Impairment Risk – R46.3** *Increased chance of skin breakdown.* **Skin Incision – R46.4** *Cutting of the integument/skin.* **Latex Allergy Response – R46.5** *Pathological reaction to latex products.* **Peripheral Alteration – R47** *Change in or modification of vascularization of the extremities.*	**Pressure Ulcer Care – R51** *Actions performed to prevent, detect, and treat skin integrity breakdown caused by pressure.* **Pressure Ulcer Stage 1 Care – R51.1** *Actions performed to prevent, detect, and treat Stage 1 skin breakdown.* **Pressure Ulcer Stage 2 Care – R51.2** *Actions performed to prevent, detect, and treat Stage 2 skin breakdown.* **Pressure Ulcer Stage 3 Care – R51.3** *Actions performed to prevent, detect, and treat Stage 3 skin breakdown.* **Pressure Ulcer Stage 4 Care – R51.4** *Actions performed to prevent, detect, and treat Stage 4 skin breakdown.* **Mouth Care – R53** *Actions performed to support oral cavity problems.* **Denture Care – R53.1** *Actions performed to control the use of artificial teeth.* **Skin Care – R54** *Actions to control the integument/skin.* **Skin Breakdown Control – R54.1** *Actions performed to support tissue integrity problems.* **Wound Care – R55** *Actions performed to support open skin areas.*

(Continued)

TABLE 13.1. CLINICAL CARE CLASSIFICATION WORKING TABLE—NURSING DIAGNOSES AND NURSING INTERVENTIONS, WITH DEFINITIONS, BY CARE COMPONENTS (CONTINUED)

Care Components	Nursing Diagnoses & Definitions	Nursing Interventions & Definitions
Coding structure consists of 5 Alphanumeric digits 1st – A to U – CCCs 2nd /3rd – Major Category 4th – SubCategory 5th – Qualifier	3 Qualifiers: 5th Digit Code **Expected Outcomes —— Actual Outcomes** To Improve (.1) or Improved (.1) To Stabilize (.2) or Stabilized (.2) To Support Deterioration (.3) or Deteriorated (.3) Example: *Activity Alteration, Improved – A01.0.1*	4 Qualifiers: 5th Digit Code **Action Type & Intervention** Assess or Monitor – (.1) Care or Perform – (.2) Teach or Instruct – (.3) Manage or Refer – (.4) Example: *Perform Activity Care – A01.0.2*
R. – SKIN INTEGRITY COMPONENT: *Cluster of elements that involve the mucous membrane, corneal, integumentary, or subcutaneous structures of the body.* **(cont.)**		**Drainage Tube Care – R55.1** *Actions performed to support drainage from tubes.* **Dressing Change – R55.2** *Actions performed to remove and replace a new bandage to a wound.* **Incision Care – R55.3** *Actions performed to support a surgical wound.*
S. – TISSUE PERFUSION COMPONENT: *Cluster of elements that involve the oxygenation of tissues, including the circulatory and neurovascular systems.*	**Tissue Perfusion Alteration – S48** *Change in or modification of the oxygenation of tissues.*	**Foot Care – S56** *Actions performed to support foot problems.* **Perineal Care – S57** *Actions performed to support perineal problems.* **Edema Control – S69** *Actions performed to control excess fluid in tissue.* **Circulatory Care – S70** *Actions performed to support the circulation of the blood (blood vessels).* **Neurovascular Care – S71** *Actions performed to control problems of the nerves and vascular systems.*

T. – URINARY ELIMINATION COMPONENT:
Cluster of elements that involve the genitourinary systems.
	Urinary Elimination Alteration – T49
	Change in or modification of excretion of the waste matter of the kidneys.
	  Functional Urinary Incontinence – T49.1
	  Involuntary, unpredictable passage of urine.
	  Reflex Urinary Incontinence – T49.2
	  Involuntary passage of urine occurring at predictable intervals.
	  Stress Urinary Incontinence – T49.3
	  Loss of urine occurring with increased abdominal pressure.
	  Total Urinary Incontinence – T49.4
	  Continuous and unpredictable loss of urine.
	  Urge Urinary Incontinence – T49.5
	  Involuntary passage of urine following a sense of urgency to void.
	  Urinary Retention – T49.6
	  Incomplete emptying of the bladder.
	Renal Alteration – T50
	Change in or modification of the kidney function.
		Bladder Care – T58
		Actions performed to control urinary drainage problems.
		  Bladder Instillation – T58.1
		  Actions performed to pour liquid through a catheter into the bladder.
		  Bladder Training – T58.2
		  Actions performed to provide instruction on the training care of urinary drainage.
		Dialysis Care – T59
		Actions performed to support dialysis treatments.
		Urinary Catheter Care – T60
		Actions performed to control the use of a urinary catheter.
		  Urinary Catheter Insertion – T60.1
		  Actions performed to place a urinary catheter in bladder.
		  Urinary Catheter Irrigation – T60.2
		  Actions performed to flush a urinary catheter.

TABLE 13.1. (CONTINUED)

Care Components	Nursing Diagnoses & Definitions	Nursing Interventions & Definitions
		Urinary Incontinence Care – T72 *Actions performed to control the inability to retain and/or involuntarily retain urine.* **Renal Care – T73** *Actions performed to control problems pertaining to the kidney.*
U. – LIFE CYCLE COMPONENT: *Cluster of elements that involve the life span of individuals.*	**Reproductive Risk – U59** *Increased chance of harm in the process of replicating or giving rise to an offspring/child.* **Fertility Risk – U59.1** *Increased chance of conception to develop an offspring/child.* **Infertility Risk – U59.2** *Increased chance of harm in preventing the development of an offspring/child.* **Contraception Risk – U59.3** *Increased chance of harm preventing the conception of an offspring/child.* **Perinatal Risk – U60** *Increased chance of harm before, during, and immediately after the creation of an offspring/child.* **Pregnancy Risk – U60.1** *Increased chance of harm during the gestational period of the formation of an offspring/child.* **Labor Risk – U60.2** *Increased chance of harm during the period supporting the bringing forth of an offspring/child.* **Delivery Risk – U60.3** *Increased chance of harm during the period supporting the expulsion of an offspring/child.* **Postpartum Risk – U60.4** *Increased chance of harm during the time period immediately following the delivery of an offspring/child.* **Growth & Development Alteration – U61** *Change in or modification of the norms for an individual's age.* **Newborn Behavior Alteration (first 30 days) – U61.1** *Change in or modification of normal standards of performing developmental skills and behavior of a typical newborn the first 30 days of life.* **Infant Behavior Alteration (31 days through 11 months) – U61.2** *Change in or modification of normal standards of performing developmental skills and behavior of a typical infant from 31 days through 11 months of age.*	**Reproductive Care – U74** *Actions performed to support the production of an offspring/child.* **Fertility Care – U74.1** *Actions performed to increase conception of an offspring/child.* **Infertility Care – U74.2** *Actions performed to support conception of the infertile client of an offspring/child.* **Contraception Care – U74.3** *Actions performed to prevent conception of an offspring/child.* **Perinatal Care – U75** *Actions performed to support perineal problems.* **Pregnancy Care – U75.1** *Actions performed to support the gestation period of the formation of an offspring/child (being with child).* **Labor Care – U75.2** *Actions performed to support the bringing forth of an offspring/child.* **Delivery Care – U75.3** *Actions performed to support the expulsion of an offspring/child at birth.* **Postpartum Care – U75.4** *Actions performed to support the time period immediately after the delivery of an offspring/child.* **Growth & Development Care – U76** *Actions performed to support normal standards of performing developmental skills and behavior of an individual of any age group.* **Newborn Care – (first 30 days) – U76.1** *Actions performed to support normal standards of performing developmental skills and behavior of an individual of a typical newborn for the first 30 days of life.* **Infant Care – (31 days through 11 months) – U76.2** *Actions performed to support normal standards of performing developmental skills and behavior of a typical infant 31 days through 11 months of age.*

(Continued)

TABLE 13.1. CLINICAL CARE CLASSIFICATION WORKING TABLE—NURSING DIAGNOSES AND NURSING INTERVENTIONS, WITH DEFINITIONS, BY CARE COMPONENTS (CONTINUED)

Care Components	Nursing Diagnoses & Definitions	Nursing Interventions & Definitions
Coding structure consists of 5 Alphanumeric digits 1st – A to U – CCCs 2nd /3rd – Major Category 4th – SubCategory 5th – Qualifier	3 Qualifiers: 5th Digit Code **Expected Outcomes ——— Actual Outcomes** To Improve (.1) or Improved (.1) To Stabilize (.2) or Stabilized (.2) To Support Deterioration (.3) or Deteriorated (.3) Example: *Activity Alteration, Improved – A01.0.1*	4 Qualifiers: 5th Digit Code **Action Type & Intervention** Assess or Monitor – (.1) Care or Perform – (.2) Teach or Instruct – (.3) Manage or Refer – (.4) Example: *Perform Activity Care – A01.0.2*
U. – LIFE CYCLE COMPONENT: *Cluster of elements that involve the life span of individuals.* **(cont.)**	**Child Behavior Alteration (1 year through 11 years) – U61.3** *Change in or modification of normal standards of performing developmental skills and behavior of a typical child from 1 year through 11 years of age.* **Adolescent Behavior Alteration (12 years through 20 years) – U61.4** *Change in or modification of normal standards of performing developmental skills and behavior of a typical adolescent from 12 years through 20 years of age.* **Adult Behavior Alteration (21 years through 64 years) – U61.5** *Change in or modification of normal standards of performing developmental skills and behavior of a typical adult from 21 years through 64 years of age.* **Older Adult Behavior Alteration (65 years & older) – U61.6** *Change in or modification of normal standards of performing developmental skills and behavior of a typical older adult from 65 years of age and over.* 1. Adapted from NANDA: *Taxonomy I: Revised 1990.* 2. Adapted with Permission from NANDA *Nursing Diagnoses & Classification 2003–2004.* 3. Clinical Care Classification System is copyrighted, placed in the Public Domain, and cannot be sold, but is available with written permission.	**Child Care – (1 year through 11 years) – U76.3** *Actions performed to support normal standards of performing developmental skills and behavior of a typical child 1 year through 11 years of age.* **Adolescent Care – (12 years through 20 years) – U76.4** *Actions performed to support normal standards of performing developmental skills and behavior of a typical adolescent 12 years through 20 years of age.* **Adult Care – U76.5 (21 years through 64 years** *Actions performed to support normal standards of performing developmental skills and behavior of a typical adult 21 years through 64 years of age.* **Older Adult Care – U76.6 (65 years and over)** *Actions performed to support normal standards of performing developmental skills and behavior of typical older adult 65 years and over.* 1. Clinical Care Classification System is copyrighted, placed in the Public Domain, and cannot be sold, but is available with written permission.

© V. K. Saba—Revised 1992, 1994, 2002, 2004/2006

REFERENCES

American Nurses Association. (1998). *Standards of clinical nursing practice.* Washington, DC: ANA.

Clark, J., & Lang, N. (1992). Nursing's next advance: An international classification for nursing practice. *International Nursing Review, 39,* 109–112.

Douglas, M. L., & Celli, M. L. (2006). Implementing and upgrading clinical information systems. In V. K. Saba & K. A. McCormick (Eds.), *Essentials of nursing informatics* (4th ed., pp. 291–309). New York: McGraw-Hill.

CLINICAL CARE CLASSIFICATION (CCC) FRAMEWORK AND TERMINOLOGY TABLES

This chapter provides the framework and structure of the Clinical Care Classification (CCC) system Version 2.0, including the Terminology Tables appropriate for documenting plans of care and/or nursing practice. The chapter also provides an in-depth description and scope of each of the CCC's six nursing process steps. Each terminology table provides a different view and approach depending on the application being configured by nursing informatics project leaders, vendors, or clinicians to use as a resource. Each table focuses on only one specific CCC Nursing Diagnosis and Outcomes or CCC of Nursing Interventions and Actions step used for documenting the nursing process. The tables are not combined as in the Working Table (Table 13.1) presented in the previous chapter.

The CCC system Version 2.0 offers a new approach for documenting patient care in an electronic health record (EHR) system. It uses a standardized framework consisting of 21 Care Components for classifying its two interrelated terminologies—(1) CCC of Nursing Diagnoses and Outcomes and (2) the CCC of Nursing Interventions and Actions. The CCC system uses a five-character alphanumeric structure to code the concepts of the two terminologies. The CCC system's standardized framework makes it possible to code, document, link, and track the patient care process for an episode of illness, as well as facilitate computer processing and statistical analyses. The system can also be used to evaluate patient care holistically, over time, across all health care settings, for population groups and geographic locations.

EXHIBIT 14.1. SIX STEPS OF THE NURSING PROCESS STANDARD OF CARE[a,b]

Assessment	Collects Patient Health Data
Diagnosis	Analyzes the Assessment Data in Determining Diagnoses
Outcome Identification	Identifies Expected Outcomes Individualized to the Patient
Planning	Develops a Plan of Care That Prescribes Interventions to Attain Expected Outcomes
Implementation	Implements the Interventions/Actions Identified in the Plan of Care
Evaluation	Evaluates the Patient's Progress Toward Attainment of Outcomes

[a] Source: *Standards of Clinical Nursing Practice,* 2nd ed. (ANA, 1998, pp. 3, 7–10).
[b] Reprinted with permission from ANA.

NURSING PROCESS

The CCC follows the six steps of the Nursing Process Standards of Care as its theoretical model. The nursing process steps focus on patient care provided by nurses and allied health personnel in clinical practice settings. The Standards of Care and the Standards of Professional Performance are both addressed in the *Standards of Clinical Nursing Practice* recommended by the American Nurses Association (1998), which identifies the specific professional responsibilities of nurses engaged in clinical practice. The nursing process operationalizes and demonstrates the art and science of nursing. The six steps of the nursing process describe the competent level of nursing care and encompass all significant actions taken by nurses to provide care to patients/clients, and forms the basis for clinical decision making. The six steps are: (1) Assessment, (2) Diagnosis, (3) Outcome Identification, (4) Planning, (5) Implementation, and (6) Evaluation. (See Exhibit 14.1 and Figure 14.1.) Each of the six steps of the nursing process also correlate with six steps of the CCC system, as shown in Exhibit 14.2 and Figure 14.2.

The CCC of Nursing Diagnoses consists of 182 (59 major categories and 123 subcategories) diagnostic concepts. This terminology expands to a second level of specificity to represent the Nursing Diagnosis Outcomes by using one of three qualifiers (Improved, Stabilized, or Deteriorated) to depict the 546 expected and actual CCC Outcomes.

The CCC of Nursing Interventions consists of 198 (72 major categories and 128 subcategories) core (atomic) concepts. It also expands to a second level of specificity to represent Action Types by using one of four qualifiers: (1) Assess or Monitor, (2) Care or Perform, (3) Teach or Instruct, or (4) Manage or Refer to depict 792 Interventions and Action Types. The two terminologies are classified by 21 Care Components that provide the standardized framework for linking the terminologies to each other and mapping them to other health-related classifications (see Figures 14.3 and 14.4).

NURSING PROCESS AND CCC SYSTEM

The Nursing Process is used as the theoretical model for documenting patient care using the CCC. Each of the six Nursing Process steps correlates with the

CCC System Framework

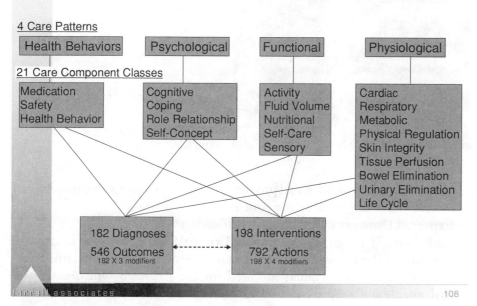

4 Care Patterns
Health Behaviors   Psychological   Functional   Physiological
21 Care Component Classes
Medication   Cognitive   Activity   Cardiac
Safety   Coping   Fluid Volume   Respiratory
Health Behavior   Role Relationship Nutritional   Metabolic
                    Self-Concept   Self-Care   Physical Regulation
                                     Sensory   Skin Integrity
                                                    Tissue Perfusion
                                                    Bowel Elimination
                                                    Urinary Elimination
                                                    Life Cycle
182 Diagnoses   198 Interventions
546 Outcomes   792 Actions
182 X 3 modifiers   198 X 4 modifiers

FIGURE 14.1. Nursing Process model.

six CCC system steps presented in Figure 14.2 and are described in detail below.

1. **Care Components: Assessment**

    Care Components provide the standardized framework for classifying the CCC's two terminologies—CCC of Nursing Diagnoses and Outcomes and CCC of Nursing Interventions and Actions. They represent four health care patterns: (1) Functional, (2) Health Behavioral, (3) Physiological, and (4) Psychological. (See Figure 14.5.) The Care Components are also used to assess patients' problems based on the signs and symptoms. The framework makes it possible to document, link, and track the six steps of the nursing process for an episode of care and provide the analyses and measures used for clinical decision making.

2. **Nursing Diagnoses: Diagnosis**

    Nursing Diagnoses are used to identify the granular atomic-level diagnostic conditions based on the analysis and synthesis of the signs and symptoms,

EXHIBIT 14.2. CCC SYSTEM FRAMEWORK BASED ON THE SIX STEPS OF THE NURSING PROCESS[a]

Standards of Care	CCC Six Documentation Steps
Assessment	CARE COMPONENTS
Diagnosis	NURSING DIAGNOSES
Outcome Identification	EXPECTED OUTCOMES
Planning	NURSING INTERVENTIONS
Implementation	ACTION TYPES
Evaluation	ACTUAL OUTCOMES

[a] *Source: Standards of Clinical Nursing Practice*, 2nd ed. (ANA, 1998, p. 3).

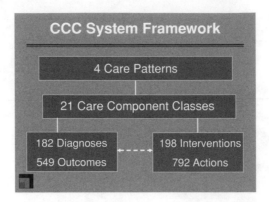

FIGURE 14.2. Nursing Process model and CCC.

assessed care components, and problems that require therapeutic nursing care to alter the health status of the patient.

3. **Expected Outcome: Outcome Identification**

   Each Nursing Diagnosis requires an **Expected Outcome** as a measurable outcome of the therapeutic nursing care that alters the health status of the patient. The three qualifiers are used for the Expected Outcomes of the patient care and are presented in the present tense as:

   - *To Improve or Resolve* patient's condition,
   - *To Stabilize or Maintain* patient's condition, or
   - To Support *Deterioration* of patient's condition.

4. **Nursing Interventions: Planning**

   Nursing Interventions are granular atomic-level services or core concepts identified to develop a plan of nursing care for the patient. They are designed to treat each diagnostic condition or patient problem assessed as requiring therapeutic nursing care.

5. **Action Types: Implementation**

   Each Nursing Intervention in the care plan requires an **Action Type** qualifier that focuses on the specific action needed to carry out the core intervention. The Action Types provide the measures used to determine status of the care process, as well as identify resources and/or cost. They also provide the evidence for clinical decision making. The four Action Types are:

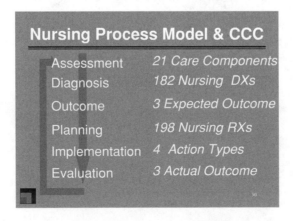

FIGURE 14.3. CCC system framework.

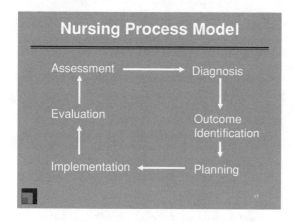

FIGURE 14.4. CCC system framework: Four health care patterns.

- *Assess/Monitor/Observe/Evaluate:* Action evaluating the health status of the patient condition.
- *Care/Perform/Provide/Assist:* Action performing therapeutic patient care (hands-on).
- *Teach/Educate/Instruct/Supervise:* Action educating patient and/or caregiver.
- *Manage/Refer/Contact/Notify:* Action coordinating the care of the patient and/or caregiver.

6. **Actual Outcome: Evaluation**

Each Nursing Diagnosis requires an **Actual Outcome** as an evaluation of the outcome of the therapeutic care or nursing interventions and action types. The same three qualifiers used to predict the Expected Outcomes for each

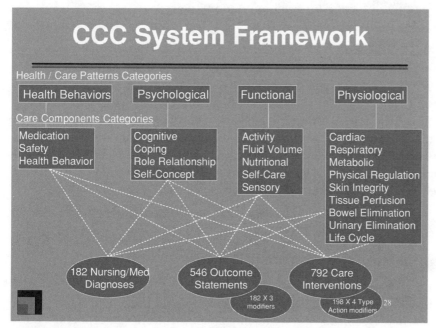

FIGURE 14.5. CCC system framework: Four health care patterns by classes.

Nursing Diagnosis are also used to evaluate whether they were met or not met as Actual Outcomes. They are presented in the past tense as:

- Improved or Resolved patient's condition,
- Stabilized or Maintained patient's condition, or
- Deteriorated or Died.

CODING STRUCTURE

The CCC system uses a five-character structure to code the two terminologies: (1) CCC of Nursing Diagnoses and Outcomes and (2) the CCC of Nursing Interventions and Actions. The coding structure is based on the format of the *International Statistical Classification of Diseases and Related Health Problems: Tenth Revision: Volume 1* (WHO, 1992). This coding structure facilitates computer processing in an EHR system, provides linkages between the two terminologies, and provides word mappings to other health-related classifications. The data elements are input only once, but used multiple times in the application, stored in a database, and retrieved to evaluate patient care. They can also be reused and aggregated for research purposes. The coding strategy for each terminology consists of the following:

- 1st position: One alphabetic character code for Care Component (A to U).
- 2nd & 3rd positions: Two-digit code for a Core Concept (major category) followed by a decimal point.
- 4th position: One-digit code for a subcategory, if available, followed by a decimal point.
- 5th position: One-digit code for:
  —one of three Expected or Actual Outcomes and/or
  —one of four Nursing Intervention Action Types.

CODING PROCESS

The coding process for each of the CCC System's two Terminologies: the CCC of Nursing Diagnoses and Outcomes and the CCC of Nursing Interventions and Actions are essential for measuring patient care. The CCC codes also make it possible to evaluate and analyze outcomes. The CCC codes and standardized framework are needed for the integration and computer processing of the plans of care applications for the EHR systems. Note: Because the two terminologies are classified by identical care components and coded using the same alphanumeric structure, they may need a special character or label to distinguish them in the EHR systems. Coding examples are presented below.

Example: Nursing Diagnosis Coding Structure

Assessed Patient Problem: *Unable to Walk* is a:
  Mobility Problem and Coded as *Activity Component (A)*.
  Physical Mobility Impairment is Nursing Diagnosis Core Concept and Coded as *(1.5)*.

Expected Outcome is added as a decimal point and fifth digit as:
To Improve Physical Activity Impairment is the Expected Outcome and Coded as *(.1)*.

Expected Outcome = *To Improve Physical Mobility Impairment (A01.5.1)* requires treatment:

Nursing Diagnosis Coding Structure:
A = *Activity* Component
  A.01.5 = *Physical Mobility Impairment* (Diagnosis—Subcategory)
    A.01.5.1 = *To Improve Physical Mobility Impairment* (To Improve—Expected Outcome)

Example of a Nursing Intervention Coding Structure

Nursing Diagnosis *Physical Mobility Impairment* requires:
A Therapeutic Action: *Teach Ambulation Therapy*
  Ambulation Therapy is coded as Activity Component (A).
  Ambulation Therapy is the Nursing Intervention Core Concept and coded as (3.1).
    Action Type is added as a decimal point and fifth digit as:
    Teach Ambulation Therapy is the Action Type Teach and coded as (.3) or
  Nursing Intervention with Action Type = *Teach Ambulation Therapy is coded as A03.1.3.*

Nursing Intervention Coding Structure
A = *Activity* (Component)
  A.03.1 = *Ambulation Therapy* (Intervention—Subcategory)
    A.03.1.3 = *Teach Ambulation Therapy* (Teach—Action Type)

Example: Nursing Diagnosis Outcomes Coding Structure

Assessed Patient Problem: *Unable to Walk* is a:
  Mobility Problem and coded as: *Activity Component (A)*.
  Physical Mobility Impairment is Nursing Diagnosis Core Concept and coded as *(1.5)*.
    Actual Outcome is added as a decimal point and a fifth digit as:
    Improved Physical Activity Impairment is the Actual Outcome and coded as *(.1)*

Nursing Diagnosis Outcome Coding Structure:
A = *Activity* Component
  A.01.5 = *Physical Mobility Impairment* (Diagnosis—Subcategory)
    A.01.5.1 = *Improved Physical Mobility Impairment (Improved*—Actual Outcome).

This coding structure facilitates computer processing and provides the linkage between the two terminologies as well as word mappings with other health care classifications. It facilitates the configuration of a plan of care, a clinical pathway, or other documentation applications. It also supports the development of decision support, evidence-based systems, and/or expert systems. Data that are not coded make it almost impossible to process, measure, and analyze patient care to develop evidence-based clinical nursing practice measures and protocols.

TERMINOLOGY TABLES

The terminology tables for the CCC Care Components; the CCC of Nursing Diagnoses; the CCC of Nursing Outcomes; and the CCC of Nursing Interventions are located at end of chapter and start on page 162.

CCC Care Components

The 21 Care Components classify the two interrelated CCC terminologies and serve as the standardized framework for them. They are used for computer processing in the EHR and analysis of clinical nursing practice. The Care Components can also be used as the framework for other patient care documentation requirements.

> A Care Component represents a cluster of elements that depict the four health care patterns: Functional, Health Behavioral, Physiological and Psychological representing a holistic approach to patient care.
>
> *Saba (1994, 1995); Saba & Sparks (1998)*

The 21 Care Components have been found to be the most clinically relevant classes, the best predictors of nursing care resource requirements, and the most appropriate framework for classifying patient care (Holzemer et al., 1997). The four Health Care Patterns provide another level of specificity for the Care Components. They categorize the care components as shown in Table 14.1 and Figure 14.1. Generally, when documenting an episode of care, four Care Components representing each of the four health care patterns, have been found to require three to five nursing diagnoses and eight to ten nursing interventions and actions to treat a patient with a specific medical condition.

The Care Components can also be used as the framework for the patient's Admission Assessment, Discharge Summary, and/or Referral for patient care to community health agencies and other organizations or settings in the Continuum of Care. By using such a framework rather than body systems, it could help focus the initial admission assessment on the patient's presenting problem and the reason for care. The Care Components can be used to aggregate patient care data elements to measure outcomes, determine resources, and costs. Three tables are presented for their use.

Care Component Tables

- Table 14.1: Clinical Care Classification 21 Care Components (Version 2.0): Coded by Four Health Care Patterns

- Table 14.2: Clinical Care Classification 21 Care Components (Version 2.0): Coded by Alphabetic Classes
- Table 14.3: Clinical Care Classification 21 Care Components (Version 2.0): Coded by Alphabetic Classes with Definitions

CCC of Nursing Diagnosis

The CCC of Nursing Diagnoses (Version 2.0) consists of 182 categories (59 two-digit major categories and 123 three digit subcategories) that depict nursing diagnoses and/or patient problems. The terminology includes the original 50 to 60 unique diagnostic concepts, several of the 104 NANDA (North American Nurses Diagnoses Association) labels derived from the *Taxonomy I: Revised– 1991,* and several from the *NANDA List of 2001/2002* (NANDA, 2001). The Nursing Diagnosis labels are structured as noun clauses, **Activity Alteration** instead of verb clauses **Altered Activity** used by NANDA, for ease of understanding and to conform to the structure of the intervention concepts. A Nursing Diagnosis is defined as:

> A clinical judgement about an individual, family, or community response to actual and potential health problems/life processes. Nursing Diagnoses provide the basis for the selection of nursing interventions to achieve outcomes which the nurse is accountable.
>
> *NANDA (1992, p. 5)*

The CCC of Nursing Diagnoses is used to label the patient problems being treated and needing clinical care by nurses and other health care providers. As in its definition, nursing diagnoses **drive** the six steps of the nursing process and justify the selection of the interventions and actions to accomplish the desired outcomes that are evaluated and measured. They identify the rationale for decision support of patient care. The tables that are included can be used for different purposes, depending on the application being configured.

Nursing Diagnoses Tables

- Table 14.4: Clinical Care Classification of 182 Nursing Diagnoses (Version 2.0): Coded and Classified by 21 Care Components
- Table 14.5: Clinical Care Classification of 182 Nursing Diagnoses (Version 2.0): Coded With Definitions and Classified by 21 Care Components
- Table 14.6: Clinical Care Classification of 182 Nursing Diagnoses (Version 2.0): Coded Alphabetically With Definitions
- Table 14.7: Clinical Care Classification of 182 Nursing Diagnoses (Version 2.0): Listed Alphabetically by Code Numbers

CCC of Nursing Outcomes

The CCC of Nursing Diagnoses is modified by using three qualifiers: (1) to **Improve**, (2) to **Stabilize**, and (3) to Support **Deterioration** to depict the results of patient care. These three qualifiers are written in the present tense, represent a second level of specificity, and are used to code the **Expected Outcomes** on initiating the care process.

The CCC of Nursing Diagnoses is also modified by the same three qualifiers: (1) **Improved**, (2) **Stabilized,** or (3) **Deteriorated** and/or died to depict when the Outcomes have been Met or Not Met or on Discharge. These three qualifiers are written in the past tense and represent a second level of specificity. They are used to code the **Actual Outcomes** of the care process.

The three qualifiers are used to code 546 possible Outcomes for the Nursing Diagnoses. The CCC Nursing Diagnosis Outcomes are presented in two separate tables: one for Expected Outcome and one for Actual Outcome. They are presented in these formats because they are used at different times during the care process and written in different tenses.

Nursing Outcome Tables

- Table 14.8: Clinical Care Classification of 182 Nursing Diagnoses (Version 2.0): Coded with Definitions, Three Expected Outcomes, and Classified by 21 Care Components
- Table 14.9: Clinical Care Classification of 182 Nursing Diagnoses (Version 2.0): Coded with Definitions, Three Actual Outcomes, and Classified by 21 Care Components.

CCC of Nursing Interventions

The CCC of Nursing Interventions (Version 2.0) consists of 198 categories (72 two-digit major categories and 126 three-digit subcategories) that depict nursing interventions, procedures, treatments, activities, and/or services. A nursing intervention is defined as:

> A single nursing action is designed to achieve an outcome for a diagnosis (medical/nursing) for which the nurse is accountable.

The CCC of Nursing Interventions is modified by using four qualifiers, each representing a specific type of intervention Action listed below:

1. **Assess or Monitor:** Collect, analyze, and monitor data on the health status.
2. **Care/Direct or Perform:** Perform a therapeutic action.
3. **Teach or Instruct:** Provide knowledge and education.
4. **Manage or Refer:** Coordinate care process.

The four Action Type qualifiers represent a second level of specificity and are used to modify each of the 198 core (atomic) concepts. Nursing Intervention with the Action Types represent a total of 792 unique intervention concepts. Such a strategy makes the terminology flexible, expandable, and easy to use to document, classify, retrieve, and analyze patient care.

Example: of the Core Atomic Concept: **Wound Care**.

Can be modified providing one of the four different Action Types: (1) **Assess** Wound Care, (2) **Perform** Wound Care, (3) **Teach** Wound Care, or (4) **Manage** Wound Care.

Each of the four Action Types utilizes different resources, nursing skills, and takes different lengths of time to perform. Action Types time, if captured, can also be used to determine care costs. Another advantage of the nursing intervention core atomic concept is its coding structure. The structure allows for not only Action Types, but also for other levels of specificity to be added. For example, if the user wants to expand **Perform Wound Care** to include supplies, or add the different catheter sizes for **Perform Bladder Installation**, then it is possible to add and code another level of specificity. The tables that are included can be used for different purposes, depending on the application being designed.

Nursing Intervention Tables

- Table 14.10: Clinical Care Classification of 198 Nursing Interventions (Version 2.0): Coded and Classified by 21 Care Components
- Table 14.11: Clinical Care Classification of 198 Nursing Interventions (Version 2.0): Coded with Definitions and Classified by 21 Care Components
- Table 14.12: Clinical Care Classification of 198 Nursing Interventions (Version 2.0): Coded Alphabetically with Definitions
- Table 14.13: Clinical Care Classification of 198 Nursing Interventions (Version 2.0): Listed Alphabetically by Code Numbers
- Table 14.14: Clinical Care Classification of 198 Nursing Interventions (Version 2.0): Coded with Definitions, Four Action Types, and Classified by 21 Care Components.

CONCLUSION

The CCC system (Version 2.0) Terminology Tables are presented for use either separately or in combination, depending on the application being designed. They can be used to link the nursing process standards of care to each other as well as map to other classifications. They serve as a resource for the configuration of any patient care documentation applications for nurses and/or allied health personnel.

TABLE 14.1. CLINICAL CARE CLASSIFICATION 21 CARE COMPONENTS (VERSION 2.0): CODED BY FOUR HEALTH CARE PATTERNS

I. **Health Behavioral Components**
1. Medication (H)
2. Safety (N)
3. Health Behavior (G)

II. **Functional Components**
4. Activity (A)
5. Fluid Volume (F)
6. Nutritional (J)
7. Self-Care (O)
8. Sensory (Q)

III. **Physiological Components**
9. Bowel/Gastric (B)
10. Cardiac (C)
11. Respiratory (L)
12. Metabolic (I)
13. Physical Regulation (K)
14. Skin Integrity (R)
15. Tissue Perfusion (S)
16. Urinary Elimination (T)
17. Life Cycle (U)

IV. **Psychological Components**
18. Cognitive (D)
19. Coping (E)
20. Role Relationship (M)
21. Self-Concept (P)

TABLE 14.2. CLINICAL CARE CLASSIFICATION 21 CARE COMPONENTS (VERSION 2.0): CODED BY ALPHABETIC CLASSES[a,b]

A   ACTIVITY COMPONENT
B   BOWEL/GASTRIC COMPONENT
C   CARDIAC COMPONENT
D   COGNITIVE COMPONENT
E   COPING COMPONENT
F   FLUID VOLUME COMPONENT
G   HEALTH BEHAVIOR COMPONENT
H   MEDICATION COMPONENT
I   METABOLIC COMPONENT
J   NUTRITIONAL COMPONENT
K   PHYSICAL REGULATION COMPONENT
L   RESPIRATORY COMPONENT
M   ROLE RELATIONSHIP COMPONENT
N   SAFETY COMPONENT
O   SELF-CARE COMPONENT
P   SELF-CONCEPT COMPONENT
Q   SENSORY COMPONENT
R   SKIN INTEGRITY COMPONENT
S   TISSUE PERFUSION COMPONENT
T   URINARY ELIMINATION COMPONENT
U   LIFE CYCLE COMPONENT

[a]Clinical Care Classification (Version 2.0) includes a new and a revised care component. See Appendix Table A.1 for revisions from Home Health Care Classification (Version 1.0).
[b]The Clinical Care Classification System is copyrighted, placed in the Public Domain, and cannot be sold, but is available with written permission.

© V. K. Saba—Revised 1992, 1994, 2002, 2004, 2006

TABLE 14.3. CLINICAL CARE CLASSIFICATION SYSTEM 21 CARE COMPONENTS (VERSION 2.0): CODED BY ALPHABETIC CLASSES WITH DEFINITIONS[a,b]

A   ACTIVITY COMPONENT
     Cluster of elements that involve the use of energy in carrying out musculoskeletal and bodily actions.

B   BOWEL/GASTRIC COMPONENT
     Cluster of elements that involve the gastrointestinal system.

C   CARDIAC COMPONENT
     Cluster of elements that involve the heart and blood vessels.

D   COGNITIVE COMPONENT
     Cluster of elements involving the mental and cerebral processes.

E   COPING COMPONENT
     Cluster of elements that involve the ability to deal with responsibilities, problems, or difficulties.

F   FLUID VOLUME COMPONENT
     Cluster of elements that involve liquid consumption.

G   HEALTH BEHAVIOR COMPONENT
     Cluster of elements that involve actions to sustain, maintain, or regain health.

H   MEDICATION COMPONENT
     Cluster of elements that involve medicinal substances.

I   METABOLIC COMPONENT
     Cluster of elements that involve the endocrine and immunological processes.

J   NUTRITIONAL COMPONENT
     Cluster of elements that involve the intake of food and nutrients.

K   PHYSICAL REGULATION COMPONENT
     Cluster of elements that involve bodily processes.

L   RESPIRATORY COMPONENT
     Cluster of elements that involve breathing and the pulmonary system.

M   ROLE RELATIONSHIP COMPONENT
     Cluster of elements involving interpersonal, work, social, family, and sexual interactions.

N   SAFETY COMPONENT
     Cluster of elements that involve prevention of injury, danger, loss, or abuse.

O   SELF-CARE COMPONENT
     Cluster of elements that involve the ability to carry out activities to maintain oneself.

P   SELF-CONCEPT COMPONENT
     Cluster of elements that involve an individual's mental image of oneself.

Q   SENSORY COMPONENT
     Cluster of elements that involve the senses including pain.

R   SKIN INTEGRITY COMPONENT
     Cluster of elements that involve the mucous membrane, corneal, integumentary, or subcutaneous structures of the body.

S   TISSUE PERFUSION COMPONENT
     Cluster of elements that involve the oxygenation of tissues, including the circulatory and neurovascular systems.

T   URINARY ELIMINATION COMPONENT
     Cluster of elements that involve the genitourinary system.

U   LIFE CYCLE COMPONENT
     Cluster of elements that involve the life span of individuals.

---

[a]Clinical Care Classification (Version 2.0) includes a new and a revised care component. See Appendix Table A.1 for revisions from Home Health Care Classification (Version 1.0).
[b]The Clinical Care Classification System is copyrighted, placed in the Public Domain, and cannot be sold, but is available with written permission.

© V. K. Saba—Revised 1992, 1994, 2002, 2004, 2006

TABLE 14.4. CLINICAL CARE CLASSIFICATION OF 182 NURSING DIAGNOSES (VERSION 2.0): CODED AND CLASSIFIED BY 21 CARE COMPONENTS[a,b,c,d]

A ACTIVITY COMPONENT
- 01 Activity Alteration
  - 01.1 Activity Intolerance
  - 01.2 Activity Intolerance Risk
  - 01.3 Diversional Activity Deficit
  - 01.4 Fatigue
  - 01.5 Physical Mobility Impairment
  - 01.6 Sleep Pattern Disturbance
  - 01.7 Sleep Deprivation
- 02 Musculoskeletal Alteration

B BOWEL/GASTRIC COMPONENT
- 03 Bowel Elimination Alteration
  - 03.1 Bowel Incontinence
  - 03.2 Colonic Constipation
  - 03.3 Diarrhea
  - 03.4 Fecal Impaction
  - 03.5 Perceived Constipation
  - 03.6 Unspecified Constipation
- 04 Gastrointestinal Alteration
- 51 Nausea

C CARDIAC COMPONENT
- 05 Cardiac Output Alteration
- 06 Cardiovascular Alteration
  - 06.1 Blood Pressure Alteration

D COGNITIVE COMPONENT
- 07 Cerebral Alteration
  - 07.1 Confusion
- 08 Knowledge Deficit
  - 08.1 Knowledge Deficit of Diagnostic Test
  - 08.2 Knowledge Deficit of Dietary Regimen
  - 08.3 Knowledge Deficit of Disease Process
  - 08.4 Knowledge Deficit of Fluid Volume
  - 08.5 Knowledge Deficit of Medication Regimen
  - 08.6 Knowledge Deficit of Safety Precautions
  - 08.7 Knowledge Deficit of Therapeutic Regimen
- 09 Thought Processes Alteration
  - 09.1 Memory Impairment

E COPING COMPONENT
- 10 Dying Process
- 52 Community Coping Impairment
- 11 Family Coping Impairment
  - 11.1 Compromised Family Coping
  - 11.2 Disabled Family Coping
- 12 Individual Coping Impairment
  - 12.1 Adjustment Impairment
  - 12.2 Decisional Conflict
  - 12.3 Defensive Coping
  - 12.4 Denial
- 13 Post-trauma Response
  - 13.1 Rape Trauma Syndrome
- 14 Spiritual State Alteration
  - 14.1 Spiritual Distress

- 53 Grieving
  - 53.1 Anticipatory Grieving
  - 53.2 Dysfunctional Grieving

F FLUID VOLUME COMPONENT
- 15 Fluid Volume Alteration
  - 15.1 Fluid Volume Deficit
  - 15.2 Fluid Volume Deficit Risk
  - 15.3 Fluid Volume Excess
  - 15.4 Fluid Volume Excess Risk

G HEALTH BEHAVIOR COMPONENT
- 17 Health Maintenance Alteration
  - 17.1 Failure to Thrive
- 18 Health-Seeking Behavior Alteration
- 19 Home Maintenance Alteration
- 20 Noncompliance
  - 20.1 Noncompliance of Diagnostic Test
  - 20.2 Noncompliance of Dietary Regimen
  - 20.3 Noncompliance of Fluid Volume
  - 20.4 Noncompliance of Medication Regimen
  - 20.5 Noncompliance of Safety Precautions
  - 20.6 Noncompliance of Therapeutic Regimen

H MEDICATION COMPONENT
- 21 Medication Risk
  - 21.1 Polypharmacy

I METABOLIC COMPONENT
- 22 Endocrine Alteration
- 23 Immunologic Alteration
  - 23.1 Protection Alteration

J NUTRITIONAL COMPONENT
- 24 Nutrition Alteration
  - 24.1 Body Nutrition Deficit
  - 24.2 Body Nutrition Deficit Risk
  - 24.3 Body Nutrition Excess
  - 24.4 Body Nutrition Excess Risk
  - 24.5 Swallowing Impairment
- 54 Infant Feeding Pattern Impairment
- 55 Breast-feeding Impairment

K PHYSICAL REGULATION COMPONENT
- 25 Physical Regulation Alteration
  - 25.1 Autonomic Dysreflexia
  - 25.2 Hyperthermia
  - 25.3 Hypothermia
  - 25.4 Thermoregulation Impairment
  - 25.5 Infection Risk
  - 25.6 Infection Unspecified
  - 25.7 Intracranial Adaptive Capacity Impairment

L RESPIRATORY COMPONENT
- 26 Respiration Alteration
  - 26.1 Airway Clearance Impairment
  - 26.2 Breathing Pattern Impairment
  - 26.3 Gas Exchange Impairment
- 56 Ventilatory Weaning Impairment

(Continued)

TABLE 14.4. (CONTINUED)

M ROLE RELATIONSHIP COMPONENT
27 Role Performance Alteration
   27.1 Parental Role Conflict
   27.2 Parenting Alteration
   27.3 Sexual Dysfunction
   27.4 Caregiver Role Strain
28 Communication Impairment
   28.1 Verbal Impairment
29 Family Processes Alteration
31 Sexuality Patterns Alteration
32 Socialization Alteration
   32.1 Social Interaction Alteration
   32.2 Social Isolation
   32.3 Relocation Stress Syndrome

N SAFETY COMPONENT
33 Injury Risk
   33.1 Aspiration Risk
   33.2 Disuse Syndrome
   33.3 Poisoning Risk
   33.4 Suffocation Risk
   33.5 Trauma Risk
34 Violence Risk
   34.1 Suicide Risk
   34.2 Self-Mutilation Risk
57 Perioperative Injury Risk
   57.1 Perioperative Positioning Injury
   57.2 Surgical Recovery Delay
58 Substance Abuse
   58.1 Tobacco Abuse
   58.2 Alcohol Abuse
   58.3 Drug Abuse

O SELF-CARE COMPONENT
35 Bathing/Hygiene Deficit
36 Dressing/Grooming Deficit
37 Feeding Deficit
38 Self-Care Deficit
   38.1 Activities of Daily Living (ADLs) Alteration
   38.2 Instrumental Activities of Daily Living (IADLs) Alteration
39 Toileting Deficit

P SELF-CONCEPT COMPONENT
40 Anxiety
41 Fear
42 Meaningfulness Alteration
   42.1 Hopelessness
   42.2 Powerlessness
43 Self-Concept Alteration
   43.1 Body Image Disturbance
   43.2 Personal Identity Disturbance
   43.3 Chronic Low Self-Esteem Disturbance
   43.4 Situational Self-Esteem Disturbance

Q SENSORY COMPONENT
44 Sensory Perceptual Alteration
   44.1 Auditory Alteration
   44.2 Gustatory Alteration
   44.3 Kinesthetic Alteration
   44.4 Olfactory Alteration
   44.5 Tactile Alteration
   44.6 Unilateral Neglect
   44.7 Visual Alteration
45 Comfort Alteration
   45.1 Acute Pain
   45.2 Chronic Pain
   45.3 Unspecified Pain

R SKIN INTEGRITY COMPONENT
46 Skin Integrity Alteration
   46.1 Oral Mucous Membranes Impairment
   46.2 Skin Integrity Impairment
   46.3 Skin Integrity Impairment Risk
   46.4 Skin Incision
   46.5 Latex Allergy Response
47 Peripheral Alteration

S TISSUE PERFUSION COMPONENT
48 Tissue Perfusion Alteration

T URINARY ELIMINATION COMPONENT
49 Urinary Elimination Alteration
   49.1 Functional Urinary Incontinence
   49.2 Reflex Urinary Incontinence
   49.3 Stress Urinary Incontinence
   49.4 Total Urinary Incontinence
   49.5 Urge Urinary Incontinence
   49.6 Urinary Retention
50 Renal Alteration

U LIFE CYCLE COMPONENT
59 Reproductive Risk
   59.1 Fertility Risk
   59.2 Infertility Risk
   59.3 Contraception Risk
60 Perinatal Risk
   60.1 Pregnancy Risk
   60.2 Labor Risk
   60.3 Delivery Risk
   60.4 Postpartum Risk
61 Growth and Development Alteration
   61.1 Newborn Behavior Alteration (first 30 days)
   61.2 Infant Behavior Alteration (31 days through 11 months)
   61.3 Child Behavior Alteration (1 year through 11 years)
   61.4 Adolescent Behavior Alteration (12 years through 20 years)
   61.5 Adult Behavior Alteration (21 years through 62 years)
   61.6 Older Adult Behavior Alteration (65 years & older)

---

[a] Adapted from NANDA (North American Nursing Diagnoses Association): *Taxonomy I: Revised 1990.*
[b] Adapted with permission from NANDA *Nursing Diagnoses & Classification, 2003–2004.*
[c] Clinical Care Classification of Nursing Diagnoses (Version 2.0) includes 9 New Major Categories and 21 Subcategories. See Appendix Table A.2 for revisions from Home Health Care Classification (Version 1.0).
[d] The Clinical Care Classification System is copyrighted, placed in the Public Domain, and cannot be sold, but is available with written permission.

© **V. K. Saba—Revised 1992, 1994, 2002, 2004, 2006**

TABLE 14.5. CLINICAL CARE CLASSIFICATION OF 182 NURSING DIAGNOSES (VERSION 2.0): CODED WITH DEFINITIONS AND CLASSIFIED BY 21 CARE COMPONENTS[a,b,c,d]

A. – ACTIVITY COMPONENT:
Cluster of elements that involve the use of energy in carrying out musculoskeletal and bodily actions.
Activity Alteration – A01
Change in or modification of energy used by the body.
  Activity Intolerance – A01.1
  Incapacity to carry out physiological or psychological daily activities.
  Activity Intolerance Risk – A01.2
  Increased chance of an incapacity to carry out physiological or psychological daily activities.
  Diversional Activity Deficit – A01.3
  Lack of interest or engagement in leisure activities.
  Fatigue – A01.4
  Exhaustion that interferes with physical and mental activities.
  Physical Mobility Impairment – A01.5
  Diminished ability to perform independent movement.
  Sleep Pattern Disturbance – A01.6
  Imbalance in the normal sleep/wake cycle.
  Sleep Deprivation – A01.7
  Lack of the normal sleep/wake cycle.
Musculoskeletal Alteration – A02
Change in or modification of the muscles, bones, or support structures.

B. – BOWEL/GASTRIC COMPONENT:
Cluster of elements that involve the gastrointestinal system.
Bowel Elimination Alteration – B03
Change in or modification of the gastrointestinal system.
  Bowel Incontinence – B03.1
  Involuntary defecation.
  Colonic Constipation – B03.2
  Infrequent or difficult passage of hard, dry feces.
  Diarrhea – B03.3
  Abnormal frequency and fluidity of feces.
  Fecal Impaction – B03.4
  Feces wedged in intestines.
  Perceived Constipation – B03.5
  Belief and treatment of infrequent or difficult passage of feces without cause.
  Unspecified Constipation B03.6
  Other forms of abnormal feces or difficult passage of feces.
  Gastrointestinal Alteration – B04
  Change in or modification of the stomach or intestines.
  Nausea – B51
  Distaste for food/fluids and an urge to vomit.

C. – CARDIAC COMPONENT:
Cluster of elements that involve the heart and blood vessels.
Cardiac Output Alteration – C05
Change in or modification of the pumping action of the heart.

Cardiovascular Alteration – C06
Change in or modification of the heart or blood vessels.
  Blood Pressure Alteration – C06.1
  Change in or modification of the systolic or diastolic pressure.

D. – COGNITIVE COMPONENT:
Cluster of elements involving the mental and cerebral processes.
Cerebral Alteration – D07
Change in or modification of thought processes or mentation.
  Confusion – D07.1
  State of being disoriented (mixed-up).
  Knowledge Deficit – D08
  Lack of information, understanding, or comprehension.
  Knowledge Deficit of Diagnostic Test – D08.1
  Lack of information on test(s) to identify disease or assess health condition.
  Knowledge Deficit Dietary Regimen – D08.2
  Lack of information on the prescribed food or fluid intake.
  Knowledge Deficit of Disease Process – D08.3
  Lack of information on the morbidity, course, or treatment of the health condition.
  Knowledge Deficit of Fluid Volume – D08.4
  Lack of information on fluid volume intake requirements.
  Knowledge Deficit of Medication Regimen – D08.5
  Lack of information on prescribed regulated course of medicinal substances.
  Knowledge Deficit of Safety Precautions – D08.6
  Lack of information on measures to prevent injury, danger, or loss.
  Knowledge Deficit of Therapeutic Regimen – D08.7
  Lack of information on regulated course of treating disease.
Thought Process Alteration – D09
Change in or modification of cognitive processes.
  Memory Impairment – D09.1
  Diminished or inability to recall past events.

E. – COPING COMPONENT:
Cluster of elements that involve the ability to deal with responsibilities, problems, or difficulties.
Dying Process – E10
Physical and behavioral responses associated with death.
Community Coping Impairment – E52
Inadequate community response to problems or difficulties.
Family Coping Impairment – E11
Inadequate family response to problems or difficulties.
  Compromised Family Coping – E11.1
  Inability of family to function optimally.
  Disabled Family Coping – E11.2
  Dysfunctional ability of family to function.

(Continued)

TABLE 14.5. (CONTINUED)

Individual Coping Impairment – E12
Inadequate personal response to problems or difficulties.
  Adjustment Impairment – E12.1
  Inadequate adjustment to condition or change in health status.
  Decisional Conflict – E12.2
  Struggle related to determining a course of action.
  Defensive Coping – E12.3
  Self-protective strategies to guard against threats to self.
  Denial – E12.4
  Attempt to reduce anxiety by refusal to accept thoughts, feelings, or facts.
Post-trauma Response – E13
Sustained behavior related to a traumatic event.
  Rape Trauma Syndrome – E13.1
  Group of symptoms related to a forced sexual act.
Spiritual State Alteration – E14
Change in or modification of the spirit or soul.
  Spiritual Distress – E14.1
  Anguish related to the spirit or soul.
Grieving – E53
Feeling of great sorrow.
  Anticipatory Grieving E53.1
  Feeling great sorrow before the event or loss.
  Dysfunctional Grieving – E53.2
  Prolonged feeling of great sorrow.

F . – FLUID VOLUME COMPONENT:
Cluster of elements that involve liquid consumption.
Fluid Volume Alteration – F15
Change in or modification of bodily fluid.
  Fluid Volume Deficit – F15.1
  Dehydration.
  Fluid Volume Deficit Risk – F15.2
  Increased chance of dehydration.
  Fluid Volume Excess – F15.3
  Fluid retention, overload, or edema.
  Fluid Volume Excess Risk – F15.4
  Increased chance of fluid retention, overload, or edema.

G. – HEALTH BEHAVIOR COMPONENT:
Cluster of elements that involve actions to sustain, maintain, or regain health.
Health Maintenance Alteration – G17
Change in or modification of ability to manage health-related needs.
  Failure to Thrive – G17.1
  Inability to grow and develop normally.
Health-Seeking Behavior Alteration – G18
Change in or modification of actions needed to improve health state.
Home Maintenance Alteration – G19
Inability to sustain a safe, healthy environment.
Noncompliance – G20
Failure to follow therapeutic recommendations.
  Noncompliance of Diagnostic Test – G20.1
  Failure to follow therapeutic recommendations on tests to identify disease or assess health condition.

Noncompliance of Dietary Regimen – G20.2
Failure to follow the prescribed food or fluid intake.
Noncompliance of Fluid Volume – G20.3
Failure to follow fluid volume intake requirements.
Noncompliance of Medication Regimen – G20.4
Failure to follow prescribed regulated course of medicinal substances.
Noncompliance of Safety Precautions – G20.5
Failure to follow measures to prevent injury, danger, or loss.
Noncompliance of Therapeutic Regimen – G20.6
Failure to follow regulated course of treating disease or health condition.

H. – MEDICATION COMPONENT:
Cluster of elements that involve medicinal substances.
Medication Risk – H21
Increased chance of negative response to medicinal substances.
  Polypharmacy – H21.1
  Use of two or more drugs together.

I. – METABOLIC COMPONENT:
Cluster of elements that involve the endocrine and immunological processes.
Endocrine Alteration – I22
Change in or modification of internal secretions or hormones.
Immunologic Alteration – I23
Change in or modification of the immune systems.
  Protection Alteration – I23.1
  Change in or modification of the ability to guard against internal or external threats to the body.

J. – NUTRITIONAL COMPONENT:
Cluster of elements that involve the intake of food and nutrients.
Nutrition Alteration – J24
Change in or modification of food and nutrients.
  Body Nutrition Deficit – J24.1
  Less than adequate intake or absorption of food or nutrients.
  Body Nutrition Deficit Risk – J24.2
  Increased chance of less than adequate intake or absorption of food or nutrients.
  Body Nutrition Excess – J24.3
  More than adequate intake or absorption of food or nutrients.
  Body Nutrition Excess Risk – J24.4
  Increased chance of more than adequate intake or absorption of food or nutrients.
  Swallowing Impairment – J24.5
  Inability to move food from mouth to stomach.
Infant Feeding Pattern Impairment – J54
Imbalance in the normal feeding habits of an infant.
Breast-feeding Impairment – J55
Diminished ability to nourish infant at the breast.

(Continued)

TABLE 14.5. CLINICAL CARE CLASSIFICATION OF 182 NURSING DIAGNOSES (VERSION 2.0): CODED WITH DEFINITIONS AND CLASSIFIED BY 21 CARE COMPONENTS[a,b,c,d] (CONTINUED)

K. – PHYSICAL REGULATION COMPONENT:
Cluster of elements that involve bodily processes.
Physical Regulation Alteration – K25
Change in or modification of somatic control.
  Autonomic Dysreflexia – K25.1
  Life-threatening inhibited sympathetic response to noxious stimuli in a person with a spinal cord injury at T7 or above.
  Hyperthermia – K25.2
  Abnormal high body temperature.
  Hypothermia – K25.3
  Abnormal low body temperature.
  Thermoregulation Impairment – K25.4
  Fluctuation of temperature between hypothermia and hyperthermia.
  Infection Risk – K25.5
  Increased chance of contamination with disease-producing germs.
  Infection Unspecified – K25.6
  Unknown contamination with disease-producing germs.
  Intracranial Adaptive Capacity Impairment – K25.7
  Intracranial fluid volumes are compromised.

L. – RESPIRATORY COMPONENT:
Cluster of elements that involve breathing and the pulmonary system.
Respiration Alteration – L26
Change in or modification of carrying out responsibilities.
  Airway Clearance Impairment – L26.1
  Inability to clear secretions/obstructions in airway.
  Breathing Pattern Impairment – L26.2
  Inadequate inhalation or exhalation.
  Gas Exchange Impairment – L26.3
  Imbalance of oxygen and carbon dioxide transfer between lung and vascular system.
Ventilatory Weaning Impairment – L56
Inability to tolerate decreased levels of ventilator support.

M. – ROLE RELATIONSHIP COMPONENT:
Cluster of elements involving interpersonal work, social, family, and sexual interactions.
Role Performance Alteration – M27
Change in or modification of carrying out responsibilities.
  Parental Role Conflict – M27.1
  Struggle with parental position and responsibilities.
  Parenting Alteration – M27.2
  Change in or modification of nurturing figures ability to promote growth.
  Sexual Dysfunction – M27.3
  Deleterious change in sex response.
  Caregiver Role Strain – M27.4
  Excessive tension of one who gives physical or emotional care and support to another person or patient.
Communication Impairment – M28
Diminished ability to exchange thoughts, opinions, or information.

  Verbal Impairment –M28.1
  Diminished ability to exchange thoughts, opinions, or information through speech.
Family Processes Alteration – M29
Change in or modification of usual functioning of a related group.
Sexuality Patterns Alteration – M31
Change in or modification of a person's sexual response.
Socialization Alteration – M32
Change in or modification of personal identity.
  Social Interaction Alteration – M32.1
  Change in or modification of inadequate quantity or quality of personal relations.
  Social Isolation – M32.2
  State of aloneness; lack of interaction with others.
  Relocation Stress Syndrome – M32.3
  Excessive tension from moving to a new location.

N. – SAFETY COMPONENT:
Cluster of elements that involve prevention of injury, danger, loss, or abuse.
Injury Risk – N33
Increased chance of danger or loss.
  Aspiration Risk – N33.1
  Increased chance of material into trachea-bronchial passages.
  Disuse Syndrome – N33.2
  Group of symptoms related to effects of immobility.
  Poisoning Risk – N33.3
  Exposure to or ingestion of dangerous products.
  Suffocation Risk – N33.4
  Increased chance of inadequate air for breathing.
  Trauma Risk – N33.5
  Increased chance of accidental tissue processes.
Violence Risk – N34
Increased chance of harming self or others.
  Suicide Risk – N34.1
  Increased chance of taking one's life intentionally.
  Self-Mutilation Risk – N34.2
  Increased chance of destroying a limb or essential part of the body.
Perioperative Injury Risk – N57
Increased chance of injury during the operative processes.
  Perioperative Positioning Injury – N57.1
  Damages from operative process positioning.
  Surgical Recovery Delay – N57.2
  Slow or delayed recovery from a surgical procedure.
Substance Abuse – N58
Excessive use of harmful bodily materials.
  Tobacco Abuse – N58.1
  Excessive use of tobacco products.
  Alcohol Abuse – N58.2
  Excessive use of distilled liquors.
  Drug Abuse – N58.3
  Excessive use of habit-forming medications.

(Continued)

TABLE 14.5. (CONTINUED)

O.– SELF-CARE COMPONENT:
Cluster of elements that involve the ability to carry out activities to maintain oneself.
Bathing/Hygiene Deficit – O35
Impaired ability to cleanse oneself.
Dressing/Grooming Deficit – O36
Inability to clothe and groom oneself.
Feeding Deficit – O37
Impaired ability to feed oneself.
Self-Care Deficit – O38
Impaired ability to maintain oneself.
   Activities of Daily Living (ADLs) Alteration – O38.1
   Change in or modification of ability to maintain oneself.
   Instrumental Activities of Daily Living (IADLs) Alteration – O38.2
   Change in or modification of more complex activities than those needed to maintain oneself.
Toileting Deficit – O39
Impaired ability to urinate or defecate for oneself.

P. – SELF-CONCEPT COMPONENT:
Cluster of elements that involve an individual's mental image of oneself.
Anxiety – P40
Feeling of distress or apprehension whose source is unknown.
Fear – P41
Feeling of dread or distress whose cause can be identified.
Meaningfulness Alteration – P42
Change in or modification of the ability to see the significance, purpose, or value in something.
   Hopelessness – P42.1
   Feeling of despair or futility and passive involvement.
   Powerlessness – P42.2
   Feeling of helplessness, or inability to act.
Self-Concept Alteration – P43
Change in or modification of ability to maintain one's image of self.
   Body Image Disturbance – P43.1
   Imbalance in the perception of the way one's body looks.
   Personal Identity Disturbance – P43.2
   Imbalance in the ability to distinguish between the self and the non-self.
   Chronic Low Self-Esteem Disturbance – P43.3
   Persistent negative evaluation of oneself.
   Situational Self-Esteem Disturbance – P43.4
   Negative evaluation of oneself in response to a loss or change.

Q. – SENSORY COMPONENT:
Cluster of elements that involve the senses, including pain.
Sensory Perceptual Alteration – Q44
Change in or modification of the response to stimuli.
   Auditory Alteration – Q44.1
   Change in or modification of diminished ability to hear.
   Gustatory Alteration – Q44.2
   Change in or modification of diminished ability to taste.

   Kinesthetic Alteration – Q44.3
   Change in or modification of diminished ability to move.
   Olfactory Alteration – Q44.4
   Change in or modification of diminished ability to smell.
   Tactile Alteration – Q44.5
   Change in or modification of diminished ability to feel.
   Unilateral Neglect – Q44.6
   Lack of awareness of one side of the body.
   Visual Alteration – Q44.7
   Change in or modification of diminished ability to see.
Comfort Alteration – Q45
Change in or modification of sensation that is distressing.
   Acute Pain – Q45.1
   Physical suffering or distress to hurt.
   Chronic Pain – Q45.2
   Pain that continues for longer than expected.
   Unspecified Pain – Q45.3
   Pain that is difficult to pinpoint.

R. – SKIN INTEGRITY COMPONENT:
Cluster of elements that involve the mucous membrane, corneal, integumentary, or subcutaneous structures of the body.
Skin Integrity Alteration – R46
Change in or modification of skin conditions.
   Oral Mucous Membranes Impairment – R46.1
   Diminished ability to maintain the tissues of the oral cavity.
   Skin Integrity Impairment – R46.2
   Decreased ability to maintain the integument.
   Skin Integrity Impairment Risk – R46.3
   Increased chance of skin breakdown.
   Skin Incision – R46.4
   Cutting of the integument/skin.
   Latex Allergy Response – R46.5
   Pathological reaction to latex products.
Peripheral Alteration – R47
Change in or modification of vascularization of the extremities.

S. – TISSUE PERFUSION COMPONENT:
Cluster of elements that involve the oxygenation of tissues, including the circulatory and neurovascular systems.
Tissue Perfusion Alteration – S48
Change in or modification of the oxygenation of tissues.

T. – URINARY ELIMINATION COMPONENT:
Cluster of elements that involve the genitourinary systems.
Urinary Elimination Alteration – T49
Change in or modification of excretion of the waste matter of the kidneys.
   Functional Urinary Incontinence – T49.1
   Involuntary, unpredictable passage of urine.
   Reflex Urinary Incontinence – T49.2
   Involuntary passage of urine occurring at predictable intervals.

(Continued)

TABLE 14.5. CLINICAL CARE CLASSIFICATION OF 182 NURSING DIAGNOSES (VERSION 2.0): CODED WITH DEFINITIONS AND CLASSIFIED BY 21 CARE COMPONENTS[a,b,c,d] (CONTINUED)

Stress Urinary Incontinence – T49.3
Loss of urine occurring with increased abdominal pressure.
Total Urinary Incontinence – T49.4
Continuous and unpredictable loss of urine.
Urge Urinary Incontinence – T49.5
Involuntary passage of urine following a sense of urgency to void.
Urinary Retention – T49.6
Incomplete emptying of the bladder.
Renal Alteration – T50
Change in or modification of the kidney function.

U. – LIFE CYCLE COMPONENT:
Cluster of elements that involve the life span of individuals.
Reproductive Risk – U59
Increased chance of harm in the process of replicating or giving rise to an offspring/child.
Fertility Risk – U59.1
Increased chance of conception to develop an offspring/child.
Infertility Risk – U59.2
Increased chance of harm on preventing the development of an offspring/child.
Contraception Risk – U59.3
Increased chance of harm preventing the conception of an offspring/child.
Perinatal Risk – U60
Increased chance of harm before, during, and immediately after the creation of an offspring/child.
Pregnancy Risk – U60.1
Increased chance of harm during the gestational period of the formation of an offspring/child.
Labor Risk – U60.2
Increased chance of harm during the period supporting the bringing forth of an offspring/child.
Delivery Risk – U60.3
Increased chance of harm during the period supporting the expulsion of an offspring/child.

Postpartum Risk – U60.4
Increased chance of harm during the time period immediately following the delivery of an offspring/child.
Growth and Development Alteration – U61
Change in or modification of the norms for an individual's age.
Newborn Behavior Alteration (first 30 days) – U61.1
Change in or modification of normal standards of performing developmental skills and behavior of a typical newborn the first 30 days of life.
Infant Behavior Alteration (31 days through 11 months) – U61.2
Change in or modification of normal standards of performing developmental skills and behavior of a typical infant from 31 days through 11 months of age.
Child Behavior Alteration (1 year through 11 years) – U61.3
Change in or modification of normal standards of performing developmental skills and behavior of a typical child from 1 year through 11 years of age.
Adolescent Behavior Alteration (12 years through 20 years) – U61.4
Change in or modification of normal standards of performing developmental skills and behavior of a typical adolescent from 12 years through 20 years of age.
Adult Behavior Alteration (21 years through 64 years) – U61.5
Change in or modification of normal standards of performing developmental skills and behavior of a typical adult from 21 years through 64 years of age.
Older Adult Behavior Alteration (65 years & older) – U61.6
Change in or modification of normal standards of performing developmental skills and behavior of a typical older adult from 65 years of age and over.

---

[a] Adapted from NANDA (North American Nursing Diagnoses Association): *Taxonomy I: Revised–1990.*
[b] Adapted with permission from NANDA *Nursing Diagnoses & Classification, 2003–2004.*
[c] Clinical Care Classification of Nursing Diagnoses (Version 2.0) includes 9 New Major Categories and 21 Subcategories. See Appendix Table A.2 for revisions from Home Health Care Classification (Version 1.0).
[d] The Clinical Care Classification System is copyrighted, placed in the Public Domain, and cannot be sold, but is available with written permission.

© V. K. Saba—Revised 1992, 1994, 2002, 2004, 2006

TABLE 14.6. CLINICAL CARE CLASSIFICATION OF 182 NURSING DIAGNOSES (VERSION 2.0): CODED ALPHABETICALLY WITH DEFINITIONS[a,b,c,d]

A01　　**Activity Alteration**
　　　　　Change in or modification of energy used by the body.

A01.1　**Activity Intolerance**
　　　　　Incapacity to carry out physiological or psychological daily activities.

A01.2　**Activity Intolerance Risk**
　　　　　Increased chance of an incapacity to carry out physiological or psychological daily activities.

O38.1　**Activities of Daily Living (ADLs) Alteration**
　　　　　Change in or modification of ability to maintain oneself.

Q45.1　**Acute Pain**
　　　　　Physical suffering or distress; to hurt.

E12.1　**Adjustment Impairment**
　　　　　Inadequate adaptation to condition or change in health status.

U61.4　**Adolescent Behavior Alteration**
　　　　　Change in or modification of normal standards of performing developmental skills and behavior of a typical adolescent from 12 years through 20 years of age.

U61.5　**Adult Behavior Alteration**
　　　　　Change in or modification of normal standards of performing developmental skills and behavior of a typical adult from 21 years through 64 years of age.

L26.1　**Airway Clearance Impairment**
　　　　　Inability to clear secretions/obstructions in airway.

N58.2　**Alcohol Abuse**
　　　　　Excessive use of distilled liquors.

E53.1　**Anticipatory Grieving**
　　　　　Feeling great sorrow before the event or loss.

P40　　**Anxiety**
　　　　　Feeling of distress or apprehension whose source is unknown.

N33.1　**Aspiration Risk**
　　　　　Increased chance of material into trachea-bronchial passages.

Q44.1　**Auditory Alteration**
　　　　　Diminished ability to hear.

K25.1　**Autonomic Dysreflexia**
　　　　　Life-threatening inhibited sympathetic response to a noxious stimuli in a person with a spinal cord injury at T7 or above.

O35　　**Bathing/Hygiene Deficit**
　　　　　Impaired ability to cleanse oneself.

C06.1　**Blood Pressure Alteration**
　　　　　Change in or modification of the systolic or diastolic pressure.

P43.1　**Body Image Disturbance**
　　　　　Imbalance in the perception of the way one's body looks.

J24.1　**Body Nutrition Deficit**
　　　　　Less than adequate intake or absorption of food or nutrients.

J24.2　**Body Nutrition Deficit Risk**
　　　　　Increased chance of less than adequate intake or absorption of food or nutrients.

J24.3　**Body Nutrition Excess**
　　　　　More than adequate intake or absorption of food or nutrients.

J24.4　**Body Nutrition Excess Risk**
　　　　　Increased chance of more than adequate intake or absorption of food or nutrients.

(Continued)

TABLE 14.6. CLINICAL CARE CLASSIFICATION OF 182 NURSING DIAGNOSES (VERSION 2.0): CODED ALPHABETICALLY WITH DEFINITIONS[a,b,c,d] **(CONTINUED)**

B03	**Bowel Elimination Alteration**
	Change in or modification of the gastrointestinal system.
B03.1	**Bowel Incontinence**
	Involuntary defecation.
J55	**Breast-feeding Impairment**
	Diminished ability to nourish infant at the breast.
L26.2	**Breathing Pattern Impairment**
	Inadequate inhalation or exhalation.
C05	**Cardiac Output Alteration**
	Change in or modification of the pumping action of the heart.
C06	**Cardiovascular Alteration**
	Change in or modification of the heart or blood vessels.
M27.4	**Caregiver Role Strain**
	Excessive tension of one who gives physical or emotional care and support to another person or patient.
D07	**Cerebral Alteration**
	Change in or modification of thought processes or mentation.
U61.3	**Child Behavior Alteration**
	Change in or modification of normal standards of performing developmental skills and behavior of a typical child from 1 year through 11 years of age.
P43.3	**Chronic Low Self-Esteem Disturbance**
	Persistent negative evaluation of oneself.
Q45.2	**Chronic Pain**
	Pain that continues for longer than expected.
B03.2	**Colonic Constipation**
	Infrequent or difficult passage of hard, dry feces.
Q45	**Comfort Alteration**
	Change in or modification of sensation that is distressing.
M28	**Communication Impairment**
	Diminished ability to exchange thoughts, opinions, or information.
E52	**Community Coping Impairment**
	Inadequate community response to problems or difficulties.
E11.1	**Compromised Family Coping**
	Inability of family to function optimally.
D07.1	**Confusion**
	State of being disoriented (mixed-up).
U59.3	**Contraception Risk**
	Increased chance of harm by preventing the conception of an offspring/child.
E12.2	**Decisional Conflict**
	Struggle related to determining a course of action.
E12.3	**Defensive Coping**
	Self-protective strategies to guard against threats to self.
U60.3	**Delivery Risk**
	Increased chance of harm during the period supporting the expulsion of an offspring/child at birth.
E12.4	**Denial**
	Attempt to reduce anxiety by refusal to accept thoughts, feelings, or facts.
B03.3	**Diarrhea**
	Abnormal frequency and fluidity of feces.

(Continued)

TABLE 14.6. (CONTINUED)

E11.2   **Disabled Family Coping**
Dysfunctional ability of family to function.

N33.2   **Disuse Syndrome**
Group of symptoms related to effects of immobility.

A01.3   **Diversional Activity Deficit**
Lack of interest or engagement in leisure activities.

O36   **Dressing/Grooming Deficit**
Impaired ability to clothe and groom oneself.

N58.3   **Drug Abuse**
Excessive use of habit-forming medications.

E10   **Dying Process**
Physical and behavioral responses associated with death.

E53.2   **Dysfunctional Grieving**
Prolonged feeling of great sorrow.

I22   **Endocrine Alteration**
Change in or modification of internal secretions or hormones.

G17.1   **Failure to Thrive**
Inability to grow and develop normally.

E11   **Family Coping Impairment**
Inadequate family response to problems or difficulties.

M29   **Family Processes Alteration**
Change in or modification of usual functioning of a related group.

A01.4   **Fatigue**
Exhaustion that interferes with physical and mental activities.

P41   **Fear**
Feeling of dread or distress whose cause can be identified.

B03.4   **Fecal Impaction**
Feces wedged in intestine.

O37   **Feeding Deficit**
Impaired ability to feed oneself.

U59.1   **Fertility Risk**
Increased chance of harm in promoting the development of an offspring/child.

F15   **Fluid Volume Alteration**
Change in or modification of bodily fluid.

F15.1   **Fluid Volume Deficit**
Dehydration

F15.2   **Fluid Volume Deficit Risk**
Increased chance of dehydration.

F15.3   **Fluid Volume Excess**
Fluid retention, overload, or edema.

F15.4   **Fluid Volume Excess Risk**
Increased chance of fluid retention, overload, or edema.

T49.1   **Functional Urinary Incontinence**
Involuntary, unpredictable passage of urine.

L26.3   **Gas Exchange Impairment**
Imbalance of oxygen and carbon dioxide transfer between lung and vascular system.

B04   **Gastrointestinal Alteration**
Change in or modification of the stomach or intestines.

E53   **Grieving**
Feeling of great sorrow.

(Continued)

TABLE 14.6. CLINICAL CARE CLASSIFICATION OF 182 NURSING DIAGNOSES (VERSION 2.0): CODED ALPHABETICALLY WITH DEFINITIONS[a,b,c,d] (CONTINUED)

U61	**Growth and Development Alteration**
	Change in or modification of the norms for an individual's age.
Q44.2	**Gustatory Alteration**
	Diminished ability to taste.
G17	**Health Maintenance Alteration**
	Change in or modification of ability to manage health-related needs.
G18	**Health-Seeking Behavior Alteration**
	Change in or modification of actions needed to improve health state.
G19	**Home Maintenance Alteration**
	Inability to sustain a safe, healthy environment.
P42.1	**Hopelessness**
	Feeling of despair or futility and passive abandonment.
K25.2	**Hyperthermia**
	Abnormal high body temperature.
K25.3	**Hypothermia**
	Subnormal low body temperature.
I23	**Immunologic Alteration**
	Change in or modification of the immune system.
E12	**Individual Coping Impairment**
	Inadequate personal response to problems or difficulties.
U61.2	**Infant Behavior Alteration**
	Change in or modification of normal standards of performing developmental skills and behavior of a typical infant from 31 days through 11 months of age.
J54	**Infant Feeding Pattern Impairment**
	Imbalance in the normal feeding habits of an infant.
K25.5	**Infection Risk**
	Increased change of contamination with disease-producing germs.
K25.6	**Infection Unspecified**
	Unknown contamination with disease-producing germs.
U59.2	**Infertility Risk**
	Increased chance of harm in preventing the development of an offspring/child.
N33	**Injury Risk**
	Increased chance of danger or loss.
O38.2	**Instrumental Activities of Daily Living (IADLs) Alteration**
	Change in or modification of more complex activities than those needed to maintain oneself.
K25.7	**Intracranial Adaptive Capacity Impairment**
	Intracranial fluid volumes are compromised.
Q44.3	**Kinesthetic Alteration**
	Diminished ability to move.
D08	**Knowledge Deficit**
	Lack of information, understanding, or comprehension.
D08.1	**Knowledge Deficit of Diagnostic Test**
	Lack of information on tests to identify disease or assess health condition.
D08.2	**Knowledge Deficit of Dietary Regimen**
	Lack of information on the prescribed food or fluid intake.
D08.3	**Knowledge Deficit of Disease Process**
	Lack of information on the morbidity, course, or treatment of the health condition.

(Continued)

TABLE 14.6. (CONTINUED)

D08.4   **Knowledge Deficit of Fluid Volume**
Lack of information on fluid volume intake requirements.

D08.5   **Knowledge Deficit of Medication Regimen**
Lack of information on prescribed regulated course of medicinal substances.

D08.6   **Knowledge Deficit of Safety Precautions**
Lack of information on measures to prevent injury, danger, or loss.

D08.7   **Knowledge Deficit of Therapeutic Regimen**
Lack of information on regulated course of treating disease.

U60.2   **Labor Risk**
Increased chance of harm during the period supporting the bringing forth of an offspring/child.

R46.5   **Latex Allergy Response**
Pathological reaction to latex products.

P42   **Meaningfulness Alteration**
Change in or modification of the ability to see the significance, purpose, or value in something.

H21   **Medication Risk**
Increased chance of negative response to medicinal substance.

D09.1   **Memory Impairment**
Diminished or inability to recall past events.

A02   **Musculoskeletal Alteration**
Change in or modification of the muscles, bones, or support structures.

B51   **Nausea**
Distaste for food/fluids and an urge to vomit.

U61.1   **Newborn Behavior Alteration**
Change in or modification of the normal standards of performing developmental skills and behavior of a typical newborn the first 30 days of life.

G20   **Noncompliance**
Failure to follow therapeutic recommendations.

G20.1   **Noncompliance of Diagnostic Test**
Failure to follow therapeutic recommendations on tests to identify disease or assess health condition.

G20.2   **Noncompliance of Dietary Regimen**
Failure to follow the prescribed food or fluid intake.

G20.3   **Noncompliance of Fluid Volume**
Failure to follow fluid volume intake requirements.

G20.4   **Noncompliance of Medication Regimen**
Failure to follow prescribed regulated course of medicinal substances.

G20.5   **Noncompliance of Safety Precautions**
Failure to follow measures to prevent injury, danger, or loss.

G20.6   **Noncompliance of Therapeutic Regimen**
Failure to follow regulated course of treating disease.

J24   **Nutrition Alteration**
Change in or modification of food or nutrients.

U61.6   **Older Adult Behavior Alteration**
Change in or modification of normal standards of performing developmental skills and behavior of a typical older adult from 65 years of age and over.

Q44.4   **Olfactory Alteration**
Diminished ability to smell.

(Continued)

TABLE 14.6. CLINICAL CARE CLASSIFICATION OF 182 NURSING DIAGNOSES (VERSION 2.0): CODED ALPHABETICALLY WITH DEFINITIONS[a,b,c,d] **(CONTINUED)**

R46.1	**Oral Mucous Membranes Impairment**
	Diminished ability to maintain the tissues of the oral cavity.
M27.1	**Parental Role Conflict**
	Struggle with parental position and responsibilities.
M27.2	**Parenting Alteration**
	Change in or modification of nurturing figure's ability to promote growth and development of infant/child.
B03.5	**Perceived Constipation**
	Belief and treatment of infrequent or difficult passage of feces without cause.
U60	**Perinatal Risk**
	Increased chance of harm before, during, and immediately after the creation of an offspring/child.
N57	**Perioperative Injury Risk**
	Increased chance of injury during the operative processes.
N57.1	**Perioperative Positioning Injury**
	Damages from operative process positioning.
R47	**Peripheral Alteration**
	Change in or modification of vascularization of the extremities.
P43.2	**Personal Identity Disturbance**
	Imbalance in the ability to distinguish between the self and the non-self.
A01.5	**Physical Mobility Impairment**
	Diminished ability to perform independent movement.
K25	**Physical Regulation Alteration**
	Change in or modification of somatic control.
N33.3	**Poisoning Risk**
	Exposure to or ingestion of dangerous products.
H21.1	**Polypharmacy**
	Use of two or more drugs together.
U60.4	**Postpartum Risk**
	Increased chance of harm during the time period immediately following the delivery of an offspring/child.
E13	**Post-trauma Response**
	Sustained behavior related to a traumatic event.
P42.2	**Powerlessness**
	Feeling of helplessness, or inability to act.
U60.1	**Pregnancy Risk**
	Increased chance of harm during the gestational period of the formation of an offspring/child.
I23.1	**Protection Alteration**
	Change in or modification of the ability to guard against internal or external threats to the body.
E13.1	**Rape Trauma Syndrome**
	Group of symptoms related to a forced sexual act.
T49.2	**Reflex Urinary Incontinence**
	Involuntary passage of urine occurring at predictable intervals.
M32.3	**Relocation Stress Syndrome**
	Excessive tension from moving to a new location.
T50	**Renal Alteration**
	Change in or modification of the kidney function.
U59	**Reproductive Risk**
	Increased chance of harm in the process of replicating or giving rise to an offspring/child.

(Continued)

TABLE 14.6. (CONTINUED)

L26	**Respiration Alteration**	Change in or modification of the breathing function.

L26 **Respiration Alteration**
Change in or modification of the breathing function.

M27 **Role Performance Alteration**
Change in or modification of carrying out responsibilities.

O38 **Self-Care Deficit**
Impaired ability to maintain oneself.

P43 **Self-Concept Alteration**
Change in or modification of ability to maintain one's image of self.

N34.2 **Self-Mutilation Risk**
Increased chance of destroying a limb or essential part of the body.

Q44 **Sensory Perceptual Alteration**
Change in or modification of the response to stimuli.

M27.3 **Sexual Dysfunction**
Deleterious change in sex response.

M31 **Sexuality Patterns Alteration**
Change in or modification of person's sexual response.

P43.4 **Situational Self-Esteem Disturbance**
Negative evaluation of oneself in response to a loss or change.

R46 **Skin Integrity Alteration**
Change in or modification of skin conditions.

R46.2 **Skin Integrity Impairment**
Diminished ability to maintain the integument.

R46.3 **Skin Integrity Impairment Risk**
Increased chance of skin breakdown.

R46.4 **Skin Incision**
Cutting of the integument/skin.

A01.7 **Sleep Deprivation**
Lack of the normal sleep/wake cycle.

A01.6 **Sleep Pattern Disturbance**
Imbalance in the normal sleep/wake cycle.

M32.1 **Social Interaction Alteration**
Inadequate quantity or quality of personal relations.

M32.2 **Social Isolation**
State of aloneness; lack of interaction with others.

M32 **Socialization Alteration**
Change in or modification of personal identity.

E14.1 **Spiritual Distress**
Anguish related to the spirit or soul.

E14 **Spiritual State Alteration**
Change in or modification of the spirit or soul.

T49.3 **Stress Urinary Incontinence**
Loss of urine occurring with increased abdominal pressure.

N58 **Substance Abuse**
Excessive use of harmful bodily materials.

N33.4 **Suffocation Risk**
Increase chance of inadequate air for breathing.

N34.1 **Suicide Risk**
Increased chance of taking one's life intentionally.

N57.2 **Surgical Recovery Delay**
Slow or delayed recovery from a surgical procedure.

J24.5 **Swallowing Impairment**
Inability to move food from mouth to stomach.

Q44.5 **Tactile Alteration**
Diminished ability to feel.

(Continued)

TABLE 14.6. CLINICAL CARE CLASSIFICATION OF 182 NURSING DIAGNOSES (VERSION 2.0): CODED ALPHABETICALLY WITH DEFINITIONS[a,b,c,d] (CONTINUED)

K25.4	**Thermoregulation Impairment**
	Fluctuation of temperature between hypothermia and hyperthermia.
S48	**Tissue Perfusion Alteration**
	Change in or modification of the oxygenation of tissues.
N58.1	**Tobacco Abuse**
	Excessive use of tobacco products.
O39	**Toileting Deficit**
	Impaired ability to urinate or defecate for oneself.
T49.4	**Total Urinary Incontinence**
	Continuous and unpredictable loss of urine.
D09	**Thought Processes Alteration**
	Change in or modification of cognitive processes.
N33.5	**Trauma Risk**
	Increased chance of accidental tissue injury.
Q44.6	**Unilateral Neglect**
	Lack of awareness of one side of the body.
B03.6	**Unspecified Constipation**
	Other forms of abnormal feces or difficult passage of feces.
Q45.3	**Unspecified Pain**
	Pain that is difficult to pinpoint.
T49	**Urinary Elimination Alteration**
	Change in or modification of excretion of the waste matter of the kidneys.
T49.6	**Urinary Retention**
	Incomplete emptying of the bladder.
T49.5	**Urge Urinary Incontinence**
	Involuntary passage of urine following a sense of urgency to void.
L56	**Ventilatory Weaning Impairment**
	Inability to tolerate decreased levels of ventilator support.
M28.1	**Verbal Impairment**
	Diminished ability to exchange thoughts, opinions, or information through speech.
N34	**Violence Risk**
	Increased chance of harming self or others.
Q44.7	**Visual Alteration**
	A diminished ability to see.

[a]Adapted from NANDA (North American Nursing Diagnoses Association): *Taxonomy I: Revised–1990.*
[b]Adapted with permission from NANDA *Nursing Diagnoses & Classification, 2003–2004.*
[c]Clinical Care Classification of Nursing Diagnoses (Version 2.0) includes 9 New Major Categories and 21 Subcategories. See Appendix Table A.2 for revisions from Home Health Care Classification (Version 1.0).
[d]The Clinical Care Classification System is copyrighted, placed in the Public Domain, and cannot be sold, but is available with written permission.

© V. K. Saba—Revised 1992, 1994, 2002, 2004, 2006

TABLE 14.7. CLINICAL CARE CLASSIFICATION OF 182 NURSING DIAGNOSES (VERSION 2.0): LISTED ALPHABETICALLY BY CODE NUMBERS[a,b,c,d]

Activity Alteration	A01
Activity Intolerance	A01.1
Activity Intolerance Risk	A01.2
Activities of Daily Living (ADLs) Alteration	O38.1
Acute Pain	Q45.1
Adjustment Impairment	E12.1
Adolescent Behavior Alteration	U61.4
Adult Behavior Alteration	U61.5
Airway Clearance Impairment	L26.1
Alcohol Abuse	N58.2
Anticipatory Grieving	E53.1
Anxiety	P40
Aspiration Risk	N33.1
Auditory Alteration	Q44.1
Autonomic Dysreflexia	K25.1
Bathing/Hygiene Deficit	O35
Blood Pressure Alteration	C06.1
Body Image Distribution	P43.1
Body Nutrition Deficit	J24.1
Body Nutrition Deficit Risk	J24.2
Body Nutrition Excess	J24.3
Body Nutrition Excess Risk	J24.4
Bowel Elimination Alteration	B03
Bowel Incontinence	B03.1
Breast-feeding Impairment	J55
Breathing Pattern Impairment	L26.2
Cardiac Output Alteration	C05
Cardiovascular Alteration	C06
Caregiver Role Strain	M27.4
Cerebral Alteration	D07
Child Behavior Alteration	U61.3
Chronic Low Self-Esteem Disturbance	P43.3
Chronic Pain	Q45.2
Colonic Constipation	B03.2
Comfort Alteration	Q45
Communication Impairment	M28
Community Coping Impairment	E52
Compromised Family Coping	E11.1
Confusion	D07.1
Contraception Risk	U59.3
Decisional Conflict	E12.2
Defensive Coping	E12.3
Delivery Risk	U60.3
Denial	E12.4
Diarrhea	B03.3
Disabled Family Coping	E11.2
Disuse Syndrome	N33.2
Diversional Activity Deficit	A01.3

(Continued)

TABLE 14.7. CLINICAL CARE CLASSIFICATION OF 182 NURSING DIAGNOSES (VERSION 2.0): LISTED ALPHABETICALLY BY CODE NUMBERS[a,b,c,d] **(CONTINUED)**

Dressing/Grooming Deficit	O36
Drug Abuse	N58.3
Dying Process	E10
Dysfunctional Grieving	E53.2
Endocrine Alteration	I22
Failure to Thrive	G17.1
Family Coping Impairment	E11
Family Process Alteration	M29
Fatigue	A01.4
Fear	P41
Fecal Impaction	B03.4
Feeding Deficit	O37
Fertility Risk	U59.1
Fluid Volume Alteration	F15
Fluid Volume Deficit	F15.1
Fluid Volume Deficit Risk	F15.2
Fluid Volume Excess	F15.3
Fluid Volume Excess Risk	F15.4
Functional Urinary Incontinence	T49.1
Gas Exchange Impairment	L26.3
Gastrointestinal Alteration	B04
Grieving	E53
Growth & Development Alteration	U61
Gustatory Alteration	Q44.2
Health Maintenance Alteration	G17
Health-Seeking Behavior Alteration	G18
Home Maintenance Alteration	G19
Hopelessness	P42.1
Hyperthermia	K25.2
Hypothermia	K25.3
Immunologic Alteration	I23
Individual Coping Impairment	E12
Infant Behavior Alteration	U61.2
Infant Feeding Pattern Impairment	J54
Infection Risk	K25.5
Infection Unspecified	K25.6
Infertility Risk	U59.2
Injury Risk	N33
Instrumental Activities of Daily Living (IADLs) Alteration	O38.2
Intracranial Adaptive Capacity Impairment	K25.7
Kinesthetic Alteration	Q44.3
Knowledge Deficit	D08
Knowledge Deficit of Diagnostic Test	D08.1
Knowledge Deficit of Dietary Regimen	D08.2
Knowledge Deficit of Disease Process	D08.3
Knowledge Deficit of Fluid Volume	D08.4
Knowledge Deficit of Medication Regimen	D08.5

(Continued)

TABLE 14.7. (CONTINUED)

Knowledge Deficit of Safety Precautions D08.6
Knowledge Deficit of Therapeutic Regimen D08.7

Labor Risk U60.2
Latex Allergy Response R46.5

Meaningfulness Alteration P42
Medication Risk H21
Memory Impairment D09.1
Musculoskeletal Alteration A02

Nausea B51
Newborn Behavior Alteration U61.1
Noncompliance G20
Noncompliance of Diagnostic Test G20.1
Noncompliance of Dietary Regimen G20.2
Noncompliance of Fluid Volume G20.3
Noncompliance of Medication Regimen G20.4
Noncompliance of Safety Precautions G20.5
Noncompliance of Therapeutic Regimen G20.6
Nutrition Alteration J24

Older Adult Behavior Alteration U61.6
Olfactory Alteration Q44.4
Oral Mucous Membranes Impairment R46.1

Parental Role Conflict M27.1
Parenting Alteration M27.2
Perceived Constipation B03.5
Perinatal Risk U60
Perioperative Injury Risk N57
Perioperative Positioning Injury N57.1
Peripheral Alteration R47
Personal Identity Disturbance P43.2
Physical Mobility Impairment A01.5
Physical Regulation Alteration K25
Poisoning Risk N33.3
Polypharmacy H21.1
Postpartum Risk U60.4
Post-trauma Response E13
Powerlessness P42.2
Pregnancy Risk U60.1
Protection Alteration I23.1

Rape Trauma Syndrome E13.1
Reflex Urinary Incontinence T49.2
Relocation Stress Syndrome M32.3
Renal Alteration T50
Reproductive Risk U59
Respiration Alteration L26
Role Performance Alteration M27

Self-Care Deficit O38
Self-Concept Alteration P43

(Continued)

TABLE 14.7. CLINICAL CARE CLASSIFICATION OF 182 NURSING DIAGNOSES (VERSION 2.0): LISTED ALPHABETICALLY BY CODE NUMBERS[a,b,c,d] (CONTINUED)

Self-Mutilation Risk	N34.2
Sensory Perceptual Alteration	Q44
Sexual Dysfunction	M27.3
Sexuality Patterns Alteration	M31
Situational Self-Esteem Disturbance	P43.4
Skin Integrity Alteration	R46
Skin Integrity Impairment	R46.2
Skin Integrity Impairment Risk	R46.3
Skin Incision	R46.4
Sleep Deprivation	A01.7
Sleep Pattern Disturbance	A01.6
Social Interaction Alteration	M32.1
Social Isolation	M32.2
Socialization Alteration	M32
Spiritual Distress	E14.1
Spiritual State Alteration	E14
Stress Urinary Incontinence	T49.3
Substance Abuse	N58
Suffocation Risk	N33.4
Suicide Risk	N34.1
Surgical Recovery Delay	N57.2
Swallowing Impairment	J24.5
Tactile Alteration	Q44.5
Thermoregulation Impairment	K25.4
Tissue Perfusion Alteration	S48
Tobacco Abuse	N58.1
Toileting Risk	O39
Total Urinary Incontinence	T49.4
Thought Processes Alteration	D09
Trauma Risk	N33.5
Unilateral Neglect	Q44.6
Unspecified Constipation	B03.6
Unspecified Pain	Q45.3
Urinary Elimination Alteration	T49
Urinary Retention	T49.6
Urge Urinary Incontinence	T49.5
Ventilatory Weaning Impairment	L56
Verbal Impairment	M28.1
Violence Risk	N34
Visual Alteration	Q44.7

[a]Adapted from NANDA (North American Nursing Diagnoses Association): *Taxonomy I Revised–1990.*
[b]Adapted with permission from NANDA *Nursing Diagnoses & Classification, 2003–2004.*
[c]Clinical Care Classification of Nursing Diagnoses (Version 2.0) includes 9 New Major Categories and 21 Subcategories. See Appendix Table A.2 for revisions from Home Health Care Classification (Version 1.0).
[d]The Clinical Care Classification System is copyrighted, placed in the Public Domain, and cannot be sold, but is available with written permission.

© **V. K. Saba–Revised 1992, 1994, 2002, 2004, 2006**

TABLE 14.8. CLINICAL CARE CLASSIFICATION OF 182 NURSING DIAGNOSES (VERSION 2.0): CODED WITH DEFINITIONS, THREE EXPECTED OUTCOMES, AND CLASSIFIED BY 21 CARE COMPONENTS[a,b,c,d]

A. – ACTIVITY COMPONENT:
Cluster of elements that involve the use of energy in carrying out musculoskeletal and bodily actions.
Activity Alteration – A01
Change in or modification of energy used by the body.
A01.0.1 Improve
A01.0.2 Stabilize
A01.0.3 Deteriorate
  Activity Intolerance – A01.1
  Incapacity to carry out physiological or psychological daily activities.
  A01.1.1. Improve
  A01.1.2. Stabilize
  A01.1.3. Deteriorate
  Activity Intolerance Risk – A01.2
  Increased chance of an incapacity to carry out physiological or psychological daily activities.
  A01.2.1. Improve
  A01.2.2. Stabilize
  A01.2.3. Deteriorate
  Diversional Activity Deficit – A01.3
  Lack of interest or engagement in leisure activities.
  A01.3.1. Improve
  A01.3.2. Stabilize
  A01.3.3. Deteriorate
  Fatigue – A01.4
  Exhaustion that interferes with physical and mental activities.
  A01.4.1. Improve
  A01.4.2. Stabilize
  A01.4.3. Deteriorate
  Physical Mobility Impairment – A01.5
  Diminished ability to perform independent movement.
  A01.5.1. Improve
  A01.5.2. Stabilize
  A01.5.3. Deteriorate
  Sleep Pattern Disturbance – A01.6
  Imbalance in the normal sleep/wake cycle.
  A01.6.1. Improve
  A01.6.2. Stabilize
  A01.6.3. Deteriorate
  Sleep Deprivation – A01.7
  Lack of the normal sleep/wake cycle.
  A01.7.1. Improve
  A01.7.2. Stabilize
  A01.7.3. Deteriorate
Musculoskeletal Alteration – A02
Change in or modification of the muscles, bones, or support structures.
A02.0.1. Improve
A02.0.2. Stabilize
A02.0.3. Deteriorate

B. – BOWEL/GASTRIC COMPONENT:
Cluster of elements that involve the gastrointestinal system.

Bowel Elimination Alteration – B03
Change in or modification of the gastrointestinal system.
B03.0.1. Improve
B03.0.2. Stabilize
B03.0.3. Deteriorate
  Bowel Incontinence – B03.1
  Involuntary defecation.
  B03.1.1. Improve
  B03.1.2. Stabilize
  B03.1.3. Deteriorate
  Colonic Constipation – B03.2
  Infrequent or difficult passage of hard, dry feces.
  B03.2.1. Improve
  B03.2.2. Stabilize
  B03.2.3. Deteriorate
  Diarrhea – B03.3
  Abnormal frequency and fluidity of feces.
  B03.2.1. Improve
  B03.2.2. Stabilize
  B03.2.3. Deteriorate
  Fecal Impaction – B03.4
  Feces wedged in intestines.
  B03.4.1. Improve
  B03.4.2. Stabilize
  B03.4.3. Deteriorate
  Perceived Constipation – B03.5
  Belief and treatment of infrequent or difficult passage of feces without cause.
  B03.5.1. Improve
  B03.5.2. Stabilize
  B03.5.3. Deteriorate
  Unspecified Constipation – B03.6
  Other forms of abnormal feces or difficult passage of feces.
  B03.6.1. Improve
  B03.6.2. Stabilize
  B03.6.3. Deteriorate
Gastrointestinal Alteration – B04
Change in or modification of the stomach or intestines.
B04.0.1. Improve
B04.0.2. Stabilize
B04.0.3. Deteriorate
Nausea – B51
Distaste for food/fluids and an urge to vomit.
B51.0.1. Improve
B51.0.2. Stabilize
B51.0.3. Deteriorate

C. – CARDIAC COMPONENT:
Cluster of elements that involve the heart and blood vessels.
Cardiac Output Alteration – C05
Change in or modification of the pumping action of the heart.
C05.0.1. Improve
C05.0.2. Stabilize
C05.0.3. Deteriorate

(Continued)

TABLE 14.8. CLINICAL CARE CLASSIFICATION OF 182 NURSING DIAGNOSES (VERSION 2.0): CODED WITH DEFINITIONS, THREE EXPECTED OUTCOMES, AND CLASSIFIED BY 21 CARE COMPONENTS[a,b,c,d] (CONTINUED)

Cardiovascular Alteration – C06
Change in or modification of the heart or blood vessels.
C06.0.1. Improve
C06.0.2. Stabilize
C06.0.3. Deteriorate
  Blood Pressure Alteration – C06.1
  Change in or modification of the systolic or diastolic pressure.
  C06.1.1. Improve
  C06.1.2. Stabilize
  C06.1.3. Deteriorate

D. – COGNITIVE COMPONENT:
Cluster of elements involving the mental and cerebral processes.
Cerebral Alteration – D07
Change in or modification of thought processes or mentation.
D07.0.1. Improve
D07.0.2. Stabilize
D07.0.3. Deteriorate
  Confusion – D07.1
  State of being disoriented (mixed-up).
  D07.1.1. Improve
  D07.1.2. Stabilize
  D07.1.3. Deteriorate
Knowledge Deficit – D08
Lack of information, understanding, or comprehension.
D08.0.1. Improve
D08.0.2. Stabilize
D08.0.3. Deteriorate
  Knowledge Deficit of Diagnostic Test – D08.1
  Lack of information on test(s) to identify disease or assess health condition.
  D08.1.1. Improve
  D08.1.2. Stabilize
  D08.1.3. Deteriorate
  Knowledge Deficit Dietary Regimen – D08.2
  Lack of information on the prescribed food or fluid intake.
  D08.2.1. Improve
  D08.2.2. Stabilize
  D08.2.3. Deteriorate
  Knowledge Deficit of Disease Process – D08.3
  Lack of information on the morbidity, course, or treatment of the health condition.
  D08.3.1. Improve
  D08.3.2. Stabilize
  D08.3.3. Deteriorate
  Knowledge Deficit of Fluid Volume – D08.4
  Lack of information on fluid volume intake requirements.
  D08.4.1. Improve
  D08.4.2. Stabilize
  D08.4.3. Deteriorate

Knowledge Deficit of Medication Regimen – D08.5
Lack of information on prescribed regulated course of medicinal substances.
D08.5.1. Improve
D08.5.2. Stabilize
D08.5.3. Deteriorate
Knowledge Deficit of Safety Precautions – D08.6
Lack of information on measures to prevent injury, danger, or loss.
D08.6.1. Improve
D08.6.2. Stabilize
D08.6.3. Deteriorate
Knowledge Deficit of Therapeutic Regimen – D08.7
Lack of information on regulated course of treating disease.
D08.7.1. Improve
D08.7.2. Stabilize
D08.7.3. Deteriorate
Thought Process Alteration – D09
Change in or modification of cognitive processes.
D09.0.1. Improve
D09.0.2. Stabilize
D09.0.3. Deteriorate
  Memory Impairment – D09.1
  Diminished or inability to recall past events.
  D09.1.1. Improve
  D09.1.2. Stabilize
  D09.1.3. Deteriorate

E. – COPING COMPONENT:
Cluster of elements that involve the ability to deal with responsibilities, problems, or difficulties.
Dying Process – E10
Physical and behavioral responses associated with death.
E10.0.1. Improve
E10.0.2. Stabilize
E10.0.3. Deteriorate
Community Coping Impairment – E52
Inadequate community response to problems or difficulties.
E52.0.1. Improve
E52.0.2. Stabilize
E52.0.3. Deteriorate
Family Coping Impairment – E11
Inadequate family response to problems or difficulties.
E11.0.1. Improve
E11.0.2. Stabilize
E11.0.3. Deteriorate
  Compromised Family Coping – E11.1
  Inability of family to function optimally.
  E11.1.1. Improve
  E11.1.2. Stabilize
  E11.1.3. Deteriorate

(Continued)

TABLE 14.8. (CONTINUED)

Disabled Family Coping – E11.2
Dysfunctional ability of family to function.
E11.2.1. Improve
E11.2.2. Stabilize
E11.2.3. Deteriorate

Individual Coping Impairment – E12
Inadequate personal response to problems or difficulties.
E12.0.1. Improve
E12.0.2. Stabilize
E12.0.3. Deteriorate

  Adjustment Impairment – E12.1
  Inadequate adjustment to condition or change in health status.
  E12.1.1. Improve
  E12.1.2. Stabilize
  E12.1.3. Deteriorate

  Decisional Conflict – E12.2
  Struggle related to determining a course of action.
  E12.2.1. Improve
  E12.2.2. Stabilize
  E12.2.3. Deteriorate

  Defensive Coping – E12.3
  Self-protective strategies to guard against threats to self.
  E12.3.1. Improve
  E12.3.2. Stabilize
  E12.3.3. Deteriorate

  Denial – E12.4
  Attempt to reduce anxiety by refusal to accept thoughts, feelings, or facts.
  E12.4.1. Improve
  E12.4.2. Stabilize
  E12.4.3. Deteriorate

Post-trauma Response – E13
Sustained behavior related to a traumatic event.
E13.0.1. Improve
E13.0.2. Stabilize
E13.0.3. Deteriorate

  Rape Trauma Syndrome – E13.1
  Group of symptoms related to a forced sexual act.
  E13.1.1. Improve
  E13.1.2. Stabilize
  E13.1.3. Deteriorate

Spiritual State Alteration – E14
Change in or modification of the spirit or soul.
E14.0.1. Improve
E14.0.2. Stabilize
E14.0.3. Deteriorate

  Spiritual Distress – E14.1
  Anguish related to the spirit or soul.
  E14.1.1. Improve
  E14.1.2. Stabilize
  E14.1.3. Deteriorate

Grieving – E53
Feeling of great sorrow.
E53.0.1. Improve
E53.0.2. Stabilize
E43.0.3. Deteriorate

  Anticipatory Grieving E53.1
  Feeling great sorrow before the event or loss.
  E53.1.1. Improve
  E.1.2. Stabilize
  E53.1.3. Deteriorate

  Dysfunctional Grieving – E53.2
  Prolonged feeling of great sorrow.
  E53.2.1. Improve
  E53.2.2. Stabilize
  E53.2.3. Deteriorate

F . – FLUID VOLUME COMPONENT:
Cluster of elements that involve liquid consumption.

Fluid Volume Alteration – F15
Change in or modification of bodily fluid
F15.0.1. Improve
F15.0.2. Stabilize
F15.0.3. Deteriorate

  Fluid Volume Deficit – F15.1
  Dehydration.
  F15.1.1. Improve
  F15.1.2. Stabilize
  F15.1.3. Deteriorate

  Fluid Volume Deficit Risk – F15.2
  Increased chance of dehydration.
  F15.2.1. Improve
  F15.2.2. Stabilize
  F15.2.3. Deteriorate

  Fluid Volume Excess – F15.3
  Fluid retention, overload, or edema.
  F15.3.1. Improve
  F15.3.2. Stabilize
  F15.3.3. Deteriorate

  Fluid Volume Excess Risk – F15.4
  Increased chance of fluid retention, overload, or edema.
  F15.4.1. Improve
  F15.4.2. Stabilize
  F15.4.3. Deteriorate

G. – HEALTH BEHAVIOR COMPONENT:
Cluster of elements that involve actions to sustain, maintain, or regain health.

Health Maintenance Alteration – G17
Change in or modification of ability to manage health-related needs.
G17.0.1. Improve
G17.0.2. Stabilize
G17.0.3. Deteriorate

(Continued)

TABLE 14.8. CLINICAL CARE CLASSIFICATION OF 182 NURSING DIAGNOSES (VERSION 2.0): CODED WITH DEFINITIONS, THREE EXPECTED OUTCOMES, AND CLASSIFIED BY 21 CARE COMPONENTS[a,b,c,d] (CONTINUED)

Failure to Thrive – G17.1
Inability to grow and develop normally.
G17.1.1. Improve
G17.1.2. Stabilize
G17.1.3. Deteriorate

Health-Seeking Behavior Alteration – G18
Change in or modification of actions needed to improve health state.
G18.0.1. Improve
G18.0.2. Stabilize
G18.0.3. Deteriorate

Home Maintenance Alteration – G19
Inability to sustain a safe, healthy environment.
G19.0.1. Improve
G19.0.2. Stabilize
G19.0.3. Deteriorate

Noncompliance – G20
Failure to follow therapeutic recommendations.
G20.0.1. Improve
G20.0.2. Stabilize
G20.0.3. Deteriorate

  Noncompliance of Diagnostic Test – G20.1
  Failure to follow therapeutic recommendations on tests to identify disease or assess health condition.
  G20.1.1. Improve
  G20.1.2. Stabilize
  G20.1.3. Deteriorate

  Noncompliance of Dietary Regimen – G20.2
  Failure to follow the prescribed food or fluid intake.
  G20.2.1. Improve
  G20.2.2. Stabilize
  G20.2.3. Deteriorate

  Noncompliance of Fluid Volume – G20.3
  Failure to follow fluid volume intake requirements.
  G20.3.1. Improve
  G20.3.2. Stabilize
  G20.3.3. Deteriorate

  Noncompliance of Medication Regimen – G20.4
  Failure to follow prescribed regulated course of medicinal substances.
  G20.4.1. Improve
  G20.4.2. Stabilize
  G20.4.3. Deteriorate

  Noncompliance of Safety Precautions – G20.5
  Failure to follow measures to prevent injury, danger, or loss.
  G20.5.1. Improve
  G20.5.2. Stabilize
  G20.5.3. Deteriorate

  Noncompliance of Therapeutic Regimen – G20.6
  Failure to follow regulated course of treating disease or health condition.
  G20.6.1. Improve
  G20.6.2. Stabilize
  G20.6.3. Deteriorate

H. – MEDICATION COMPONENT:
Cluster of elements that involve medicinal substances.
Medication Risk – H21
Increased chance of negative response to medicinal substances.
H21.0.1. Improve
H21.0.2. Stabilize
H21.0.3. Deteriorate

  Polypharmacy – H21.1
  Use of two or more drugs together.
  H21.1.1. Improve
  H21.1.2. Stabilize
  H21.1.3. Deteriorate

I. – METABOLIC COMPONENT:
Cluster of elements that involve the endocrine and immunological processes.
Endocrine Alteration – I22
Change in or modification of internal secretions or hormones.
I22.0.1. Improve
I22.0.2. Stabilize
I22.0.3. Deteriorate

Immunologic Alteration – I23
Change in or modification of the immune systems.
I23.0.1. Improve
I23.0.2. Stabilize
I23.0.3. Deteriorate

  Protection Alteration – I23.1
  Change in or modification of the ability to guard against internal or external threats to the body.
  I23.1.1. Improve
  I23.1.2. Stabilize
  I23.1.3. Deteriorate

J. – NUTRITIONAL COMPONENT:
Cluster of elements that involve the intake of food and nutrients.
Nutrition Alteration – J24
Change in or modification of food and nutrients.
J24.0.1. Improve
J24.0.2. Stabilize
J24.0.3. Deteriorate

  Body Nutrition Deficit – J24.1
  Less than adequate intake or absorption of food or nutrients.
  J24.1.1. Improve
  J24.1.2. Stabilize
  J24.1.3. Deteriorate

  Body Nutrition Deficit Risk – J24.2
  Increased chance of less than adequate intake or absorption of food or nutrients.
  J24.2.1. Improve
  J24.2.2. Stabilize
  J24.2.3. Deteriorate

(Continued)

TABLE 14.8. (CONTINUED)

Body Nutrition Excess – J24.3
More than adequate intake or absorption of food or nutrients.
J24.3.1. Improve
J24.3.2. Stabilize
J24.3.3. Deteriorate
Body Nutrition Excess Risk – J24.4
Increased chance of more than adequate intake or absorption of food or nutrients.
J24.4.1. Improve
J24.4.2. Stabilize
J24.4.3. Deteriorate
Swallowing Impairment – J24.5
Inability to move food from mouth to stomach.
J24.5.1. Improve
J24.5.2. Stabilize
J24.5.3. Deteriorate
Infant Feeding Pattern Impairment – J54
Imbalance in the normal feeding habits of an infant.
J54.0.1. Improve
J54.0.2. Stabilize
J54.0.3. Deteriorate
Breast-feeding Impairment – J55
Diminished ability to nourish infant at the breast.
J55.0.1. Improve
J55.0.2. Stabilize
J55.0.3. Deteriorate

K. – PHYSICAL REGULATION COMPONENT:
Cluster of elements that involve bodily processes.
Physical Regulation Alteration – K25
Change in or modification of somatic control.
K25.0.1. Improve
K25.0.2. Stabilize
K25.0.3. Deteriorate
Autonomic Dysreflexia – K25.1
Life-threatening inhibited sympathetic response to noxious stimuli in a person with a spinal cord injury at T7 or above.
K25.1.1. Improve
K25.1.2. Stabilize
K25.1.3. Deteriorate
Hyperthermia – K25.2
Abnormal high body temperature.
K25.2.1. Improve
K25.2.2. Stabilize
K25.2.3. Deteriorate
Hypothermia – K25.3
Abnormal low body temperature.
K25.3.1. Improve
K25.3.2. Stabilize
K25.3.3. Deteriorate

Thermoregulation Impairment – K25.4
Fluctuation of temperature between hypothermia and hyperthermia.
K25.4.1. Improve
K25.4.2. Stabilize
K25.4.3. Deteriorate
Infection Risk – K25.5
Increased chance of contamination with disease-producing germs.
K25.5.1. Improve
K25.5.2. Stabilize
K25.5.3. Deteriorate
Infection Unspecified – K25.6
Unknown contamination with disease-producing germs.
K25.6.1. Improve
K25.6.2. Stabilize
K25.6.3. Deteriorate
Intracranial Adaptive Capacity Impairment – K25.7
Intracranial fluid volumes are compromised.
K25.7.1. Improve
K25.7.2. Stabilize
K25.7.3. Deteriorate

L. – RESPIRATORY COMPONENT:
Cluster of element that involve breathing and the pulmonary system.
Respiration Alteration – L26
Change in or modification of carrying out responsibilities.
L26.0.1. Improve
L26.0.2. Stabilize
L26.0.3. Deteriorate
Airway Clearance Impairment – L26.1
Inability to clear secretions/obstructions in airway.
L26.1.1. Improve
L26.1.2. Stabilize
L26.1.3. Deteriorate
Breathing Pattern Impairment – L26.2
Inadequate inhalation or exhalation.
L26.2.1. Improve
L26.2.2. Stabilize
L26.2.3. Deteriorate
Gas Exchange Impairment – L26.3
Imbalance of oxygen and carbon dioxide transfer between lung and vascular system.
L26.3.1. Improve
L26.3.2. Stabilize
L26.3.3. Deteriorate
Ventilatory Weaning Impairment – L56
Inability to tolerate decreased levels of ventilator support.
L56.0.1. Improve
L56.0.2. Stabilize
L56.0.3. Deteriorate

(Continued)

TABLE 14.8. CLINICAL CARE CLASSIFICATION OF 182 NURSING DIAGNOSES (VERSION 2.0): CODED WITH DEFINITIONS, THREE EXPECTED OUTCOMES, AND CLASSIFIED BY 21 CARE COMPONENTS[a,b,c,d] (CONTINUED)

M. – ROLE RELATIONSHIP COMPONENT:
Cluster of elements involving interpersonal work, social, family, and sexual interactions.
Role Performance Alteration – M27
Change in or modification of carrying out responsibilities.
M.27.0.1. Improve
M.27.0.2. Stabilize
M.27.0.3. Deteriorate
   Parental Role Conflict – M27.1
   Struggle with parental position and responsibilities.
   M.27.1.1. Improve
   M.27.1.2. Stabilize
   M.27.1.3. Deteriorate
   Parenting Alteration – M27.2
   Change in or modification of nurturing figure's ability to promote growth.
   M.27.2.1. Improve
   M.27.2.2. Stabilize
   M.27.2.3. Deteriorate
   Sexual Dysfunction – M27.3
   Deleterious change in sex response.
   M.27.3.1. Improve
   M.27.3.2. Stabilize
   M.27.3.3. Deteriorate
   Caregiver Role Strain – M27.4
   Excessive tension of one who gives physical or emotional care and support to another person or patient.
   M.27.4.1. Improve
   M.27.4.2. Stabilize
   M.27.4.3. Deteriorate
Communication Impairment – M28
Diminished ability to exchange thoughts, opinions, or information.
M.28.0.1. Improve
M.28.0.2. Stabilize
M.28.0.3. Deteriorate
   Verbal Impairment –M28.1
   Diminished ability to exchange thoughts, opinions, or information through speech.
   M.28.1.1. Improve
   M.28.1.2. Stabilize
   M.28.1.3. Deteriorate
Family Processes Alteration – M29
Change in or modification of usual functioning of a related group.
M.29.0.1. Improve
M.29.0.2. Stabilize
M.29.0.3. Deteriorate
Sexuality Patterns Alteration – M31
Change in or modification of person's sexual response.
M.31.0.1. Improve
M.31.0.2. Stabilize
M.31.0.3. Deteriorate

Socialization Alteration – M32
Change in or modification of personal identity.
M.32.0.1. Improve
M.32.0.2. Stabilize
M.32.0.3. Deteriorate
   Social Interaction Alteration – M32.1
   Change in or modification of inadequate quantity or quality of personal relations.
   M.32.1.1. Improve
   M.32.1.2. Stabilize
   M.32.1.3. Deteriorate
   Social Isolation – M32.2
   State of aloneness; lack of interaction with others.
   M.32.2.1. Improve
   M.32.2.2. Stabilize
   M.32.2.3. Deteriorate
   Relocation Stress Syndrome – M32.3
   Excessive tension from moving to a new location.
   M.32.3.1. Improve
   M.32.3.2. Stabilize
   M.32.3.3. Deteriorate

N. – SAFETY COMPONENT:
Cluster of elements that involve prevention of injury, danger, loss, or abuse.
Injury Risk – N33
Increased chance of danger or loss.
N.33.0.1. Improve
N.33.0.2. Stabilize
N.33.0.3. Deteriorate
   Aspiration Risk – N33.1
   Increased chance of material into trachea-bronchial passages.
   N33.1.1. Improve
   N.33.1.2. Stabilize
   N.33.1.3. Deteriorate
   Disuse Syndrome – N33.2
   Group of symptoms related to effects of immobility.
   N.33.2.1. Improve
   N.33.2.2. Stabilize
   N.33.2.3. Deteriorate
   Poisoning Risk – N33.3
   Exposure to or ingestion of dangerous products.
   N.33.3.1. Improve
   N.33.3.2. Stabilize
   N.33.3.3. Deteriorate
   Suffocation Risk – N33.4
   Increased chance of inadequate air for breathing.
   N.33.4.1. Improve
   N.33.4.2. Stabilize
   N.33.4.3. Deteriorate

(Continued)

TABLE 14.8. (CONTINUED)

Trauma Risk – N33.5
Increased chance of accidental tissue processes.
N33.5.1. Improve
N33.5.2. Stabilize
N33.5.3. Deteriorate
Violence Risk – N34
Increased chance of harming self or others.
N34.0.1. Improve
N34.0.2. Stabilize
N34.0.3. Deteriorate
Suicide Risk – N34.1
Increased chance of taking one's life intentionally.
N34.1.1. Improve
N34.1.2. Stabilize
N34.1.3. Deteriorate
Self-Mutilation Risk – N34.2
Increased chance of destroying a limb or essential part of the body.
N34.2.1. Improve
N34.2.2. Stabilize
N34.2.3. Deteriorate
Perioperative Injury Risk – N57
Increased chance of injury during the operative processes.
N57.0.1. Improve
N57.0.2. Stabilize
N57.0.3. Deteriorate
Perioperative Positioning Injury – N57.1
Damages from operative process positioning.
N57.1.1. Improve
N57.1.2. Stabilize
N57.1.3. Deteriorate
Surgical Recovery Delay – N57.2
Slow or delayed recovery from a surgical procedure.
N57.2.1. Improve
N57.2.2. Stabilize
N57.2.3. Deteriorate
Substance Abuse – N58
Excessive use of harmful bodily materials.
N58.0.1. Improve
N58.0.2. Stabilize
N58.0.3. Deteriorate
Tobacco Abuse – N58.1
Excessive use of tobacco products.
N58.1.1. Improve
N58.1.2. Stabilize
N58.1.3. Deteriorate
Alcohol Abuse – N58.2
Excessive use of distilled liquors.
N58.2.1. Improve
N58.2.2. Stabilize
N58.2.3. Deteriorate
Drug Abuse – N58.3
Excessive use of habit-forming medications.
N58.3.1. Improve
N58.3.2. Stabilize
N58.3.3. Deteriorate

O. – SELF-CARE COMPONENT:
Cluster of elements that involve the ability to carry out activities to maintain oneself.
Bathing/Hygiene Deficit – O35
Impaired ability to cleanse oneself.
O35.0.1. Improve
O35.0.2. Stabilize
O35.0.3. Deteriorate
Dressing/Grooming Deficit - O36
Inability to clothe and groom oneself.
O36.0.1. Improve
O36.0.2. Stabilize
O36.0.3. Deteriorate
Feeding Deficit – O37
Impaired ability to feed oneself.
O37.0.1. Improve
O37.0.2. Stabilize
O37.0.3. Deteriorate
Self-Care Deficit – O38
Impaired ability to maintain oneself.
O38.0.1. Improve
O38.0.2. Stabilize
O38.0.3. Deteriorate
Activities of Daily Living (ADLs) Alteration – O38.1
Change in or modification of ability to maintain oneself.
O38.1.1. Improve
O38.1.2. Stabilize
O38.1.3. Deteriorate
Instrumental Activities of Daily Living (IADLs) Alteration – O38.2
Change in or modification of more complex activities than than those needed to maintain oneself.
O38.2.1. Improve
O38.2.2. Stabilize
O38.2.3. Deteriorate
Toileting Deficit – O39
Impaired ability to urinate or defecate for oneself.
O39.0.1. Improve
O39.0.2. Stabilize
O39.0.3. Deteriorate

P. – SELF-CONCEPT COMPONENT:
Cluster of elements that involve an individual's mental image of oneself.
Anxiety – P40
Feeling of distress or apprehension whose source is unknown.
P40.0.1. Improve
P40.0.2. Stabilize
P40.0.3. Deteriorate
Fear – P41
Feeling of dread or distress whose cause can be identified.
P41.0.1. Improve
P41.0.2. Stabilize
P41.0.3. Deteriorate

(Continued)

TABLE 14.8. CLINICAL CARE CLASSIFICATION OF 182 NURSING DIAGNOSES (VERSION 2.0): CODED WITH DEFINITIONS, THREE EXPECTED OUTCOMES, AND CLASSIFIED BY 21 CARE COMPONENTS[a,b,c,d] (CONTINUED)

Meaningfulness Alteration – P42
Change in or modification of the ability to see the significance, purpose, or value in something.
P42.0.1. Improve
P42.0.2. Stabilize
P42.0.3. Deteriorate
   Hopelessness – P42.1
   Feeling of despair or futility and passive involvement.
   P42.1.1. Improve
   P42.1.2. Stabilize
   P42.1.3. Deteriorate
   Powerlessness – P42.2
   Feeling of helplessness, or inability to act.
   P42.2.1. Improve
   P42.2.2. Stabilize
   P42.2.3. Deteriorate
Self-Concept Alteration – P43
Change in or modification of ability to maintain one's image of self.
P43.0.1. Improve
P43.0.2. Stabilize
P43.0.3. Deteriorate
   Body Image Disturbance – P43.1
   Imbalance in the perception of the way one's body looks.
   P43.1.1. Improve
   P43.1.2. Stabilize
   P43.1.3. Deteriorate
   Personal Identity Disturbance – P43.2
   Imbalance in the ability to distinguish between the self and the non-self.
   P43.2.1. Improve
   P43.2.2. Stabilize
   P43.2.3. Deteriorate
   Chronic Low Self-Esteem Disturbance – P43.3
   Persistent negative evaluation of oneself.
   P43.3.1. Improve
   P43.3.2. Stabilize
   P43.3.3. Deteriorate
   Situational Self-Esteem Disturbance – P43.4
   Negative evaluation of oneself in response to a loss or change.
   P43.4.1. Improve
   P43.4.2. Stabilize
   P43.4.3. Deteriorate

Q. – SENSORY COMPONENT:
Cluster of elements that involve the senses, including pain.
Sensory Perceptual Alteration – Q44
Change in or modification of the response to stimuli.
Q44.0.1. Improve
Q44.0.2. Stabilize
Q44.0.3. Deteriorate
   Auditory Alteration – Q44.1
   Change in or modification of diminished ability to hear.

Q44.1.1. Improve
Q44.1.2. Stabilize
Q44.1.3. Deteriorate
Gustatory Alteration – Q44.2
Change in or modification of diminished ability to taste.
Q44.2.1. Improve
Q44.2.2. Stabilize
Q44.2.3. Deteriorate
Kinesthetic Alteration – Q44.3
Change in or modification of diminished ability to move.
Q44.3.1. Improve
Q44.3.2. Stabilize
Q44.3.3. Deteriorate
Olfactory Alteration – Q44.4
Change in or modification of diminished ability to smell.
Q44.4.1. Improve
Q44.4.2. Stabilize
Q44.4.3. Deteriorate
Tactile Alteration – Q44.5
Change in or modification of diminished ability to feel.
Q44.5.1. Improve
Q44.5.2. Stabilize
Q44.5.3. Deteriorate
Unilateral Neglect – Q44.6
Lack of awareness of one side of the body.
Q44.6.1. Improve
Q44.6.2. Stabilize
Q44.6.3. Deteriorate
Visual Alteration – Q44.7
Change in or modification of diminished ability to see.
Q44.7.1. Improve
Q44.7.2. Stabilize
Q44.7.3. Deteriorate
Comfort Alteration – Q45
Change in or modification of sensation that is distressing.
Q45.0.1. Improve
Q45.0.2. Stabilize
Q45.0.3. Deteriorate
   Acute Pain – Q45.1
   Physical suffering or distress to hurt.
   Q45.1.1. Improve
   Q45.1.2. Stabilize
   Q45.1.3. Deteriorate
   Chronic Pain – Q45.2
   Pain that continues for longer than expected.
   Q45.2.1. Improve
   Q45.2.2. Stabilize
   Q45.2.3. Deteriorate
   Unspecified Pain – Q45.3
   Pain that is difficult to pinpoint.
   Q45.3.1. Improve
   Q45.3.2. Stabilize
   Q45.3.3. Deteriorate

(Continued)

TABLE 14.8. (CONTINUED)

R. – SKIN INTEGRITY COMPONENT:
Cluster of elements that involve the mucous membrane, corneal, integumentary, or subcutaneous structures of the body.
Skin Integrity Alteration – R46
Change in or modification of skin conditions.
R46.0.1. Improve
R46.0.2. Stabilize
R46.0.3. Deteriorate
  Oral Mucous Membranes Impairment – R46.1
  Diminished ability to maintain the tissues of the oral cavity.
  R46.1.1. Improve
  R46.1.2. Stabilize
  R46.1.3. Deteriorate
  Skin Integrity Impairment – R46.2
  Decreased ability to maintain the integument.
  R46.2.1. Improve
  R46.2.2. Stabilize
  R46.2.3. Deteriorate
  Skin Integrity Impairment Risk – R46.3
  Increased chance of skin breakdown.
  R46.3.1. Improve
  R46.3.2. Stabilize
  R46.3.3. Deteriorate
  Skin Incision – R46.4
  Cutting of the integument.
  R46.4.1. Improve
  R46.4.2. Stabilize
  R46.4.3. Deteriorate
  Latex Allergy Response – R46.5
  Pathological reaction to latex products.
  R46.5.1. Improve
  R46.5.2. Stabilize
  R46.5.3. Deteriorate
Peripheral Alteration – R47
Change in or modification of vascularization of the extremities.
R47.0.1. Improve
R47.0.2. Stabilize
R47.0.3. Deteriorate

S. – TISSUE PERFUSION COMPONENT:
Cluster of elements that involve the oxygenation of tissues, including the circulatory and neurovascular systems.
Tissue Perfusion Alteration – S48
Change in or modification of the oxygenation of tissues.
S48.0.1. Improve
S48.0.2. Stabilize
S48.0.3. Deteriorate

T. – URINARY ELIMINATION COMPONENT:
Cluster of elements that involve the genitourinary systems.
Urinary Elimination Alteration – T49
Change in or modification of excretion of the waste matter of the kidneys.

T49.0.1. Improve
T49.0.2. Stabilize
T49.0.3. Deteriorate
  Functional Urinary Incontinence – T49.1
  Involuntary, unpredictable passage of urine.
  T49.1.1. Improve
  T49.1.2. Stabilize
  T49.1.3. Deteriorate
  Reflex Urinary Incontinence – T49.2
  Involuntary passage of urine occurring at predictable intervals.
  T49.2.1. Improve
  T49.2.2. Stabilize
  T49.2.3. Deteriorate
  Stress Urinary Incontinence – T49.3
  Loss of urine occurring with increased abdominal pressure.
  T49.3.1. Improve
  T49.3.2. Stabilize
  T49.3.3. Deteriorate
  Total Urinary Incontinence – T49.4
  Continuous and unpredictable loss of urine.
  T49.4.1. Improve
  T49.4.2. Stabilize
  T49.4.3. Deteriorate
  Urge Urinary Incontinence – T49.5
  Involuntary passage of urine following a sense of urgency to void.
  T49.5.1. Improve
  T49.5.2. Stabilize
  T49.5.3. Deteriorate
  Urinary Retention – T49.6
  Incomplete emptying of the bladder.
  T49.6.1. Improve
  T49.6.2. Stabilize
  T49.6.3. Deteriorate
Renal Alteration – T50
Change in or modification of the kidney function.
T50.0.1. Improve
T50.0.2. Stabilize
T50.0.3. Deteriorate

U. – LIFE CYCLE COMPONENT
Cluster of elements that involve the life span of individuals.
Reproductive Risk – U59
Increased chance of harm in the process of replicating or giving rise to an offspring/child.
U59.0.1. Improve
U59.0.2. Stabilize
U59.0.3. Deteriorate
  Fertility Risk – U59.1
  Increased chance of conception to develop an offspring/child.
  U59.1.1. Improve
  U59.1.2. Stabilize
  U59.1.3. Deteriorate

(Continued)

TABLE 14.8. CLINICAL CARE CLASSIFICATION OF 182 NURSING DIAGNOSES (VERSION 2.0): CODED WITH DEFINITIONS, THREE EXPECTED OUTCOMES, AND CLASSIFIED BY 21 CARE COMPONENTS[a,b,c,d] (CONTINUED)

Infertility Risk – U59.2
Increased chance of harm on preventing the development of an offspring/child.
U59.2.1. Improve
U59.2.2. Stabilize
U59.2.3. Deteriorate
Contraception Risk – U59.3
Increased chance of harm preventing the conception of an offspring/child.
U59.3.1. Improve
U59.3.2. Stabilize
U59.3.3. Deteriorate
Perinatal Risk – U60
Increased chance of harm before, during, and immediately after the creation of an offspring/child.
U60.1.1. Improve
U60.1.2. Stabilize
U60.1.3. Deteriorate
Pregnancy Risk – U60.1
Increased chance of harm during the gestational period of the formation of an offspring/child.
U60.1.1. Improve
U60.1.2. Stabilize
U60.1.3. Deteriorate
Labor Risk – U60.2
Increased chance of harm during the period supporting the bringing forth of an offspring/child.
U60.2.1. Improve
U60.2.2. Stabilize
U60.2.3. Deteriorate
Delivery Risk – U60.3
Increased chance of harm during the period supporting the expulsion of an offspring/child.
U60.3.1. Improve
U60.3.2. Stabilize
U60.3.3. Deteriorate
Postpartum Risk – U60.4
Increased chance of harm during the time period immediately following the delivery of an offspring/child.
U60.4.1. Improve
U60.4.2. Stabilize
U60.4.3. Deteriorate
Growth & Development Alteration – U61
Change in or modification of the norms for an individual's age.
U61.0.1. Improve
U61.0.2. Stabilize
U61.0.3. Deteriorate

Newborn Behavior Alteration (first 30 days) – U61.1
Change in or modification of normal standards of performing developmental skills and behavior of a typical newborn the first 30 days of life.
U61.1.1. Improve
U61.1.2. Stabilize
U61.1.3. Deteriorate
Infant Behavior Alteration (31 days through 11 months) – U61.2
Change in or modification of normal standards of performing developmental skills and behavior of a typical infant from 31 days through 11 months of age.
U61.2.1. Improve
U61.2.2. Stabilize
U61.2.3. Deteriorate
Child Behavior Alteration (1 year through 11 years) – U61.3
Change in or modification of normal standards of performing developmental skills and behavior of a typical child from 1 year through 11 years of age.
U61.3.1. Improve
U61.3.2. Stabilize
U61.3.3. Deteriorate
Adolescent Behavior Alteration (12 years through 20 years) – U61.4
Change in or modification of normal standards of performing developmental skills and behavior of a typical adolescent from 12 years through 20 years of age.
U61.4.1. Improve
U61.4.2. Stabilize
U61.4.3. Deteriorate
Adult Behavior Alteration (21 years through 64 years) – U61.5
Change in or modification of normal standards of performing developmental skills and behavior of a typical adult from 21 years through 64 years of age.
U61.5.1. Improve
U61.5.2. Stabilize
U61.5.3. Deteriorate
Older Adult Behavior Alteration (64 years & older) – U61.6
Change in or modification of normal standards of performing developmental skills and behavior of a typical older adult from 65 years of age and over.
U61.6.1. Improve
U61.6.2. Stabilize
U61.6.3. Deteriorate

[a]Adapted from NANDA (North American Nursing Diagnoses Association): *Taxonomy I: Revised–1990.*
[b]Adapted with permission from NANDA *Nursing Diagnoses & Classification, 2003–2004.*
[c]Clinical Care Classification of Nursing Diagnoses (Version 2.0) includes 9 New Major Categories and 21 Subcategories. See Appendix Table A.2 for revisions from Home Health Care Classification (Version 1.0).
[d]The Clinical Care Classification System is copyrighted, placed in the Public Domain, and cannot be sold, but is available with written permission.

© V. K. Saba—Revised 1992, 1994, 2002, 2004, 2006

TABLE 14.9. CLINICAL CARE CLASSIFICATION OF 182 NURSING DIAGNOSES (VERSION 2.0): CODES WITH DEFINITIONS, THREE ACTUAL OUTCOMES, AND CLASSIFIED BY 21 CARE COMPONENTS[a,b,c,d]

A. – ACTIVITY COMPONENT:
Cluster of elements that involve the use of energy in carrying out musculoskeletal and bodily actions.
Activity Alteration – A01
Change in or modification of energy used by the body.
A01.0.1 Improved
A01.0.2 Stabilized
A01.0.3 Deteriorated
  Activity Intolerance – A01.1
  Incapacity to carry out physiological or psychological daily activities.
  A01.1.1. Improved
  A01.1.2. Stabilized
  A01.1.3. Deteriorated
  Activity Intolerance Risk – A01.2
  Increased chance of an incapacity to carry out physiological or psychological daily activities.
  A01.2.1. Improved
  A01.2.2. Stabilized
  A01.2.3. Deteriorated
  Diversional Activity Deficit – A01.3
  Lack of interest or engagement in leisure activities.
  A01.3.1. Improved
  A01.3.2. Stabilized
  A01.3.3. Deteriorated
  Fatigue – A01.4
  Exhaustion that interferes with physical and mental activities.
  A01.4.1. Improved
  A01.4.2. Stabilized
  A01.4.3. Deteriorated
  Physical Mobility Impairment – A01.5
  Diminished ability to perform independent movement.
  A01.5.1. Improved
  A01.5.2. Stabilized
  A01.5.3. Deteriorated
  Sleep Pattern Disturbance – A01.6
  Imbalance in the normal sleep/wake cycle.
  A01.6.1. Improved
  A01.6.2. Stabilized
  A01.6.3. Deteriorated
  Sleep Deprivation – A01.7
  Lack of the normal sleep/wake cycle.
  A01.7.1. Improved
  A01.7.2. Stabilized
  A01.7.3. Deteriorated
Musculoskeletal Alteration – A02
Change in or modification of the muscles, bones, or support structures.
A02.0.1. Improved
A02.0.2. Stabilized
A02.0.3. Deteriorated

B. – BOWEL/GASTRIC COMPONENT:
Cluster of elements that involve the gastrointestinal system.
Bowel Elimination Alteration – B03
Change in or modification of the gastrointestinal system.
B03.0.1. Improved
B03.0.2. Stabilized
B03.0.3. Deteriorated
  Bowel Incontinence – B03.1
  Involuntary defecation.
  B03.1.1. Improved
  B03.1.2. Stabilized
  B03.1.3. Deteriorated
  Colonic Constipation – B03.2
  Infrequent or difficult passage of hard, dry feces.
  B03.2.1. Improved
  B03.2.2. Stabilized
  B03.2.3. Deteriorated
  Diarrhea – B03.3
  Abnormal frequency and fluidity of feces.
  B03.2.1. Improved
  B03.2.2. Stabilized
  B03.2.3. Deteriorated
  Fecal Impaction – B03.4
  Feces wedged in intestines.
  B03.4.1. Improved
  B03.4.2. Stabilized
  B03.4.3. Deteriorated
  Perceived Constipation – B03.5
  Belief and treatment of infrequent or difficult passage of feces without cause.
  B03.5.1. Improved
  B03.5.2. Stabilized
  B03.5.3. Deteriorated
  Unspecified Constipation B03.6
  Other forms of abnormal feces or difficult passage of feces.
  B03.6.1. Improved
  B03.6.2. Stabilized
  B03.6.3. Deteriorated
Gastrointestinal Alteration – B04
Change in or modification of the stomach or intestines.
B04.0.1. Improved
B04.0.2. Stabilized
B04.0.3. Deteriorated
Nausea – B51
Distaste for food/fluids and an urge to vomit.
B51.0.1. Improved
B51.0.2. Stabilized
B51.0.3. Deteriorated

(Continued)

TABLE 14.9. CLINICAL CARE CLASSIFICATION OF 182 NURSING DIAGNOSES (VERSION 2.0): CODES WITH DEFINITIONS, THREE ACTUAL OUTCOMES, AND CLASSIFIED BY 21 CARE COMPONENTS[a,b,c,d] (CONTINUED)

C. – CARDIAC COMPONENT:
Cluster of elements that involve the heart and blood vessels.
Cardiac Output Alteration – C05
Change in or modification of the pumping action of the heart.
C05.0.1. Improved
C05.0.2. Stabilized
C05.0.3. Deteriorated
Cardiovascular Alteration – C06
Change in or modification of the heart or blood vessels.
C06.0.1. Improved
C06.0.2. Stabilized
C06.0.3. Deteriorated
  Blood Pressure Alteration – C06.1
  Change in or modification of the systolic or diastolic pressure.
  C06.1.1. Improved
  C06.1.2. Stabilized
  C06.1.3. Deteriorated

D. – COGNITIVE COMPONENT:
Cluster of elements involving the mental and cerebral processes.
Cerebral Alteration – D07
Change in or modification of thought processes or mentation.
D07.0.1. Improved
D07.0.2. Stabilized
D07.0.3. Deteriorated
  Confusion – D07.1
  State of being disoriented (mixed-up).
  D07.1.1. Improved
  D07.1.2. Stabilized
  D07.1.3. Deteriorated
Knowledge Deficit – D08
Lack of information, understanding, or comprehension.
D08.0.1. Improved
D08.0.2. Stabilized
D08.0.3. Deteriorated
  Knowledge Deficit of Diagnostic Test – D08.1
  Lack of information on test(s) to identify disease or assess health condition.
  D08.1.1. Improved
  D08.1.2. Stabilized
  D08.1.3. Deteriorated
  Knowledge Deficit Dietary Regimen – D08.2
  Lack of information on the prescribed food or fluid intake.
  D08.2.1. Improved
  D08.2.2. Stabilized
  D08.2.3. Deteriorated
  Knowledge Deficit of Disease Process – D08.3
  Lack of information on the morbidity, course, or treatment of the health condition.
  D08.3.1. Improved
  D08.3.2. Stabilized
  D08.3.3. Deteriorated

Knowledge Deficit of Fluid Volume – D08.4
Lack of information on fluid volume intake requirements.
D08.4.1. Improved
D08.4.2. Stabilized
D08.4.3. Deteriorated
Knowledge Deficit of Medication Regimen – D08.5
Lack of information on prescribed regulated course of medicinal substances.
D08.5.1. Improved
D08.5.2. Stabilized
D08.5.3. Deteriorated
Knowledge Deficit of Safety Precautions – D08.6
Lack of information on measures to prevent injury, danger, or loss.
D08.6.1. Improved
D08.6.2. Stabilized
D08.6.3. Deteriorated
Knowledge Deficit of Therapeutic Regimen – D08.7
Lack of information on regulated course of treating disease.
D08.7.1. Improved
D08.7.2. Stabilized
D08.7.3. Deteriorated
Thought Process Alteration – D09
Change in or modification of cognitive processes.
D09.0.1. Improved
D09.0.2. Stabilized
D09.0.3. Deteriorated
  Memory Impairment – D09.1
  Diminished or inability to recall past events.
  D09.1.1. Improved
  D09.1.2. Stabilized
  D09.1.3. Deteriorated

E. – COPING COMPONENT:
Cluster of elements that involve the ability to deal with responsibilities, problems, or difficulties.
Dying Process – E10
Physical and behavioral responses associated with death.
E10.0.1. Improved
E10.0.2. Stabilized
E10.0.3. Deteriorated
Community Coping Impairment – E52
Inadequate community response to problems or difficulties.
E52.0.1. Improved
E52.0.2. Stabilized
E52.0.3. Deteriorated
Family Coping Impairment – E11
Inadequate family response to problems or difficulties.
E11.0.1. Improved
E11.0.2. Stabilized
E11.0.3. Deteriorated

(Continued)

TABLE 14.9. (CONTINUED)

Compromised Family Coping – E11.1
Inability of family to function optimally.
E11.1.1. Improved
E11.1.2. Stabilized
E11.1.3. Deteriorated
Disabled Family Coping – E11.2
Dysfunctional ability of family to function.
E11.2.1. Improved
E11.2.2. Stabilized
E11.2.3. Deteriorated
Individual Coping Impairment – E12
Inadequate personal response to problems or difficulties.
E12.0.1. Improved
E12.0.2. Stabilized
E12.0.3. Deteriorated
    Adjustment Impairment – E12.1
    Inadequate adjustment to condition or change in health
      status.
    E12.1.1. Improved
    E12.1.2. Stabilized
    E12.1.3. Deteriorated
    Decisional Conflict – E12.2
    Struggle related to determining a course of action.
    E12.2.1. Improved
    E12.2.2. Stabilized
    E12.2.3. Deteriorated
    Defensive Coping – E12.3
    Self-protective strategies to guard against threats to self.
    E12.3.1. Improved
    E12.3.2. Stabilized
    E12.3.3. Deteriorated
    Denial – E12.4
    Attempt to reduce anxiety by refusal to accept thoughts,
      feelings, or facts.
    E12.4.1. Improved
    E12.4.2. Stabilized
    E12.4.3. Deteriorated
Post-trauma Response – E13
Sustained behavior related to a traumatic event.
E13.0.1. Improved
E13.0.2. Stabilized
E13.0.3. Deteriorated
    Rape Trauma Syndrome – E13.1
    Group of symptoms related to a forced sexual act.
    E13.1.1. Improved
    E13.1.2. Stabilized
    E13.1.3. Deteriorated
Spiritual State Alteration – E14
Change in or modification of the spirit or soul.
E14.0.1. Improved
E14.0.2. Stabilized
E14.0.3. Deteriorated
    Spiritual Distress – E14.1
    Anguish related to the spirit or soul.
    E14.1.1. Improved

    E14.1.2. Stabilized
    E14.1.3. Deteriorated
Grieving – E53
Feeling of great sorrow.
E53.0.1. Improved
E53.0.2. Stabilized
E43.0.3. Deteriorated
    Anticipatory Grieving – E53.1
    Feeling great sorrow before the event or loss.
    E53.1.1. Improved
    E53.1.2. Stabilized
    E53.1.3. Deteriorated
    Dysfunctional Grieving – E53.2
    Prolonged feeling of great sorrow.
    E53.2.1. Improved
    E53.2.2. Stabilized
    E53.2.3. Deteriorated

F. – FLUID VOLUME COMPONENT:
Cluster of elements that involve liquid consumption.
Fluid Volume Alteration – F15
Change in or modification of bodily fluid.
F15.0.1. Improved
F15.0.2. Stabilized
F15.0.3. Deteriorated
    Fluid Volume Deficit – F15.1
    Dehydration.
    F15.1.1. Improved
    F15.1.2. Stabilized
    F15.1.3. Deteriorated
    Fluid Volume Deficit Risk – F15.2
    Increased chance of dehydration.
    F15.2.1. Improved
    F15.2.2. Stabilized
    F15.2.3. Deteriorated
    Fluid Volume Excess – F15.3
    Fluid retention, overload, or edema.
    F15.3.1. Improved
    F15.3.2. Stabilized
    F15.3.3. Deteriorated
    Fluid Volume Excess Risk – F15.4
    Increased chance of fluid retention, overload, or edema.
    F15.4.1. Improved
    F15.4.2. Stabilized
    F15.4.3. Deteriorated

G. – HEALTH BEHAVIOR COMPONENT:
Cluster of elements that involve actions to sustain, maintain,
  or regain health.
Health Maintenance Alteration – G17
Change in or modification of ability to manage
  health-related needs.
G17.0.1. Improved
G17.0.2. Stabilized
G17.0.3. Deteriorated

(Continued)

TABLE 14.9. CLINICAL CARE CLASSIFICATION OF 182 NURSING DIAGNOSES (VERSION 2.0): CODES WITH DEFINITIONS, THREE ACTUAL OUTCOMES, AND CLASSIFIED BY 21 CARE COMPONENTS[a,b,c,d] (CONTINUED)

Failure to Thrive – G17.1
Inability to grow and develop normally.
G17.1.1. Improved
G17.1.2. Stabilized
G17.1.3. Deteriorated

Health-Seeking Behavior Alteration – G18
Change in or modification of actions needed to improve health state.
G18.0.1. Improved
G18.0.2. Stabilized
G18.0.3. Deteriorated

Home Maintenance Alteration – G19
Inability to sustain a safe, healthy environment.
G19.0.1. Improved
G19.0.2. Stabilized
G19.0.3. Deteriorated

Noncompliance – G20
Failure to follow therapeutic recommendations.
G20.0.1. Improved
G20.0.2. Stabilized
G20.0.3. Deteriorated

  Noncompliance of Diagnostic Test – G20.1
  Failure to follow therapeutic recommendations on tests to identify disease or assess health condition.
  G20.1.1. Improved
  G20.1.2. Stabilized
  G20.1.3. Deteriorated

  Noncompliance of Dietary Regimen – G20.2
  Failure to follow the prescribed food or fluid intake.
  G20.2.1. Improved
  G20.2.2. Stabilized
  G20.2.3. Deteriorated

  Noncompliance of Fluid Volume – G20.3
  Failure to follow fluid volume intake requirements.
  G20.3.1. Improved
  G20.3.2. Stabilized
  G20.3.3. Deteriorated

  Noncompliance of Medication Regimen – G20.4
  Failure to follow prescribed regulated course of medicinal substances.
  G20.4.1. Improved
  G20.4.2. Stabilized
  G20.4.3. Deteriorated

  Noncompliance of Safety Precautions – G20.5
  Failure to follow measures to prevent injury, danger, or loss.
  G20.5.1. Improved
  G20.5.2. Stabilized
  G20.5.3. Deteriorated

  Noncompliance of Therapeutic Regimen – G20.6
  Failure to follow regulated course of treating disease or health condition.
  G20.6.1. Improved
  G20.6.2. Stabilized
  G20.6.3. Deteriorated

H. – MEDICATION COMPONENT:
Cluster of elements that involve medicinal substances.

Medication Risk – H21
Increased chance of negative response to medicinal substances.
H21.0.1. Improved
H21.0.2. Stabilized
H21.0.3. Deteriorated

  Polypharmacy – H21.1
  Use of two or more drugs together.
  H21.1.1. Improved
  H21.1.2. Stabilized
  H21.1.3. Deteriorated

I. – METABOLIC COMPONENT:
Cluster of elements that involve the endocrine and immunological processes.

Endocrine Alteration – I22
Change in or modification of internal secretions or hormones.
I22.0.1. Improved
I22.0.2. Stabilized
I22.0.3. Deteriorated

Immunologic Alteration – I23
Change in or modification of the immune systems.
I23.0.1. Improved
I23.0.2. Stabilized
I23.0.3. Deteriorated

  Protection Alteration – I23.1
  Change in or modification of the ability to guard against internal or external threats to the body.
  I23.1.1. Improved
  I23.1.2. Stabilized
  I23.1.3. Deteriorated

J. – NUTRITIONAL COMPONENT:
Cluster of elements that involve the intake of food and nutrients.

Nutrition Alteration – J24
Change in or modification of food and nutrients.
J24.0.1. Improved
J24.0.2. Stabilized
J24.0.3. Deteriorated

  Body Nutrition Deficit – J24.1
  Less than adequate intake or absorption of food or nutrients.
  J24.1.1. Improved
  J24.1.2. Stabilized
  J24.1.3. Deteriorated

  Body Nutrition Deficit Risk – J24.2
  Increased chance of less than adequate intake or absorption of food or nutrients.
  J24.2.1. Improved
  J24.2.2. Stabilized
  J24.2.3. Deteriorated

(Continued)

TABLE 14.9. (CONTINUED)

Body Nutrition Excess – J24.3
More than adequate intake or absorption of food or nutrients.
J24.3.1. Improved
J24.3.2. Stabilized
J24.3.3. Deteriorated
Body Nutrition Excess Risk – J24.4
Increased chance of more than adequate intake or absorption of food or nutrients.
J24.4.1. Improved
J24.4.2. Stabilized
J24.4.3. Deteriorated
Swallowing Impairment – J24.5
Inability to move food from mouth to stomach.
J24.5.1. Improved
J24.5.2. Stabilized
J24.5.3. Deteriorated
Infant Feeding Pattern Impairment – J54
Imbalance in the normal feeding habits of an infant.
J54.0.1. Improved
J54.0.2. Stabilized
J54.0.3. Deteriorated
Breast-feeding Impairment – J55
Diminished ability to nourish infant at the breast.
J55.0.1. Improved
J55.0.2. Stabilized
J55.0.3. Deteriorated

K. – PHYSICAL REGULATION COMPONENT:
Cluster of elements that involve bodily processes.
Physical Regulation Alteration – K25
Change in or modification of somatic control.
K25.0.1. Improved
K25.0.2. Stabilized
K25.0.3. Deteriorated
  Autonomic Dysreflexia – K25.1
  Life-threatening inhibited sympathetic response to noxious stimuli in a person with a spinal cord injury at T7 or above.
  K25.1.1. Improved
  K25.1.2. Stabilized
  K25.1.3. Deteriorated
  Hyperthermia – K25.2
  Abnormal high body temperature.
  K25.2.1. Improved
  K25.2.2. Stabilized
  K25.2.3. Deteriorated
  Hypothermia – K25.3
  Abnormal low body temperature.
  K25.3.1. Improved
  K25.3.2. Stabilized
  K25.3.3. Deteriorated

Thermoregulation Impairment – K25.4
Fluctuation of temperature between hypothermia and hyperthermia.
K25.4.1. Improved
K25.4.2. Stabilized
K25.4.3. Deteriorated
Infection Risk – K25.5
Increased chance of contamination with disease-producing germs.
K25.5.1. Improved
K25.5.2. Stabilized
K25.5.3. Deteriorated
Infection Unspecified – K25.6
Unknown contamination with disease-producing germs.
K25.6.1. Improved
K25.6.2. Stabilized
K25.6.3. Deteriorated
Intracranial Adaptive Capacity Impairment – K25.7
Intracranial fluid volumes are compromised.
K25.7.1. Improved
K25.7.2. Stabilized
K25.7.3. Deteriorated

L. – RESPIRATORY COMPONENT
Cluster of elements that involve breathing and the pulmonary system.
Respiration Alteration – L26
Change in or modification of carrying out responsibilities.
L26.0.1. Improved
L26.0.2. Stabilized
L26.0.3. Deteriorated
  Airway Clearance Impairment – L26.1
  Inability to clear secretions/obstructions in airway.
  L26.1.1. Improved
  L26.1.2. Stabilized
  L26.1.3. Deteriorated
  Breathing Pattern Impairment – L26.2
  Inadequate inhalation or exhalation.
  L26.2.1. Improved
  L26.2.2. Stabilized
  L26.2.3. Deteriorated
  Gas Exchange Impairment – L26.3
  Imbalance of oxygen and carbon dioxide transfer between lung and vascular system.
  L26.3.1. Improved
  L26.3.2. Stabilized
  L26.3.3. Deteriorated
Ventilatory Weaning Impairment – L56
Inability to tolerate decreased levels of ventilator support.
L56.0.1. Improved
L56.0.2. Stabilized
L56.0.3. Deteriorated

(Continued)

TABLE 14.9. CLINICAL CARE CLASSIFICATION OF 182 NURSING DIAGNOSES (VERSION 2.0): CODES WITH DEFINITIONS, THREE ACTUAL OUTCOMES, AND CLASSIFIED BY 21 CARE COMPONENTS[a,b,c,d] (CONTINUED)

M. – ROLE RELATIONSHIP COMPONENT:
Cluster of elements involving interpersonal work, social, family, and sexual interactions.
Role Performance Alteration – M27
Change in or modification of carrying out responsibilities.
M.27.0.1. Improved
M.27.0.2. Stabilized
M.27.0.3. Deteriorated
 Parental Role Conflict – M27.1
 Struggle with parental position and responsibilities.
 M.27.1.1. Improved
 M.27.1.2. Stabilized
 M.27.1.3. Deteriorated
 Parenting Alteration – M27.2
 Change in or modification of nurturing figure's ability to promote growth.
 M.27.2.1. Improved
 M.27.2.2. Stabilized
 M.27.2.3. Deteriorated
 Sexual Dysfunction – M27.3
 Deleterious change in sex response.
 M.27.3.1. Improved
 M.27.3.2. Stabilized
 M.27.3.3. Deteriorated
 Caregiver Role Strain – M27.4
 Excessive tension of one who gives physical or emotional care and support to another person or patient.
 M.27.4.1. Improved
 M.27.4.2. Stabilized
 M.27.4.3. Deteriorated
Communication Impairment – M28
Diminished ability to exchange thoughts, opinions, or information.
M.28.0.1. Improved
M.28.0.2. Stabilized
M.28.0.3. Deteriorated
 Verbal Impairment –M28.1
 Diminished ability to exchange thoughts, opinions, or information through speech.
 M.28.1.1. Improved
 M.28.1.2. Stabilized
 M.28.1.3. Deteriorated
Family Processes Alteration – M29
Change in or modification of usual functioning of a related group.
M.29.0.1. Improved
M.29.0.2. Stabilized
M.29.0.3. Deteriorated
Sexuality Patterns Alteration – M31
Change in or modification of person's sexual response.
M.31.0.1. Improved
M.31.0.2. Stabilized
M.31.0.3. Deteriorated
Socialization Alteration – M32
Change in or modification of personal identity.

M.32.0.1. Improved
M.32.0.2. Stabilized
M.32.0.3. Deteriorated
 Social Interaction Alteration – M32.1
 Change in or modification of inadequate quantity or quality of personal relations.
 M.32.1.1. Improved
 M.32.1.2. Stabilized
 M.32.1.3. Deteriorated
 Social Isolation – M32.2
 State of aloneness, lack of interaction with others.
 M.32.2.1. Improved
 M.32.2.2. Stabilized
 M.32.2.3. Deteriorated
 Relocation Stress Syndrome – M32.3
 Excessive tension from moving to a new location.
 M.32.3.1. Improved
 M.32.3.2. Stabilized
 M.32.3.3. Deteriorated

N. – SAFETY COMPONENT:
Cluster of elements that involve prevention of injury, danger, loss, or abuse.
Injury Risk – N33
Increased chance of danger or loss.
N.33.0.1. Improved
N.33.0.2. Stabilized
N.33.0.3. Deteriorated
 Aspiration Risk – N33.1
 Increased chance of material into trachea-bronchial passages.
 N33.1.1. Improved
 N33.1.2. Stabilized
 N33.1.3. Deteriorated
 Disuse Syndrome – N33.2
 Group of symptoms related to effects of immobility.
 N33.2.1. Improved
 N33.2.2. Stabilized
 N33.2.3. Deteriorated
 Poisoning Risk – N33.3
 Exposure to or ingestion of dangerous products.
 N33.3.1. Improved
 N33.3.2. Stabilized
 N33.3.3. Deteriorated
 Suffocation Risk – N33.4
 Increased chance of inadequate air for breathing.
 N33.4.1. Improved
 N33.4.2. Stabilized
 N33.4.3. Deteriorated
 Trauma Risk – N33.5
 Increased chance of accidental tissue processes.
 N33.5.1. Improved
 N33.5.2. Stabilized
 N33.5.3. Deteriorated

(Continued)

TABLE 14.9. (CONTINUED)

Violence Risk – N34
Increased chance of harming self or others.
N34.0.1. Improved
N34.0.2. Stabilized
N34.0.3. Deteriorated

Suicide Risk – N34.1
Increased chance of taking one's life intentionally.
N34.1.1. Improved
N34.1.2. Stabilized
N34.1.3. Deteriorated

Self-Mutilation Risk – N34.2
Increased chance of destroying a limb or essential part of the body.
N34.2.1. Improved
N34.2.2. Stabilized
N34.2.3. Deteriorated

Perioperative Injury Risk – N57
Increased chance of injury during the operative processes.
N57.0.1. Improved
N57.0.2. Stabilized
N57.0.3. Deteriorated

Perioperative Positioning Injury – N57.1
Damages from operative process positioning.
N57.1.1. Improved
N57.1.2. Stabilized
N57.1.3. Deteriorated

Surgical Recovery Delay – N57.2
Slow or delayed recovery from a surgical procedure.
N57.2.1. Improved
N57.2.2. Stabilized
N57.2.3. Deteriorated

Substance Abuse – N58
Excessive use of harmful bodily materials.
N58.0.1. Improved
N58.0.2. Stabilized
N58.0.3. Deteriorated

Tobacco Abuse – N58.1
Excessive use of tobacco products.
N58.1.1. Improved
N58.1.2. Stabilized
N58.1.3. Deteriorated

Alcohol Abuse – N58.2
Excessive use of distilled liquors.
N58.2.1. Improved
N58.2.2. Stabilized
N58.2.3. Deteriorated

Drug Abuse – N58.3
Excessive use of habit-forming medications.
N58.3.1. Improved
N58.3.2. Stabilized
N58.3.3. Deteriorated

O.– SELF-CARE COMPONENT:
Cluster of elements that involve the ability to carry out activities to maintain oneself.

Bathing/Hygiene Deficit – O35
Impaired ability to cleanse oneself.
O35.0.1. Improved
O35.0.2. Stabilized
O35.0.3. Deteriorated

Dressing/Grooming Deficit - O36
Inability to clothe and groom oneself.
O36.0.1. Improved
O36.0.2. Stabilized
O36.0.3. Deteriorated

Feeding Deficit – O37
Impaired ability to feed oneself.
O37.0.1. Improved
O37.0.2. Stabilized
O37.0.3. Deteriorated

Self-Care Deficit – O38
Impaired ability to maintain oneself.
O38.0.1. Improved
O38.0.2. Stabilized
O38.0.3. Deteriorated

Activities of Daily Living (ADLs) Alteration – O38.1
Change in or modification of ability to maintain oneself.
O38.1.1. Improved
O38.1.2. Stabilized
O38.1.3. Deteriorated

Instrumental Activities of Daily Living (IADLs) Alteration – O38.2
Change in or modification of more complex activities than those needed to maintain oneself.
O38.2.1. Improved
O38.2.2. Stabilized
O38.2.3. Deteriorated

Toileting Deficit – O39
Impaired ability to urinate or defecate for oneself.
O39.0.1. Improved
O39.0.2. Stabilized
O39.0.3. Deteriorated

P. – SELF-CONCEPT COMPONENT:
Cluster of elements that involve an individual's mental image of oneself.

Anxiety – P40
Feeling of distress or apprehension whose source is unknown.
P40.0.1. Improved
P40.0.2. Stabilized
P40.0.3. Deteriorated

Fear – P41
Feeling of dread or distress whose cause can be identified.
P41.0.1. Improved
P41.0.2. Stabilized
P41.0.3. Deteriorated

(Continued)

TABLE 14.9. CLINICAL CARE CLASSIFICATION OF 182 NURSING DIAGNOSES (VERSION 2.0): CODES WITH DEFINITIONS, THREE ACTUAL OUTCOMES, AND CLASSIFIED BY 21 CARE COMPONENTS[a,b,c,d] (CONTINUED)

Meaningfulness Alteration – P42
Change in or modification of the ability to see the significance, purpose, or value in something.
P42.0.1. Improved
P42.0.2. Stabilized
P42.0.3. Deteriorated
   Hopelessness – P42.1
   Feeling of despair or futility and passive involvement.
   P42.1.1. Improved
   P42.1.2. Stabilized
   P42.1.3. Deteriorated
   Powerlessness – P42.2
   Feeling of helplessness, or inability to act.
   P42.2.1. Improved
   P42.2.2. Stabilized
   P42.2.3. Deteriorated

Self Concept Alteration – P43
Change in or modification of ability to maintain one's image of self.
P43.0.1. Improved
P43.0.2. Stabilized
P43.0.3. Deteriorated
   Body Image Disturbance – P43.1
   Imbalance in the perception of the way one's body looks.
   P43.1.1. Improved
   P43.1.2. Stabilized
   P43.1.3. Deteriorated
   Personal Identity Disturbance – P43.2
   Imbalance in the ability to distinguish between the self and the non-self.
   P43.2.1. Improved
   P43.2.2. Stabilized
   P43.2.3. Deteriorated
   Chronic Low Self-Esteem Disturbance – P43.3
   Persistent negative evaluation of oneself.
   P43.3.1. Improved
   P43.3.2. Stabilized
   P43.3.3. Deteriorated
   Situational Self-Esteem Disturbance – P43.4
   Negative evaluation of oneself in response to a loss or change.
   P43.4.1. Improved
   P43.4.2. Stabilized
   P43.4.3. Deteriorated

Q. – SENSORY COMPONENT:
Cluster of elements that involve the senses including pain.
Sensory Perceptual Alteration – Q44
Change in or modification of the response to stimuli.
Q44.0.1. Improved
Q44.0.2. Stabilized
Q44.0.3. Deteriorated
   Auditory Alteration – Q44.1
   Change in or modification of diminished ability to hear.
   Q44.1.1. Improved
   Q44.1.2. Stabilized
   Q44.1.3. Deteriorated

   Gustatory Alteration – Q44.2
   Change in or modification of diminished ability to taste.
   Q44.2.1. Improved
   Q44.2.2. Stabilized
   Q44.2.3. Deteriorated
   Kinesthetic Alteration – Q44.3
   Change in or modification of diminished ability to move.
   Q44.3.1. Improved
   Q44.3.2. Stabilized
   Q44.3.3. Deteriorated
   Olfactory Alteration – Q44.4
   Change in or modification of diminished ability to smell.
   Q44.4.1. Improved
   Q44.4.2. Stabilized
   Q44.4.3. Deteriorated
   Tactile Alteration – Q44.5
   Change in or modification of diminished ability to feel.
   Q44.5.1. Improved
   Q44.5.2. Stabilized
   Q44.5.3. Deteriorated
   Unilateral Neglect – Q44.6
   Lack of awareness of one side of the body.
   Q44.6.1. Improved
   Q44.6.2. Stabilized
   Q44.6.3. Deteriorated
   Visual Alteration – Q44.7
   Change in or modification of diminished ability to see.
   Q44.7.1. Improved
   Q44.7.2. Stabilized
   Q44.7.3. Deteriorated

Comfort Alteration – Q45
Change in or modification of sensation that is distressing.
Q45.0.1. Improved
Q45.0.2. Stabilized
Q45.0.3. Deteriorated
   Acute Pain – Q45.1
   Physical suffering or distress to hurt.
   Q45.1.1. Improved
   Q45.1.2. Stabilized
   Q45.1.3. Deteriorated
   Chronic Pain – Q45.2
   Pain that continues for longer than expected.
   Q45.2.1. Improved
   Q45.2.2. Stabilized
   Q45.2.3. Deteriorated
   Unspecified Pain – Q45.3
   Pain that is difficult to pinpoint.
   Q45.3.1. Improved
   Q45.3.2. Stabilized
   Q45.3.3. Deteriorated

R. – SKIN INTEGRITY COMPONENT:
Cluster of elements that involve the mucous membrane, corneal, integumentary, or subcutaneous structures of the body.

(Continued)

TABLE 14.9. (CONTINUED)

Skin Integrity Alteration – R46
Change in or modification of skin conditions.
R46.0.1. Improved
R46.0.2. Stabilized
R46.0.3. Deteriorated

  Oral Mucous Membranes Impairment – R46.1
  Diminished ability to maintain the tissues of the oral cavity.
  R46.1.1. Improved
  R46.1.2. Stabilized
  R46.1.3. Deteriorated

  Skin Integrity Impairment – R46.2
  Decreased ability to maintain the integument.
  R46.2.1. Improved
  R46.2.2. Stabilized
  R46.2.3. Deteriorated

  Skin Integrity Impairment Risk – R46.3
  Increased chance of skin breakdown.
  R46.3.1. Improved
  R46.3.2. Stabilized
  R46.3.3. Deteriorated

  Skin Incision – R46.4
  Cutting of the integument/skin.
  R46.4.1. Improved
  R46.4.2. Stabilized
  R46.4.3. Deteriorated

  Latex Allergy Response – R46.5
  Pathological reaction to latex products.
  R46.5.1. Improved
  R46.5.2. Stabilized
  R46.5.3. Deteriorated

Peripheral Alteration – R47
Change in or modification of vascularization of the extremities.
R47.0.1. Improved
R47.0.2. Stabilized
R47.0.3. Deteriorated

S. – TISSUE PERFUSION COMPONENT:
Cluster of elements that involve the oxygenation of tissues including the circulatory and neurovascular systems.

Tissue Perfusion Alteration – S48
Change in or modification of the oxygenation of tissues.
S48.0.1. Improved
S48.0.2. Stabilized
S48.0.3. Deteriorated

T. – URINARY ELIMINATION COMPONENT:
Cluster of elements that involve the genitourinary systems.

Urinary Elimination Alteration – T49
Change in or modification of excretion of the waste matter of the kidneys.
T49.0.1. Improved
T49.0.2. Stabilized
T49.0.3. Deteriorated

  Functional Urinary Incontinence – T49.1
  Involuntary, unpredictable passage of urine.
  T49.1.1. Improved
  T49.1.2. Stabilized
  T49.1.3. Deteriorated

  Reflex Urinary Incontinence – T49.2
  Involuntary passage of urine occurring at predictable intervals.
  T49.2.1. Improved
  T49.2.2. Stabilized
  T49.2.3. Deteriorated

  Stress Urinary Incontinence – T49.3
  Loss of urine occurring with increased abdominal pressure.
  T49.3.1. Improved
  T49.3.2. Stabilized
  T49.3.3. Deteriorated

  Total Urinary Incontinence – T49.4
  Continuous and unpredictable loss of urine.
  T49.4.1. Improved
  T49.4.2. Stabilized
  T49.4.3. Deteriorated

  Urge Urinary Incontinence – T49.5
  Involuntary passage of urine following a sense of urgency to void.
  T49.5.1. Improved
  T49.5.2. Stabilized
  T49.5.3. Deteriorated

  Urinary Retention – T49.6
  Incomplete emptying of the bladder.
  T49.6.1. Improved
  T49.6.2. Stabilized
  T49.6.3. Deteriorated

Renal Alteration – T50
Change in or modification of the kidney function.
T50.0.1. Improved
T50.0.2. Stabilized
T50.0.3. Deteriorated

U. – LIFE CYCLE COMPONENT:
Cluster of elements that involve the life span of individuals.

Reproductive Risk – U59
Increased chance of harm in the process of replicating or giving rise to an offspring/child.
U59.0.1. Improved
U59.0.2. Stabilized
U59.0.3. Deteriorated

  Fertility Risk – U59.1
  Increased chance of conception to develop an offspring/child.
  U59.1.1. Improved
  U59.1.2. Stabilized
  U59.1.3. Deteriorated

(Continued)

TABLE 14.9. CLINICAL CARE CLASSIFICATION OF 182 NURSING DIAGNOSES (VERSION 2.0): CODES WITH DEFINITIONS, THREE ACTUAL OUTCOMES, AND CLASSIFIED BY 21 CARE COMPONENTS[a,b,c,d] (CONTINUED)

Infertility Risk – U59.2
Increased chance of harm on preventing the development of an offspring/child.
U59.2.1. Improved
U59.2.2. Stabilized
U59.2.3. Deteriorated
Contraception Risk – U59.3
Increased chance of harm preventing the conception of an offspring/child.
U59.3.1. Improved
U59.3.2. Stabilized
U59.3.3. Deteriorated
Perinatal Risk – U60
Increased chance of harm before, during, and immediately after the creation of an offspring/child.
U60.1.1. Improved
U60.1.2. Stabilized
U60.1.3. Deteriorated
Pregnancy Risk – U60.1
Increased chance of harm during the gestational period of the formation of an offspring/child.
U60.1.1. Improved
U60.1.2. Stabilized
U60.1.3. Deteriorated
Labor Risk – U60.2
Increased chance of harm during the period supporting the bringing forth of an offspring/child.
U60.2.1. Improved
U60.2.2. Stabilized
U60.2.3. Deteriorated
Delivery Risk – U60.3
Increased chance of harm during the period supporting the expulsion of an offspring/child.
U60.3.1. Improved
U60.3.2. Stabilized
U60.3.3. Deteriorated
Postpartum Risk – U60.4
Increased chance of harm during the time period immediately following the delivery of an offspring/child.
U60.4.1. Improved
U60.4.2. Stabilized
U60.4.3. Deteriorated
Growth & Development Alteration – U61
Change in or modification of the norms for an individual's age.
U61.0.1. Improved
U61.0.2. Stabilized
U61.0.3. Deteriorated

Newborn Behavior Alteration (first 30 days) – U61.1
Change in or modification of normal standards of performing developmental skills and behavior of a typical newborn the first 30 days of life.
U61.1.1. Improved
U61.1.2. Stabilized
U61.1.3. Deteriorated
Infant Behavior Alteration (31 days through 11 months) – U61.2
Change in or modification of normal standards of performing developmental skills and behavior of a typical infant from 31 days through 11 months of age.
U61.2.1. Improved
U61.2.2. Stabilized
U61.2.3. Deteriorated
Child Behavior Alteration (1 year through 11 years) – U61.3
Change in or modification of normal standards of performing developmental skills and behavior of a typical child from 1 year through 11 years of age.
U61.3.1. Improved
U61.3.2. Stabilized
U61.3.3. Deteriorated
Adolescent Behavior Alteration (12 years through 20 years) – U61.4
Change in or modification of normal standards of performing developmental skills and behavior of a typical adolescent from 12 years through 20 years of age.
U61.4.1. Improved
U61.4.2. Stabilized
U61.4.3. Deteriorated
Adult Behavior Alteration (21 years through 64 years) – U61.5
Change in or modification of normal standards of performing developmental skills and behavior of a typical adult from 21 years through 64 years of age.
U61.5.1. Improved
U61.5.2. Stabilized
U61.5.3. Deteriorated
Older Adult Behavior Alteration (65 years & older) – U61.6
Change in or modification of normal standards of performing developmental skills and behavior of a typical older adult from 65 years of age and over.
U61.6.1. Improved
U61.6.2. Stabilized
U61.6.3. Deteriorated

---

[a]Adapted from NANDA (North American Nursing Diagnoses Association): *Taxonomy I: Revised–1990.*
[b]Adapted with permission from NANDA *Nursing Diagnoses & Classification, 2003–2004.*
[c]Clinical Care Classification of Nursing Diagnoses (Version 2.0) includes 9 New Major Categories and 21 Subcategories. See Appendix Table A.2 for revisions from Home Health Care Classification (Version 1.0).
[d]The Clinical Care Classification System is copyrighted, placed in the Public Domain & cannot be sold, but is available with written permission.

© V. K. Saba—Revised 1992, 1994, 2002, 2004, 2006

TABLE 14.10. CLINICAL CARE CLASSIFICATION OF 198 NURSING INTERVENTIONS (VERSION 2.0): CODED AND CLASSIFIED BY 21 CARE COMPONENTS[a,b]

A. ACTIVITY COMPONENT
01 Activity Care
   01.2 Energy Conservation
02 Fracture Care
   02.1 Cast Care
   02.2 Immobilizer Care
03 Mobility Therapy
   03.1 Ambulation Therapy
   03.2 Assistive Device Therapy
   03.3 Transfer Care
04 Sleep Pattern Control
05 Musculoskeletal Care
   05.1 Range of Motion
   05.2 Rehabilitation Exercise
61 Bedbound Care
   61.1 Positioning Therapy

B. BOWEL/GASTRIC COMPONENT
06 Bowel Care
   06.1 Bowel Training
   06.2 Disimpaction
   06.3 Enema
   06.4 Diarrhea Care
07 Ostomy Care
   07.1 Ostomy Irrigation
62 Gastric Care
   62.1 Nausea Care

C. CARDIAC COMPONENT
08 Cardiac Care
   08.1 Cardiac Rehabilitation
09 Pacemaker Care

D. COGNITIVE COMPONENT
10 Behavior Care
11 Reality Orientation
63 Wandering Control
64 Memory Loss Care

E. COPING COMPONENT
12 Counseling Service
   12.1 Coping Support
   12.2 Stress Control
   12.3 Crisis Therapy
13 Emotional Support
   13.1 Spiritual Comfort
14 Terminal Care
   14.1 Bereavement Support
   14.2 Dying/Death Measures
   14.3 Funeral Arrangements

F. FLUID VOLUME COMPONENT
15 Fluid Therapy
   15.1 Hydration Control
   15.2 Intake/Output
16 Infusion Care
   16.1 Intravenous Care
   16.2 Venous Catheter Care

G. HEALTH BEHAVIOR COMPONENT
17 Community Special Services
   17.1 Adult Day Center
   17.2 Hospice
   17.3 Meals-on-Wheels
18 Compliance Care
   18.1 Compliance with Diet
   18.2 Compliance with Fluid Volume
   18.3 Compliance with Medical Regimen
   18.4 Compliance with Medication Regimen
   18.5 Compliance with Safety Precautions
   18.6 Compliance with Therapeutic Regimen
19 Nursing Contact
   19.1 Bill of Rights
   19.2 Nursing Care Coordination
   19.3 Nursing Status Report
20 Physician Contact
   20.1 Medical Regimen Orders
   20.2 Physician Status Report
21 Professional/Ancillary Services
   21.1 Health Aide Service
   21.2 Medical Social Worker Service
   21.3 Nurse Specialist Service
   21.4 Occupational Therapist Service
   21.5 Physical Therapist Service
   21.6 Speech Therapist Service

H. MEDICATION COMPONENT
22 Chemotherapy Care
23 Injection Administration
   23.1 Insulin Injection
   23.2 Vitamin B12 Injection
24 Medication Care
   24.1 Medication Actions
   24.2 Medication Prefill Preparation
   24.3 Medication Side Effects
   24.4 Medication Treatment
25 Radiation Therapy Care

(Continued)

TABLE 14.10. CLINICAL CARE CLASSIFICATION OF 198 NURSING INTERVENTIONS (VERSION 2.0): CODED AND CLASSIFIED BY 21 CARE COMPONENTS[a,b] (CONTINUED)

I. METABOLIC COMPONENT
26 Allergic Reaction Control
27 Diabetic Care
65 Immunological Care

J. NUTRITIONAL COMPONENT
28 Enteral Tube Care
   28.1 Enteral Tube Insertion
   28.2 Enteral Tube Irrigation
29 Nutrition Care
   29.2 Feeding Technique
   29.3 Regular Diet
   29.4 Special Diet
   29.5 Enteral Feeding
   29.6 Parenteral Feeding
66 Breast-feeding Support
67 Weight Control

K. PHYSICAL REGULATION COMPONENT
30 Infection Control
   30.1 Universal Precautions
31 Physical Health Care
   31.1 Health History
   31.2 Health Promotion
   31.3 Physical Examination
   31.4 Clinical Measurements
32 Specimen Care
   32.1 Blood Specimen Care
   32.2 Stool Specimen Care
   32.3 Urine Specimen Care
   32.5 Sputum Specimen Care
33 Vital Signs
   33.1 Blood Pressure
   33.2 Temperature
   33.3 Pulse
   33.4 Respiration

L. RESPIRATORY COMPONENT
35 Oxygen Therapy Care
36 Pulmonary Care
   36.1 Breathing Exercises
   36.2 Chest Physiotherapy
   36.3 Inhalation Therapy
   36.4 Ventilator Care
37 Tracheostomy Care

M. ROLE RELATIONSHIP COMPONENT
38 Communication Care
39 Psychosocial Care
   39.1 Home Situation Analysis
   39.2 Interpersonal Dynamics Analysis
   39.3 Family Process Analysis
   39.4 Sexual Behavior Analysis
   39.5 Social Network Analysis

N. SAFETY COMPONENT
40 Substance Abuse Control
   40.1 Tobacco Abuse Control
   40.2 Alcohol Abuse Control
   40.3 Drug Abuse Control
41 Emergency Care
42 Safety Precautions
   42.1 Environmental Safety
   42.2 Equipment Safety
   42.3 Individual Safety
68 Violence Control

O. SELF-CARE COMPONENT
43 Personal Care
   43.1 Activities of Daily Living (ADLs)
   43.2 Instrumental Activities of Daily Living (IADLs)

P. SELF-CONCEPT COMPONENT
45 Mental Health Care
   45.1 Mental Health History
   45.2 Mental Health Promotion
   45.3 Mental Health Screening
   45.4 Mental Health Treatment

Q. SENSORY COMPONENT
47 Pain Control
   47.1 Acute Pain Control
   47.2 Chronic Pain Control
48 Comfort Care
49 Ear Care
   49.1 Hearing Aid Care
   49.2 Wax Removal
50 Eye Care
   50.1 Cataract Care
   50.2 Vision Care

(Continued)

TABLE 14.10. (CONTINUED)

R. SKIN INTEGRITY COMPONENT
  51 Pressure Ulcer Care
      51.1 Pressure Ulcer Stage 1 Care
      51.2 Pressure Ulcer Stage 2 Care
      51.3 Pressure Ulcer Stage 3 Care
      51.4 Pressure Ulcer Stage 4 Care
  53 Mouth Care
      53.1 Denture Care
  54 Skin Care
      54.1 Skin Breakdown Control
  55 Wound Care
      55.1 Drainage Tube Care
      55.2 Dressing Change
      55.3 Incision Care

S. TISSUE PERFUSION COMPONENT
  56 Foot Care
  57 Perineal Care
  69 Edema Control
  70 Circulatory Care
  71 Neurovascular Care

T. URINARY ELIMINATION COMPONENT
  58 Bladder Care
      58.1 Bladder Instillation
      58.2 Bladder Training
  59 Dialysis Care
  60 Urinary Catheter Care
      60.1 Urinary Catheter Insertion
      60.2 Urinary Catheter Irrigation
  72 Urinary Incontinence Care
  73 Renal Care

U. LIFE CYCLE COMPONENT
  74 Reproductive Care
      74.1 Fertility Care
      74.2 Infertility Care
      74.3 Contraception Care
  75 Perinatal Care
      75.1 Pregnancy Care
      75.2 Labor Care
      75.3 Delivery Care
      75.4 Postpartum Care
  76 Growth & Development Care
      76.1 Newborn Care (first 30 days)
      76.2 Infant Care (31 days through 11 months)
      76.3 Child Care (1 year through 11 years)
      76.4 Adolescent Care (12 years through 20 years)
      76.5 Adult Care (21 years through 64 years)
      76.6 Older Adult Care (65 years and over)

[a]Clinical Care Classification of Nursing Interventions (Version 2.0) includes 12 New Major Categories and 24 Subcategories. See Appendix Table A.3 for revisions from Home Health Care Classification (Version 1.0).
[b]The Clinical Care Classification System is copyrighted, placed in the Public Domain, and cannot be sold, but is available with written permission.

© V. K. Saba—Revised 1992, 1994, 2002, 2004, 2006

TABLE 14.11. CLINICAL CARE CLASSIFICATION OF 198 NURSING INTERVENTIONS (VERSION 2.0): CODED WITH DEFINITIONS AND CLASSIFIED BY 21 CARE COMPONENTS[a,b]

A. – ACTIVITY COMPONENT:
Cluster of elements that involve the use of energy in carrying out musculoskeletal and bodily actions.
Activity Care – A01
Activities performed to carry out physiological or psychological daily activities.
   Energy Conservation – A01.2
   Actions performed taken to preserve energy.
Fracture Care – A02
Actions performed to control broken bones.
   Cast Care – A02.1
   Actions performed to control a rigid dressing.
   Immobilizer Care – A02.2
   Actions performed to control a splint, cast, or prescribed bed rest.
Mobility Therapy – A03
Actions performed to advise and instruct on mobility deficits.
   Ambulation Therapy – A03.1
   Actions performed to promote walking.
   Assistive Device Therapy – A03.2
   Actions performed to support the use of products to aid in caring for oneself.
   Transfer Care – A03.3
   Actions performed to assist in moving from one place to another.
Sleep Pattern Control – A04
Actions performed to support the sleep and wake cycles.
Musculosketal Care – A05
Actions performed to restore physical functioning.
   Range of Motion – A05.1
   Actions performed to provide the active and passive exercises to maintain joint function.
   Rehabilitation Exercise – A05.2
   Actions performed to promote physical functioning.
Bedbound Care – A61
Actions performed to support an individual confined to bed.
   Positioning Therapy – A61.1
   Process to support changes in body positioning.

B. – BOWEL/GASTRIC COMPONENT:
Cluster of elements that involve the gastrointestinal system.
Bowel Care – B06
Actions performed to control and restore the functioning of the bowel.
   Bowel Training – B06.1
   Actions performed to provide instruction on bowel elimination conditions.
   Disimpaction – B06.2
   Actions performed to manually remove feces.
   Enema – B06.3
   Actions performed to administer fluid rectally.
   Diarrhea Care – B06.4
   Actions performed to control the abnormal frequency and fluidity of feces.
Ostomy Care – B07
Actions performed to control the artificial opening that removes waste products.
   Ostomy Irrigation – B07.1
   Actions performed to flush or wash out an ostomy.

(Continued)

TABLE 14.11. (CONTINUED)

Gastric Care – B62
Actions performed to control changes in the stomach and intestines.
  Nausea Care – B62.1
  Actions performed to control the distaste for food and desire to vomit.

C. – CARDIAC COMPONENT:
Cluster of elements that involve the heart and blood vessels.
Cardiac Care – C08
Actions performed to control changes in the heart or blood vessels.
  Cardiac Rehabilitation – C08.1
  Actions performed to restore cardiac health.
Pacemaker Care – C09
Actions performed to control the use of an electronic device that provides a normal heartbeat.

D. – COGNITIVE COMPONENT:
Cluster of elements involving the mental and cerebral processes.
Behavior Care – D10
Actions performed to support observable responses to internal and external stimuli.
Reality Orientation – D11
Actions performed to promote the ability to locate oneself in an environment.
Wandering Control – D63
Actions performed to control abnormal movability.
Memory Loss Care –D64
Actions performed to control a person's inability to recall ideas and/or events.

E. – COPING COMPONENT
Cluster of elements that involve the ability to deal with responsibilities, problems, or difficulties.
Counseling Service – E12
Actions performed to provide advice or instruction to help another.
  Coping Support – E12.1
  Actions performed to sustain a person dealing with responsibilities, problems, or difficulties.
  Stress Control – E12.2
  Actions performed to support the physiological response of the body to a stimulus.
  Crisis Therapy – E12.3
  Actions performed to sustain a person dealing with a condition, event, or radical change in status.
Emotional Support – E13
Actions performed to maintain a positive affective state.
  Spiritual Comfort – E13.1
  Actions performed to console, restore, or promote spiritual health.
Terminal Care – E14
Actions performed in the period surrounding death.
  Bereavement Support – E14.1
  Actions performed to provide comfort to the family/friends of the person who died.
  Dying/Death Measures – E14.2
  Actions performed to support the dying process.
  Funeral Arrangements – E14.3
  Actions performed to direct the preparatory for burial.

F. – FLUID VOLUME COMPONENT:
Cluster of elements that involve liquid consumption.
Fluid Therapy – F15.0
Actions performed to provide liquid volume intake.

(Continued)

TABLE 14.11. CLINICAL CARE CLASSIFICATION OF 198 NURSING INTERVENTIONS (VERSION 2.0): CODED WITH DEFINITIONS AND CLASSIFIED BY 21 CARE COMPONENTS[a,b] (CONTINUED)

Hydration Control – F15.1
Actions performed to control the state of fluid balance.
Intake/Output – F15.2
Actions performed to measure the amount of fluid/food and excretion of waste.
Infusion Care – F16
Actions performed to support solutions given through the vein.
Intravenous Care – F16.1
Actions performed to administer an infusion through a vein.
Venous Catheter Care – F16.2
Actions performed to control the use of infusion equipment.

G. – HEALTH BEHAVIOR COMPONENT:
Cluster of elements that involve actions to sustain, maintain, or regain health.
Community Special Services – G17
Actions performed to provide advice or information about special community services.
Adult Day Center – G17.1
Actions performed to direct the provision of a day program for adults in a specific location.
Hospice – G17.2
Actions performed to support the provision of offering and/or providing care for terminally ill persons.
Meals-on-Wheels – G17.3
Actions performed to direct the provision of community program of meals delivered to the home.
Compliance Care – G18
Actions performed to encourage conformity in therapeutic recommendations.
Compliance with Diet – G18.1
Actions performed to encourage conformity to food or fluid intake.
Compliance with Fluid Volume – G18.2
Actions performed to encourage conformity to therapeutic intake of liquids.
Compliance with Medical Regimen – G18.3
Actions performed to encourage conformity to physician's plan of care.
Compliance with Medication Regimen – G18.4
Actions performed to encourage conformity to follow prescribed course of medicinal substances.
Compliance with Safety Precaution – G18.5
Actions performed to encourage conformity with measures to protect self or others from injury, danger, or loss.
Compliance with Therapeutic Regimen – G18.6
Actions performed to encourage conformity with the health team's plan of care.
Nursing Contact – G19
Actions performed to communicate with another nurse.
Bill of Rights – G19.1
Statements related to entitlements during an episode of illness.
Nursing Care Coordination – G19.2
Actions performed to synthesize all plans of care by a nurse.
Nursing Status Report – G19.3
Actions performed to document patient condition by a nurse.
Physician Contact – G20
Actions performed to communicate with a physician.
Medical Regimen Orders – G20.1
Actions performed to support the physician's plan of treatment.
Physician Status Report – G20.2
Actions performed to document patient condition by a physician.

(Continued)

TABLE 14.11. (CONTINUED)

Professional/Ancillary Services – G21
Actions performed to support the duties performed by health team members.
   Health Aide Service – G21.1
   Actions performed to support care services by a health aide.
   Medical Social Worker Service – G21.2
   Actions performed to provide advice or instruction by a medical social worker.
   Nurse Specialist Service – G21.3
   Actions performed to provide advice or instruction by an advanced practice nurse or nurse practitioner.
   Occupational Therapist Service – G21.4
   Actions performed to provide advice or instruction by an occupational therapist.
   Physical Therapist Service – G21.5
   Actions performed to provide advice or instruction by a physical therapist.
   Speech Therapist Service – G21.6
   Actions performed to provide advice or instruction by a speech therapist.

H. – MEDICATION COMPONENT:
Cluster of elements that involve medicinal substances.
Chemotherapy Care – H22
Actions performed to control and monitor antineoplastic agents.
Injection Administration – H23
Actions performed to dispense a medication by a hypodermic.
   Insulin Injection – H23.1
   Actions performed to administer a hypodermic administration of insulin.
   Vitamin B12 Injection – H23.2
   Actions performed to administer a hypodermic administration of vitamin B12.
Medication Care – H24
Actions performed to direct the dispensing of prescribed drugs.
   Medication Actions – H24.1
   Actions performed to support and monitor the use of medicinal substances.
   Medication Prefill Preparation – H24.2
   Actions performed to ensure the continued supply of prescribed drugs.
   Medication Side Effects – H24.3
   Actions performed to control untoward reaction or conditions to prescribed drugs.
   Medication Treatment – H24.4
   Actions performed to administer drugs or remedies regardless of route.
Radiation Therapy Care – H25
Actions performed to control and monitor radiation therapy.

I. – METABOLIC COMPONENT:
Cluster of elements that involve the endocrine and immunological processes.
Allergic Reaction Care – I26.0
Actions performed to reduce symptoms or precautions to reduce allergies.
Diabetic Care – I27
Actions performed to support the control of diabetic conditions.
Immunological Care – I65
Actions performed to protect against a particular disease.

J. – NUTRITIONAL COMPONENT:
Cluster of elements that involve the intake of food and nutrients.
Enteral Tube Care – J28
Actions performed to control the use on an enteral drainage tube.
   Enteral Tube Insertion – J28.1
   Actions performed to support the placement of an enteral drainage tube.
   Enteral Tube Irrigation – J28.2
   Actions performed to flush or wash out an enteral tube.

(Continued)

TABLE 14.11. CLINICAL CARE CLASSIFICATION OF 198 NURSING INTERVENTIONS (VERSION 2.0): CODED WITH DEFINITIONS AND CLASSIFIED BY 21 CARE COMPONENTS[a,b] (CONTINUED)

Nutrition Care – J29
Actions performed to support the intake of food and nutrients.
  Feeding Technique – J29.2
  Actions performed to provide special measures to provide nourishment.
  Regular Diet – J29.3
  Actions performed to support the ingestion of food and nutrients from established nutrition standards.
  Special Diet – J29.4
  Actions performed to support the ingestion of food and nutrients prescribed for a specific purpose.
  Enteral Feeding – J29.5
  Actions performed to provide nourishment through a gastrointestinal route.
  Parenteral Feeding – J29.6
  Actions performed to provide nourishment through intravenous or subcutaneous routes.
Breast-feeding Support – J66
Actions performed to provide nourishment of an infant at the breast.
Weight Control – J67
Actions performed to control obesity or debilitation.

K. – PHYSICAL REGULATION COMPONENT:
Cluster of elements that involve bodily processes.
Infection Control – K30
Actions performed to contain a communicable disease.
  Universal Precautions – K30.1
  Practices to prevent the spread of infections and infectious diseases.
Physical Health Care – K31
Actions performed to support somatic problems.
  Health History – K31.1
  Actions performed to obtain information about past illness and health status.
  Health Promotion – K31.2
  Actions performed to encourage behaviors to enhance health state.
  Physical Examination – K31.3
  Actions performed to observe somatic events.
  Clinical Measurements – K31.4
  Actions performed to conduct procedures to evaluate somatic events.
Specimen Care – K32
Actions performed to direct the collection and/or the examination of a bodily specimen.
  Blood Specimen Care – K32.1
  Actions performed to collect and/or examine a sample of blood.
  Stool Specimen Care – K32.2
  Actions performed to collect and/or examine a sample of feces.
  Urine Specimen Care – K32.3
  Actions performed to collect and/or examine a sample of urine.
  Sputum Specimen Care – K32.5
  Actions performed to collect and/or examine a sample of sputum.
Vital Signs – K33
Actions performed to measure temperature, respiration, pulse, and blood pressure.
  Blood Pressure – K33.1
  Actions performed to measure the diastolic and systolic pressure of the blood.
  Temperature – K33.2
  Actions performed to measure body temperature.
  Pulse – K33.3
  Actions performed to measure rhythmical beats of the heart.
  Respiration – K33.4
  Actions performed to measure the function of breathing.

(Continued)

TABLE 14.11. (CONTINUED)

L. – RESPIRATORY COMPONENT:
Cluster of elements that involve breathing and the pulmonary system.
Oxygen Therapy Care – L35
Actions performed to support the administration of oxygen treatment.
Pulmonary Care – L36
Actions performed to support pulmonary hygiene.
   Breathing Exercises – L36.1
   Actions performed to provide therapy on respiratory or lung exertion.
   Chest Physiotherapy – L36.2
   Actions performed to provide exercises to provide postural drainage of lungs.
   Inhalation Therapy – L36.3
   Actions performed to support breathing treatments.
   Ventilator Care – L36.4
   Actions performed to control and monitor the use of a ventilator.
Tracheostomy Care – L37
Actions performed to support a tracheostomy.

M. – ROLE RELATIONSHIP COMPONENT:
Cluster of elements involving interpersonal, work, social, family, and sexual interactions.
Communication Care – M38
Actions performed to exchange verbal information.
Psychosocial Care – M39
Actions performed to support the study of psychological and social factors.
   Home Situation Analysis – M39.1
   Actions performed to analyze the living environment.
   Interpersonal Dynamics Analysis – M39.2
   Actions performed to support the analysis of the driving forces in a relationship between people.
   Family Process Analysis – M39.3
   Actions performed to support the change and/or modification of a related group.
   Sexual Behavior Analysis – M39.4
   Actions performed to support the change and/or modification of a person's sexual response.
   Social Network Analysis – M39.5
   Actions performed to improve the quantity or quality of personal relationships.

N. – SAFETY COMPONENT:
Cluster of elements that involve prevention of injury, danger, loss, or abuse.
Substance Abuse Control – N40
Actions performed to control situations to avoid, detect, or minimize harm.
   Tobacco Abuse Control – N40.1
   Actions performed to avoid, minimize, or control the use of tobacco.
   Alcohol Abuse Control – N40.2
   Actions performed to avoid, minimize, or control the use of distilled liquors.
   Drug Abuse Control – N40.3
   Actions performed to avoid, minimize, or control the use of any habit-forming medication.
Emergency Care – N41
Actions performed to support a sudden or unexpected occurrence.
Safety Precautions – N42
Actions performed to advance measures to avoid, danger, or harm.
   Environmental Safety – N42.1
   Precautions recommended to prevent or reduce environmental injury.

(Continued)

TABLE 14.11. CLINICAL CARE CLASSIFICATION OF 198 NURSING INTERVENTIONS (VERSION 2.0): CODED WITH DEFINITIONS AND CLASSIFIED BY 21 CARE COMPONENTS[a,b] (CONTINUED)

Equipment Safety – N42.2
Precautions recommended to prevent or reduce equipment injury.
Individual Safety – N42.3
Precautions to reduce individual injury.
Violence Control – N68
Actions performed to control behaviors that may cause harm to oneself or others.

O. – SELF-CARE COMPONENT:
Cluster of elements that involve the ability to carry out activities to maintain oneself.
Personal Care – O43
Actions performed to care for oneself.
  Activities of Daily Living (ADLs) – O43.1
  Actions performed to support personal activities to maintain oneself.
  Instrumental Activities of Daily Living (IADLs) – 043.2
  Complex activities performed to support basic life skills.

P. – SELF-CONCEPT COMPONENT:
Cluster of elements that involve an individual's mental image of oneself.
Mental Health Care – P45
Actions taken to promote emotional well-being.
  Mental Health History – P45.1
  Actions performed to obtain information about past or present emotional well-being.
  Mental Health Promotion – P45.2
  Actions performed to encourage or further emotional well-being.
  Mental Health Screening – P45.3
  Actions performed to systematically examine the emotional well-being.
  Mental Health Treatment – P45.4
  Actions performed to support protocols used to treat emotional problems.

Q. – SENSORY COMPONENT:
Cluster of elements that involve the senses including pain.
Pain Control – Q47
Actions performed to support responses to injury or damage.
  Acute Pain Control – Q47.1
  Actions performed to control physical suffering, hurting, or distress.
  Chronic Pain Control – Q47.2
  Actions performed to control physical suffering, hurting, or distress that continues longer than expected.
Comfort Care – Q48
Actions performed to enhance or improve well-being.
Ear Care – Q49
Actions performed to support ear problems.
  Hearing Aid Care – Q49.1
  Actions performed to control the use of a hearing aid.
  Wax Removal – Q49.2
  Actions performed to remove cerumen from ear.
Eye Care – Q50
Actions performed to support eye problems.
  Cataract Care – Q50.1
  Actions performed to control cataract conditions.
  Vision Care – Q50.2
  Actions performed to control vision problems.

R. – SKIN INTEGRITY COMPONENT:
Cluster of elements that involve the mucous membrane, corneal, integumentary, or subcutaneous structures of the body.

(Continued)

TABLE 14.11. (CONTINUED)

Pressure Ulcer Care – R51
Actions performed to prevent, detect, and treat skin integrity breakdown caused by pressure.
   Pressure Ulcer Stage 1 Care – R51.1
   Actions performed to prevent, detect, and treat Stage 1 skin breakdown.
   Pressure Ulcer Stage 2 Care – R51.2
   Actions performed to prevent, detect, and treat Stage 2 skin breakdown.
   Pressure Ulcer Stage 3 Care – R51.3
   Actions performed to prevent, detect, and treat Stage 3 skin breakdown.
   Pressure Ulcer Stage 4 Care – R51.4
   Actions performed to prevent, detect, and treat Stage 4 skin breakdown.
Mouth Care – R53
Actions performed to support oral cavity problems.
   Denture Care – R53.1
   Actions performed to control the use of artificial teeth.
Skin Care – R54
Actions to control the integument/skin.
   Skin Breakdown Control – R54.1
   Actions performed to support integument/skin problems.
Wound Care – R55
Actions performed to support open skin areas.
   Drainage Tube Care – R55.1
   Actions performed to support drainage from tubes.
   Dressing Change – R55.2
   Actions performed to remove and replace a new bandage to a wound.
   Incision Care – R55.3
   Actions performed to support a surgical wound.

S. – TISSUE PERFUSION COMPONENT:
Cluster of elements that involve the oxygenation of tissues including the circulatory and neurovascular systems.
Foot Care – S56
Actions performed to support foot problems.
Perineal Care – S57
Actions performed to support perineal problems.
Edema Control – S69
Actions performed to control excess fluid in tissue.
Circulatory Care – S70
Actions performed to support the circulation of the blood (blood vessels).
Neurovascular Care – S71
Actions performed to control problems of the nerves and vascular systems.

T. – URINARY ELIMINATION COMPONENT:
Cluster of elements that involve the genitourinary system.
Bladder Care – T58
Actions performed to control urinary drainage problems.
   Bladder Instillation – T58.1
   Actions performed to pour liquid through a catheter into the bladder.
   Bladder Training – T58.2
   Actions performed to provide instruction on the training care of urinary drainage.
Dialysis Care – T59
Actions performed to support dialysis treatments.
Urinary Catheter Care – T60
Actions performed to control the use of a urinary catheter.
   Urinary Catheter Insertion – T60.1
   Actions performed to place a urinary catheter in the bladder.

(Continued)

TABLE 14.11. CLINICAL CARE CLASSIFICATION OF 198 NURSING INTERVENTIONS (VERSION 2.0): CODED WITH DEFINITIONS AND CLASSIFIED BY 21 CARE COMPONENTS[a,b] (CONTINUED)

Urinary Catheter Irrigation – T60.2
Actions performed to flush a urinary catheter.
Urinary Incontinence Care – T72
Actions performed to control the inability to retain and/or involuntary retain urine.
Renal Care – T73
Actions performed to control problems pertaining to the kidney.

U. – LIFE CYCLE COMPONENT:
Cluster of elements that involve the life span of individuals.
Reproductive Care – U74
Actions performed to support the production of an offspring/child.
   Fertility Care – U74.1
   Actions performed to increase conception of an offspring/child.
   Infertility Care – U74.2
   Actions performed to support conception of the infertile client of an offspring/child.
   Contraception Care – U74.3
   Actions performed to prevent conception of an offspring/child.
Perinatal Care – U75
Actions performed to support perineal problems.
   Pregnancy Care – U75.1
   Actions performed to support the gestation period of the formation of an offspring/child (being with child).
   Labor Care – U75.2
   Actions performed to support the bringing forth of an offspring/child.
   Delivery Care – U75.3
   Actions performed to support the expulsion of an offspring/child at birth.
   Postpartum Care – U75.4
   Actions performed to support the time period immediately after the delivery of an offspring/child.
Growth & Development Care – U76
Actions performed to support normal standards of performing developmental skills and behavior of an individual of any age group.
   Newborn Care – U76.1 (first 30 days)
   Actions performed to support normal standards of performing developmental skills and behavior of an individual of a typical newborn for the first 30 days of life.
   Infant Care – U76.2 (31 days through 11 months)
   Actions performed to support normal standards of performing developmental skills and behavior of a typical infant 31 days through 11 months of age.
   Child Care – U76.3 (1 year through 11 years)
   Actions performed to support normal standards of performing developmental skills and behavior of a typical child 1 year through 11 years of age.
   Adolescent Care – U76.4 (12 years through 20 years)
   Actions performed to support normal standards of performing developmental skills and behavior of a typical adolescent 12 years through 20 years of age.
   Adult Care – U76.5 (21 years through 64 years)
   Actions performed to support normal standards of performing developmental skills and behavior of a typical adult 21 years through 64 years of age.
   Older Adult Care – U76.6 (65 years and over)
   Actions performed to support normal standards of performing developmental skills and behavior of typical older adult 65 years and over.

---

[a]Clinical Care Classification of Nursing Interventions (Version 2.0) includes 12 New Major Categories and 24 Subcategories. See Appendix Table A.3 for revisions from Home Health Care Classification (Version 1.0).
[b]The Clinical Care Classification System is copyrighted, placed in the Public Domain and cannot be sold, but is available with written permission.

TABLE 14.12. CLINICAL CARE CLASSIFICATION OF 198 NURSING INTERVENTIONS (VERSION 2.0): CODED ALPHABETICALLY WITH DEFINITIONS[a,b]

A01   Activity Care
  Actions performed to carry out physiological or psychological daily activities.

O43.1   Activities of Daily Living (ADLs)
  Personal activities to maintain oneself.

Q47.1   Acute Pain Control
  Actions performed to control physical suffering, hurting, or distress.

U76.4   Adolescent Care
  Actions performed to support the normal standards of performing developmental skills and behavior of a typical adolescent 12 years through 20 years of age.

U76.5   Adult Care
  Actions performed to support the normal standards of performing developmental skills and behavior of a typical adult 21 years through 64 years of age.

G17.1   Adult Day Center
  Actions performed to direct the provision of a day program for adults in a specific location.

N40.2   Alcohol Abuse Control
  Actions performed to avoid, minimize, or control the use of distilled liquors.

I26   Allergic Reaction Control
  Actions performed to reduce symptoms or precautions to reduce allergies.

A03.1   Ambulation Therapy
  Actions performed to promote walking.

A03.2   Assistive Device Therapy
  Actions performed to support the use of products to aid in caring for oneself.

A61   Bedbound Care
  Actions performed to support an individual confined to bed.

D10   Behavior Care
  Actions performed to support observable responses to internal and external stimuli.

E14.1   Bereavement Support
  Actions performed to provide comfort to the family/friends of the person who died.

G19.1   Bill of Rights
  Statements related to entitlement during an episode of illness.

T58   Bladder Care
  Actions performed to control urinary drainage problems.

T58.1   Bladder Instillation
  Actions performed to pour liquid into a catheter.

T58.2   Bladder Training
  Actions performed to provide instruction on the care of urinary drainage problems.

K33.1   Blood Pressure
  Actions performed to measure the diastolic and systolic pressure of the blood.

K32.1   Blood Specimen Care
  Actions performed to collect and/or examine a sample of blood.

B06   Bowel Care
  Actions performed to control or restore the functioning of the bowel.

B06.1   Bowel Training
  Actions performed to provide instruction on bowel elimination conditions.

J66   Breast-feeding Support
  Actions performed to support nourishment of an infant at the breast.

L36.1   Breathing Exercises
  Actions performed to provide therapy on respiratory or lung exertion.

C08   Cardiac Care
  Actions performed to control changes in the heart or blood vessels.

C08.1   Cardiac Rehabilitation
  Actions performed to restore cardiac health.

A02.1   Cast Care
  Actions performed to control a rigid dressing.

(Continued)

TABLE 14.12. CLINICAL CARE CLASSIFICATION OF 198 NURSING INTERVENTIONS (VERSION 2.0): CODED ALPHABETICALLY WITH DEFINITIONS[a,b] (CONTINUED)

Q50.1   Cataract Care
       Actions performed to control cataract conditions.

H22   Chemotherapy Care
       Actions performed to control and monitor antineoplastic agents.

L36.2   Chest Physiotherapy
       Exercises to provide postural drainage of lungs.

U76.3   Child Care
       Actions performed to support the normal standards of performing developmental skills and behavior of a typical child 1 year through 11 years of age.

Q47.2   Chronic Pain Control
       Actions performed to control physical suffering, hurting, or distress that continues longer than expected.

S70   Circulatory Care
       Actions performed to support the circulation of the blood (blood vessels).

K31.4   Clinical Measurements
       Actions performed to conduct procedures to evaluate somatic events.

Q48   Comfort Care
       Actions performed to enhance or improve well-being.

G18   Compliance Care
       Actions performed to encourage conformity to therapeutic recommendations.

G18.1   Compliance with Diet
       Actions performed to encourage conformity to food or fluid intake.

G18.2   Compliance with Fluid Volume
       Actions performed to encourage conformity to therapeutic intake of liquids.

G18.3   Compliance with Medical Regimen
       Actions performed to encourage conformity to physician's plan of care.

G18.4   Compliance with Medication Regimen
       Actions performed to encourage conformity to follow prescribed course of medicinal substances.

G18.5   Compliance with Safety Precautions
       Actions performed to encourage conformity with measures to protect the self or others from injury, danger, or loss.

G18.6   Compliance with Therapeutic Regimen
       Actions performed to encourage conformity with the health team's plan of care.

M38   Communication Care
       Actions performed to exchange verbal information.

G17   Community Special Services
       Actions performed to provide advice or information about special community services.

U74.3   Contraception Care
       Actions performed to prevent conception of an offspring/child.

E12.1   Coping Support
       Actions performed to sustain a person dealing with responsibilities, problems, or difficulties.

E12   Counseling Service
       Actions performed to provide advice or instruction to help another.

E12.3   Crisis Therapy
       Actions performed to sustain a person dealing with a condition, event, or radical change in status.

U75.3   Delivery Care
       Actions performed to support the expulsion of an offspring/child at birth.

R53.1   Denture Care
       Actions performed to control the use of artificial teeth.

I27   Diabetic Care
       Actions performed to control diabetic conditions.

T59   Dialysis Care
       Actions performed to support dialysis treatments.

(Continued)

TABLE 14.12. (CONTINUED)

B06.4	Diarrhea Care
	Actions performed to control the abnormal frequency and fluidity of feces.
B06.2	Disimpaction
	Actions performed to manually remove feces.
R55.1	Drainage Tube Care
	Actions performed to control drainage from tubes.
R55.2	Dressing Change
	Actions performed to remove and replace new bandage(s) to a wound.
N40.3	Drug Abuse Control
	Actions performed to avoid, minimize, or control the use of any habit-forming medication.
E14.2	Dying/Death Measures
	Actions performed to support the dying process.
Q49	Ear Care
	Actions performed to support ear problems.
S69	Edema Control
	Actions performed to control excess fluid in tissue.
N41	Emergency Care
	Actions performed to support a sudden or unexpected occurrence.
E13	Emotional Support
	Actions performed to sustain a positive affective state.
B06.3	Enema
	Actions performed to administer fluid rectally.
A01.2	Energy Conservation
	Actions performed taken to preserve energy.
J29.5	Enteral Feeding
	Actions performed to provide nourishment through a gastrointestinal route.
J28	Enteral Tube Care
	Actions performed to control the use of an enteral drainage tube.
J28.1	Enteral Tube Insertion
	Actions performed in the placement of an enteral drainage tube.
J28.2	Enteral Tube Irrigation
	Actions performed to flush or wash out an enteral tube.
N42.1	Environmental Safety
	Precautions recommended to prevent or reduce environmental injury.
N42.2	Equipment Safety
	Precautions recommended to prevent or reduce equipment injury.
Q50	Eye Care
	Actions performed to support eye problems.
M39.3	Family Process Analysis
	Actions performed to support the change and/or modification of a related group.
J29.2	Feeding Technique
	Actions performed to provide special measures to provide nourishment.
U74.1	Fertility Care
	Actions performed to promote the development of an offspring/child.
F15	Fluid Therapy
	Actions performed to provide liquid volume intake.
S56	Foot Care
	Actions performed to support foot problems.
A02	Fracture Care
	Actions performed to control broken bones.
E14.3	Funeral Arrangements
	Actions performed to direct the preparatory measures for burial.
B62	Gastric Care
	Actions performed to control changes in the stomach or intestines.

(Continued)

TABLE 14.12. CLINICAL CARE CLASSIFICATION OF 198 NURSING INTERVENTIONS (VERSION 2.0): CODED ALPHABETICALLY WITH DEFINITIONS[a,b] **(CONTINUED)**

U76	Growth & Development Care	
	Actions performed to support the normal standards of performing developmental skills and behavior of an individual typical of any age group.	
G21.1	Health Aide Service	
	Actions performed to support the provision of home care services by a home health aide.	
K31.1	Health History	
	Actions performed to obtain information about past illness and health status.	
K31.2	Health Promotion	
	Actions performed to encourage behaviors to enhance health state.	
Q49.1	Hearing Aid Care	
	Actions performed to control the use of a hearing aid.	
M39.1	Home Situation Analysis	
	Analysis of living environment.	
G17.2	Hospice	
	Actions performed to support the provision of offering and/or providing care for terminally ill persons.	
F15.1	Hydration Control	
	Actions performed to control the state of fluid balance.	
A02.2	Immobilizer Care	
	Actions performed to control a splint, cast, or prescribed bed rest.	
I65	Immunologic Care	
	Actions performed to protect against a particular disease.	
R55.3	Incision Care	
	Actions performed to support a surgical wound.	
N42.3	Individual Safety	
	Precautions to reduce individual injury.	
U76.2	Infant Care	
	Actions performed to support the normal standards of performing developmental skills and behavior of a typical infant 31 days through 11 month of age.	
K30	Infection Control	
	Actions performed to contain a communicable illness.	
U74.2	Infertility Care	
	Actions performed to prevent the development of an offspring/child (promote barreness).	
F16	Infusion Care	
	Actions performed to support solutions given via vein.	
L36.3	Inhalation Therapy	
	Actions performed to support breathing treatments.	
H23	Injection Administration	
	Actions performed to dispense a medication by a hypodermic.	
O43.2	Instrumental Activities of Daily Living (IADLs)	
	Complex activities performed to support basic life skills.	
H23.1	Insulin Injection	
	Actions performed to dispense a hypodermic administration of insulin.	
F15.2	Intake/Output	
	Actions performed to measure the amount of fluids/food and excretion of waste.	
M39.2	Interpersonal Dynamics Analysis	
	Analysis of the driving forces in a relationship between people.	
F16.1	Intravenous Care	
	Actions performed to administer an infusion via a vein.	
U75.2	Labor Care	
	Actions performed to support the bringing forth of an offspring/child.	
G17.3	Meals-on-Wheels	
	Actions performed to direct the provision of community program of meals delivered to the home.	
G20.1	Medical Regimen Orders	
	Actions performed to support the physician's plan of treatment.	

(Continued)

TABLE 14.12. (CONTINUED)

G21.2   Medical Social Worker Service
         Actions performed to provide advice or instruction by medical social worker.

H24.1   Medication Actions
         Activities related to monitor the use of medicinal substances.

H24   Medication Care
         Actions performed to direct the dispensing of prescribed drugs.

H24.2   Medication Pre-fill Preparation
         Activities to ensure the continued supply of prescribed drugs.

H24.3   Medication Side Effects
         Actions performed to control untoward reactions or conditions to prescribed drugs.

H24.4   Medication Treatment
         Actions performed to administer drugs or remedies regardless of route.

D64   Memory Loss Care
         Actions performed to control a person's inability to recall ideas and/or events.

P45   Mental Health Care
         Actions taken to promote emotional well-being.

P45.1   Mental Health History
         Actions performed to obtain information about past and present emotional well-being.

P45.2   Mental Health Promotion
         Actions performed to encourage or further emotional well-being.

P45.3   Mental Health Screening
         Actions performed to systematically examine the emotional well-being.

P45.4   Mental Health Treatment
         Actions performed to support protocols used to treat emotional problems.

A03   Mobility Therapy
         Actions performed to advise and instruct on mobility deficits.

R53   Mouth Care
         Actions performed to support oral cavity problems.

A05   Musculosketal Care
         Actions performed to restore physical functioning.

B62.1   Nausea Care
         Actions performed to control the distaste for food and desire to vomit.

S71   Neurovascular Care
         Actions performed to control problems of the nerves and vascular systems.

U76.1   Newborn Care
         Actions performed to support the normal standards of performing development skills and behavior of a typical newborn for the first 30 days of life.

G21.3   Nurse Specialist Service
         Actions performed to obtain advice or instruction by advanced nurse specialists or nurse practitioners.

G19.2   Nursing Care Coordination
         Actions performed to synthesize all plans of care.

G19   Nursing Contact
         Actions performed to communicate with another nurse.

G19.3   Nursing Status Report
         Actions performed to document condition by nurse.

J29   Nutrition Care
         Actions performed to support the intake of food and nutrients.

G21.4   Occupational Therapist Service
         Actions performed to provide advice or instruction by occupational therapist.

U76.6   Older Adult Care
         Actions performed to support the normal standards of performing developmental skills and behavior of a typical older adult 65 years of age and over.

(Continued)

TABLE 14.12. CLINICAL CARE CLASSIFICATION OF 198 NURSING INTERVENTIONS (VERSION 2.0): CODED ALPHABETICALLY WITH DEFINITIONS[a,b] (CONTINUED)

B07	Ostomy Care	
	Actions performed to control the artificial opening that removes waste products.	
B07.1	Ostomy Irrigation	
	Actions performed to flush or wash out an ostomy.	
L35	Oxygen Therapy Care	
	Actions performed to support the administration of oxygen treatment.	
C09	Pacemaker Care	
	Actions performed to control the use of an electronic device that provides a normal heartbeat.	
Q47	Pain Control	
	Actions performed to support responses to injury or damage.	
J29.6	Parenteral Feeding	
	Actions performed to provide nourishment through intravenous or subcutaneous routes.	
U75	Perinatal Care	
	Actions performed to support the period before, during, and immediately after the creation of an offspring/child.	
S57	Perineal Care	
	Actions performed to support perineal problems.	
O43	Personal Care	
	Actions performed to care for oneself.	
K31.3	Physical Examination	
	Actions performed to observe somatic events.	
K31	Physical Health Care	
	Actions performed to support somatic problems.	
G21.5	Physical Therapist Service	
	Actions performed to obtain advice or instruction by physical therapist.	
G20	Physician Contact	
	Actions performed to communicate with a physician.	
G20.2	Physician Status Report	
	Actions performed to document condition by physician.	
A61.1	Positioning Therapy	
	Process to support changes in body position.	
U75.4	Postpartum Care	
	Actions performed to support the time period immediately after delivery of an offspring/child.	
U75.1	Pregnancy Care	
	Actions performed to support the gestation period of the formation of an offspring/child (being with child).	
R51	Pressure Ulcer Care	
	Actions performed to prevent, detect, and treat skin integrity breakdown caused by pressure.	
R51.1	Pressure Ulcer Stage 1 Care	
	Actions performed to prevent Stage 1 skin breakdown.	
R51.2	Pressure Ulcer Stage 2 Care	
	Actions performed to prevent Stage 2 skin breakdown.	
R51.3	Pressure Ulcer Stage 3 Care	
	Actions performed to prevent Stage 3 skin breakdown.	
R1.4	Pressure Ulcer Stage 4 Care	
	Actions performed to prevent Stage 4 skin breakdown.	
G21	Professional/Ancillary Services	
	Actions performed to support the duties performed by health team members.	
M39	Psychosocial Care	
	Study of psychological and social factors.	
L36	Pulmonary Care	
	Actions performed to support pulmonary hygiene.	
K33.3	Pulse	
	Actions performed to measure rhythmical beats of the heart.	
H25	Radiation Therapy Care	
	Actions performed to control and monitor radiation therapy.	

(Continued)

TABLE 14.12. (CONTINUED)

A05.1	Range of Motion	

Actions performed to provide the active or passive exercises to maintain joint function.

D11   Reality Orientation
Actions performed to promote the ability to locate oneself in environment.

J29.3   Regular Diet
Actions performed to support the ingestion of food and nutrients from established nutrition standards.

A05.2   Rehabilitation Exercise
Activities to promote physical functioning.

T73   Renal Care
Actions performed to control problems pertaining to the kidney.

U74   Reproductive Care
Actions performed to support the production of an offspring child.

K33.4   Respiration
Actions performed to measure the function of breathing.

N42   Safety Precautions
Actions performed to advance measures to avoid injury, danger, or harm.

M39.4   Sexual Behavior Analysis
Actions performed to support the change and/or modification of a person's sexual response.

R54.1   Skin Breakdown Control
Actions performed to support integument/skin problems.

R54   Skin Care
Actions performed to control the integument/skin.

A04   Sleep Pattern Control
Actions performed to support the sleep and wake cycles.

M39.5   Social Network Analysis
Actions performed to improve the quantity or quality of personal relationships.

J29.4   Special Diet
Actions performed to support the ingestion of food and nutrients prescribed for a specific purpose.

K32   Specimen Care
Actions performed to direct the collection and/or examination of a bodily specimen.

G21.6   Speech Therapist Service
Actions performed to provide advice or instruction by speech therapist.

E13.1   Spiritual Comfort
Actions performed to console, restore, or promote spiritual health.

K32.5   Sputum Specimen Care
Actions performed to collect and/or examine a sample of sputum.

K32.2   Stool Specimen Care
Actions performed to collect and/or examine a sample of feces.

E12.2   Stress Control
Actions performed to support the physiological response of the body to a stimulus.

N40   Substance Abuse Control
Actions performed to control situations to avoid, detect, or minimize harm.

K33.2   Temperature
Actions performed to measure body temperature.

E14   Terminal Care
Actions performed in the period of time surrounding death.

N40.1   Tobacco Abuse Control
Actions performed to avoid, minimize, or control the use of tobacco products.

L37   Tracheostomy Care
Actions performed to support a tracheostomy.

A03.3   Transfer Care
Actions performed to assist in moving from one place to another.

T60   Urinary Catheter Care
Actions performed to control the use of a urinary catheter.

(Continued)

TABLE 14.12. CLINICAL CARE CLASSIFICATION OF 198 NURSING INTERVENTIONS (VERSION 2.0): CODED ALPHABETICALLY WITH DEFINITIONS[a,b] (CONTINUED)

T60.1	Urinary Catheter Insertion	
	Actions performed to place a urinary catheter in bladder.	
T60.2	Urinary Catheter Irrigation	
	Actions performed to flush out a urinary catheter.	
T72	Urinary Incontinence Care	
	Actions performed to control the inability to retain and/or involuntary retain urine.	
K32.3	Urine Specimen Care	
	Actions performed to collect and/or examine a sample of urine.	
K30.1	Universal Precautions	
	Practices to prevent spread of infection and infectious diseases.	
F16.2	Venous Catheter Care	
	Actions performed to control the use of infusion equipment.	
L36.4	Ventilator Care	
	Actions performed to control and monitor the use of a ventilator.	
N68	Violence Control	
	Actions performed to control behaviors that may cause harm to oneself or others.	
Q50.2	Vision Care	
	Actions performed to control vision problems.	
K33	Vital Signs	
	Actions performed to measure temperature, pulse, respirations, and blood pressure.	
H23.2	Vitamin B12 Injection	
	Actions performed to administer a hypodermic of Vitamin B12.	
D63	Wandering Control	
	Actions performed to control abnormal movability.	
Q49.2	Wax Removal	
	Actions performed to remove cerumen from the ear.	
J67	Weight Control	
	Actions performed to control obesity or debilitation.	
R55	Wound Care	
	Actions performed to support open skin areas.	

[a]Clinical Care Classification of Nursing Interventions (Version 2.0) includes 12 New Major Categories and 24 Subcategories. See Appendix Table A.3 for revisions from Home Health Care Classification (Version 1.0).
[b]The Clinical Care Classification System is copyrighted, placed in the Public Domain, and cannot be sold, but is available with written permission.

TABLE 14.13. CLINICAL CARE CLASSIFICATION OF 198 NURSING INTERVENTIONS (VERSION 2.0): LISTED ALPHABETICALLY BY CODE NUMBERS[a,b]

Activity Care	A01
Activities of Daily Living (ADLs)	O43.1
Acute Pain Control	Q47.1
Adolescent Care	U76.4
Adult Care	U76.5
Adult Day Center	G17.1
Alcohol Abuse Control	N40.2
Allergic Reaction Analysis	I26
Ambulation Therapy	A03.1
Assistive Device Therapy	A03.2
Bedbound Care	A61
Behavior Care	D10
Bereavement Support	E14.1
Bill of Rights	G19.1
Bladder Care	T58
Bladder Instillation	T58.1
Bladder Training	T58.2
Blood Pressure	K33.1
Blood Specimen Care	K32.1
Bowel Care	B06
Bowel Training	B06.1
Breast-feeding Support	J66
Breathing Exercises	L36.1
Cardiac Care	C08
Cardiac Rehabilitation	C08.1
Cast Care	A02.1
Cataract Care	Q50.1
Chemotherapy Care	H22
Chest Physiotherapy	L36.2
Child Care	U76.3
Chronic Pain Control	Q47.2
Circulatory Care	S70
Clinical Measurements	K31.4
Comfort Care	Q48
Compliance Care	G18
Compliance with Diet	G18.1
Compliance with Fluid Volume	G18.2
Compliance with Medical Regimen	G18.3
Compliance with Medication Regimen	G18.4
Compliance with Safety Precautions	G18.5
Compliance with Therapeutic Regimen	G18.6
Communication Care	M38
Community Special Services	G17
Contraception Care	U74.3
Coping Support	E12.1
Counseling Services	E12
Crisis Therapy	E12.3
Delivery Care	U75.3
Denture Care	R53.1
Diabetic Care	I27

(Continued)

TABLE 14.13. CLINICAL CARE CLASSIFICATION OF 198 NURSING INTERVENTIONS (VERSION 2.0): LISTED ALPHABETICALLY BY CODE NUMBERS[a,b] (CONTINUED)

Dialysis Care T60
Diarrhea Care B06.4
Disimpaction B06.2
Drainage Tube Care R55.1
Dressing Change R55.2
Drug Abuse Control N40.3
Dying/Death Measures E14.2

Ear Care Q49
Edema Control S69
Emergency Care N41
Emotional Support E13
Enema B06.3
Energy Conservation A01.2
Enteral Feeding J29.5
Enteral Tube Care J28
Enteral Tube Insertion J28.1
Enteral Tube Irrigation J28.2
Environmental Safety N42.1
Equipment Safety N42.2
Eye Care Q50

Family Process Analysis M39.3
Feeding Technique J29.2
Fertility Care U74.1
Fluid Therapy F15
Foot Care S56
Fracture Care A02
Funeral Arrangements E14.3

Gastric Care B62
Growth & Development Care U76

Health Aide Service G21.1
Health History K31.1
Health Promotion K31.2
Hearing Aid Care Q49.1
Home Situation Analysis M39.1
Hospice G17.2
Hydration Control F15.1

Immobilizer Care A02.2
Immunological Care I65
Incision Care R55.3
Individual Safety N42.3
Infant Care U76.2
Infection Control K30
Infertility Care U74.2
Infusion Care F16
Inhalation Therapy L36.3
Injection Administration H23
Instrumental Activities of Daily Living (IADLs) O43.2
Insulin Injection H23.1
Intake/Output F15.2
Interpersonal Dynamics Analysis M39.2
Intravenous Care F16.1

Labor Care U75.2

(Continued)

TABLE 14.13. (CONTINUED)

Meals-on-Wheels G17.3
Medical Regimen Orders G20.1
Medical Social Worker Service G21.2
Medication Actions H24.1
Medication Care H24
Medication Pre-fill Preparation H24.2
Medication Side Effects H24.3
Medication Treatment H24.4
Memory Loss Care D64
Mental Health Care P45
Mental Health History P45.1
Mental Health Promotion P45.2
Mental Health Screening P45.3
Mental Health Treatment P45.4
Mobility Therapy A03
Mouth Care R53
Musculosketal Care A05

Nausea Care B62.1
Neurovascular Care S71
Newborn Care U76.1
Nurse Specialist Service G21.3
Nursing Care Coordination G19.2
Nursing Contact G19
Nursing Status Report G19.3
Nutrition Care J29

Occupational Therapist Service G21.4
Older Adult Care U76.6
Ostomy Care B07
Ostomy Irrigation B07.1
Oxygen Therapy Care L35

Pacemaker Care C09
Pain Control Q47
Parenteral Feeding J29.6
Perinatal Care U75
Perineal Care S57
Personal Care O43
Physical Examination K31.3
Physical Health Care K31
Physical Therapist Services G21.5
Physician Contact G20
Physician Status Report G20.2
Positioning Therapy A61.1
Postpartum Care U75.4
Pregnancy Care U75.1
Pressure Ulcer Care R51
Pressure Ulcer Stage 1 Care R51.1
Pressure Ulcer Stage 2 Care R51.2
Pressure Ulcer Stage 3 Care R51.3
Pressure Ulcer Stage 4 Care R51.4
Professional/Ancillary Services G21
Psychosocial Care M39
Pulmonary Care L36
Pulse K33.3

(Continued)

TABLE 14.13. CLINICAL CARE CLASSIFICATION OF 198 NURSING INTERVENTIONS (VERSION 2.0): LISTED ALPHABETICALLY BY CODE NUMBERS[a,b] (CONTINUED)

Radiation Therapy Care H25
Range of Motion A05.1
Reality Orientation D11
Regular Diet J29.3
Rehabilitation Exercise A05.2
Renal Care T73
Reproductive Care U74
Respiration K33.4

Safety Precautions N42
Sexual Behavior Analysis M39.4
Skin Breakdown Control R54.1
Skin Care R54
Sleep Pattern Control A04
Social Network Analysis M39.5
Special Diet J29.4
Specimen Care K32
Speech Therapist Service G21.6
Spiritual Comfort E13.1
Sputum Specimen Care K32.5
Stool Specimen Care K32.2
Stress Control E12.2
Substance Abuse Control N40

Temperature K33.2
Terminal Care E14
Tobacco Abuse Control N40.1
Tracheostomy Care L37
Transfer Care A03.3

Urinary Catheter Care T60
Urinary Catheter Insertion T60.1
Urinary Catheter Irrigation T60.2
Urinary Incontinence Care T72
Urine Specimen Care K23.3
Universal Precautions K30.1

Venous Catheter Care F16.2
Ventilator Care L36.4
Violence Control N68
Vision Care Q50.2
Vital Signs K33
Vitamin B12 Injection H23.2

Wandering Control D63
Wax Removal Q.49.2
Weight Control J67
Wound Care R55

[a]Clinical Care Classification of Nursing Interventions (Version 2.0) includes 12 New Major Categories and 24 Subcategories. See Appendix Table A.3 for revisions from Home Health Care Classification (Version 1.0).
[b]The Clinical Care Classification System is copyrighted, placed in the Public Domain, and cannot be sold, but is available with written permission.

TABLE 14.14. CLINICAL CARE CLASSIFICATION OF 198 NURSING INTERVENTIONS (VERSION 2.0): CODED WITH DEFINITIONS, FOUR ACTION TYPES, AND CLASSIFIED BY 21 CARE COMPONENTS[a,b]

Assess/Monitor – *Collect and analyze data on the health status*
Care/Perform – *Perform a therapeutic action*
Teach/Instruct – *Provide knowledge and skill*
Manage/Refer – *Coordinate and refer*

A. – ACTIVITY COMPONENT:
Cluster of elements that involve the use of energy in carrying out musculoskeletal and bodily actions.

Activity Care – A01
Activities performed to carry out physiological or psychological daily activities.
A01.0.1. Assess Activity Care
A01.0.2. Care Activity Care
A01.0.3. Teach Activity Care
A01.0.4. Manage Activity Care
  Energy Conservation – A01.2
  Actions performed to preserve energy.
  A01.2.1. Assess Energy Conservation
  A01.2.2. Care Energy Conservation
  A01.2.3. Teach Energy Conservation
  A01.2.4. Manage Energy Conservation

Fracture Care – A02
Actions performed to control broken bones.
A02.0.1. Assess Fracture Care
A02.0.2. Care Fracture Care
A02.0.3. Teach Fracture Care
A02.0.4. Manage Fracture Care
  Cast Care – A02.1
  Actions performed to control a rigid dressing.
  A02.1.1. Assess Cast Care
  A02.1.2. Care Cast Care
  A02.1.3. Teach Cast Care
  A02.1.4. Manage Cast Care
  Immobilizer Care – A02.2
  Actions performed to control a splint, cast, or prescribed bed rest.
  A02.2.1. Assess Immobilizer Care
  A02.2.2. Care Immobilizer Care
  A02.2.3. Teach Immobilizer Care
  A02.2.4. Manage Immobilizer Care

Mobility Therapy – A03
Actions performed to advise and instruct on mobility deficits.
A03.0.1. Assess Mobility Therapy
A03.0.2. Care Mobility Therapy
A03.0.3. Teach Mobility Therapy
A03.0.4. Manage Mobility Therapy
  Ambulation Therapy – A03.1
  Actions performed to promote walking.
  A03.1.1. Assess Ambulation Therapy
  A03.1.2. Care Ambulation Therapy
  A03.1.3. Teach Ambulation Therapy
  A03.1.4. Manage Ambulation Therapy
  Assistive Device Therapy – A03.2
  Actions performed to support the use of products to aid in caring for oneself.

A03.2.1. Assess Assistive Device Therapy
A03.2.2. Care Assistive Device Therapy
A03.2.3. Teach Assistive Device Therapy
A03.2.4. Manage Assistive Device Therapy
  Transfer Care – A03.3
  Actions performed to assist in moving from one place to another.
  A03.3.1. Assess Transfer Care
  A03.3.2. Care Transfer Care
  A03.3.3. Teach Transfer Care
  A03.3.4. Manage Transfer Care

Sleep Pattern Control – A04
Actions performed to support the sleep and wake cycles.
A04.0.1. Assess Sleep Pattern Control
A04.0.2. Care Sleep Pattern Control
A04.0.3. Teach Sleep Pattern Control
A04.0.4. Manage Sleep Pattern Control

Musculosketal Care – A05
Actions performed to restore physical functioning.
A05.0.1. Assess Rehabilitation Care
A05.0.2. Care Rehabilitation Care
A05.0.3. Teach Rehabilitation Care
A05.0.4. Manage Rehabilitation Care
  Range of Motion – A05.1
  Actions performed to provide the active and passive exercises to maintain joint function.
  A05.1.1. Assess Range of Motion
  A05.1.2. Care Range of Motion
  A05.1.3. Teach Range of Motion
  A05.1.4. Manage Range of Motion
  Rehabilitation Exercise – A05.2
  Actions performed to promote physical functioning.
  A05.2.1. Assess Rehabilitation Exercise
  A05.2.2. Care Rehabilitation Exercise
  A05.2.3. Teach Rehabilitation Exercise
  A05.2.4. Manage Rehabilitation Exercise

Bedbound Care – A61
Actions performed to support an individual confined to bed.
A61.0.1. Assess Bedbound Care
A61.0.2. Care Bedbound Care
A61.0.3. Teach Bedbound Care
A61.0.4. Manage Bedbound Care
  Positioning Therapy – A61.1
  Process to support changes in body positioning.
  A61.1.1. Assess Positioning Therapy
  A61.1.2. Care Positioning Therapy
  A61.1.3. Teach Positioning Therapy
  A61.1.4. Manage Positioning Therapy

(Continued)

TABLE 14.14. CLINICAL CARE CLASSIFICATION OF 198 NURSING INTERVENTIONS (VERSION 2.0): CODED WITH DEFINITIONS, FOUR ACTION TYPES, AND CLASSIFIED BY 21 CARE COMPONENTS[a,b] (CONTINUED)

B. – BOWEL/GASTRIC COMPONENT:
Cluster of elements that involve the gastrointestinal system.
Bowel Care – B06
Actions performed to control and restore the functioning of the bowel.
B06.0.1. Assess Bowel Care
B06.0.2. Care Bowel Care
B06.0.3. Teach Bowel Care
B06.0.4. Manage Bowel Care
Bowel Training – B06.1
Actions performed to provide instruction on bowel elimination conditions.
B06.1.1. Assess Bowel Training
B06.1.2. Care Bowel Training
B06.1.3. Teach Bowel Training
B06.1.4. Manage Bowel Training
Disimpaction – B06.2
Actions performed to manually remove feces.
B06.2.1. Assess Disimpaction
B06.2.2. Care Disimpaction
B06.2.3. Teach Disimpaction
B06.2.4. Manage Disimpaction
Enema – B06.3
Actions performed to administer fluid rectally.
B06.3.1. Assess Enema
B06.3.2. Care Enema
B06.3.3. Teach Enema
B06.3.4. Manage Enema
Diarrhea Care – B06.4
Actions performed to control the abnormal frequency and fluidity of feces.
B06.4.1. Assess Diarrhea Care
B06.4.2. Care Diarrhea Care
B06.4.3. Teach Diarrhea Care
B06.4.4. Manage Diarrhea Care
Ostomy Care – B07
Actions performed to control the artificial opening that removes waste products.
B07.0.1. Assess Ostomy Care
B07.0.2. Care Ostomy Care
B07.0.3. Teach Ostomy Care
B07.0.4. Manage Ostomy Care
Ostomy Irrigation – B07.1
Actions performed to flush or wash out an ostomy.
B07.1.1. Assess Ostomy Irrigation
B07.1.2. Care Ostomy Irrigation
B07.1.3. Teach Ostomy Irrigation
B07.1.4. Manage Ostomy Irrigation
Gastric Care – B62
Actions performed to control changes in the stomach and intestines.
B62.0.1. Assess Gastric Care
B62.0.2. Care Gastric Care
B62.0.3. Teach Gastric Care
B62.0.4. Manage Gastric Care

Nausea Care – B62.1
Actions performed to control the distaste for food and desire to vomit.
B62.1.1. Assess Nausea Care
B62.1.2. Care Nausea Care
B62.1.3. Teach Nausea Care
B62.1.4. Manage Nausea Care

C. – CARDIAC COMPONENT:
Cluster of elements that involve the heart and blood vessels.
Cardiac Care – C08
Actions performed to control changes in the heart or blood vessels.
C08.0.1. Assess Cardiac Care
C08.0.2. Care Cardiac Care
C08.0.3. Teach Cardiac Care
C08.0.4. Manage Cardiac Care
Cardiac Rehabilitation – C08.1
Actions performed to restore cardiac health.
C08.1.1. Assess Cardiac Rehabilitation
C08.1.2. Care Cardiac Rehabilitation
C08.1.3. Teach Cardiac Rehabilitation
C08.1.4. Manage Cardiac Rehabilitation
Pacemaker Care – C09
Actions performed to control the use of an electronic device that provides a normal heartbeat.
C09.0.1. Assess Pacemaker Care
C09.0.2. Care Pacemaker Care
C09.0.3. Teach Pacemaker Care
C09.0.4. Manage Pacemaker Care

D. – COGNITIVE COMPONENT:
Cluster of elements involving the mental and cerebral processes.
Behavior Care – D10
Actions performed to support observable responses to internal and external stimuli.
D10.0.1. Assess Behavior Care
D10.0.2. Care Behavior Care
D10.0.3. Teach Behavior Care
D10.0.4. Manage Behavior Care
Reality Orientation – D11
Actions performed to promote the ability to locate oneself in an environment.
D11.0.1. Assess Reality Orientation
D11.0.2. Care Reality Orientation
D11.0.3. Teach Reality Orientation
D11.0.4. Manage Reality Orientation
Wandering Control – D63
Actions performed to control abnormal movability.
D63.0.1. Assess Wandering Control
D63.0.2. Care Wandering Control
D63.0.3. Teach Wandering Control
D63.0.4. Manage Wandering Control
Memory Loss Care –D64
Actions performed to control a person's inability to recall ideas and/or events.

(Continued)

TABLE 14.14. (CONTINUED)

D64.0.1. Assess Memory Loss Care
D64.0.2. Care Memory Loss Care
D64.0.3. Teach Memory Loss Care
D64.0.4. Manage Memory Loss Care

E. – COPING COMPONENT:
Cluster of elements that involve the ability to deal with responsibilities, problems, or difficulties.
Counseling Service – E12
Actions performed to provide advice or instruction to help another.
E12.0.1. Assess Counseling Service
E12.0.2. Care Counseling Service
E12.0.3. Teach Counseling Service
E12.0.4. Manage Counseling Service

  Coping Support – E12.1
  Actions performed to sustain a person dealing with responsibilities, problems, or difficulties.
  E12.1.1. Assess Coping Support
  E12.1.2. Care Coping Support
  E12.1.3. Teach Coping Support
  E12.1.4. Manage Coping Support

  Stress Control – E12.2
  Actions performed to support the physiological response of the body to a stimulus.
  E12.2.1. Assess Stress Control
  E12.2.2. Care Stress Control
  E12.2.3. Teach Stress Control
  E12.2.4. Manage Stress Control

  Crisis Therapy – E12.3
  Actions performed to sustain a person dealing with a condition, event, or radical change in status.
  E12.3.1. Assess Crisis Therapy
  E12.3.2. Care Crisis Therapy
  E12.3.3. Teach Crisis Therapy
  E12.3.4. Manage Crisis Therapy

Emotional Support – E13
Actions performed to maintain a positive affective state.
E13.0.1. Assess Emotional Support
E13.0.2. Care Emotional Support
E13.0.3. Teach Emotional Support
E13.0.4. Manage Emotional Support

  Spiritual Comfort – E13.1
  Actions performed to console, restore, or promote spiritual health.
  E13.1.1. Assess Spiritual Comfort
  E13.1.2. Care Spiritual Comfort
  E13.1.3. Teach Spiritual Comfort
  E13.1.4. Manage Spiritual Comfort

Terminal Care – E14
Actions performed in the period surrounding death.
E14.0.1. Assess Terminal Care – *Collect and analyze data on the health status*
E14.0.2. Care Terminal Care
E14.0.3. Teach Terminal Care
E14.0.4. Manage Terminal Care

Bereavement Support – E14.1
Actions performed to provide comfort to the family/friends of the person who died.
E14.1.1. Assess Bereavement Support
E14.1.2. Care Bereavement Support
E14.1.3. Teach Bereavement Support
E14.1.4. Manage Bereavement Support
Dying/Death Measures – E14.2
Actions performed to support the dying process.
E14.2.1. Assess Dying/Death Measures
E14.2.2. Care Dying/Death Measures
E14.2.3. Teach Dying/Death Measures
E14.2.4. Manage Dying/Death Measures
Funeral Arrangements – E14.3
Actions performed to direct the preparatory for burial.
E14.3.1. Assess Funeral Arrangements
E14.3.2. Care Funeral Arrangements
E14.3.3. Teach Funeral Arrangements
E14.3.4. Manage Funeral Arrangements

F. – FLUID VOLUME COMPONENT:
Cluster of elements that involve liquid consumption.
Fluid Therapy – F15.0
Actions performed to provide liquid volume intake.
F15.0.1. Assess Fluid Therapy
F15.0.2. Care Fluid Therapy
F15.0.3. Teach Fluid Therapy
F15.0.4. Manage Fluid Therapy

  Hydration Control – F15.1
  Actions performed to control the state of fluid balance.
  F15.1.1. Assess Hydration Control
  F15.1.2. Care Hydration Control
  F15.1.3. Teach Hydration Control
  F15.1.4. Manage Hydration Control

  Intake/Output – F15.2
  Actions performed to measure the amount of fluid/food and excretion of waste.
  F15.2.1. Assess Intake/Output
  F15.2.2. Care Intake/Output
  F15.2.3. Teach Intake/Output
  F15.2.4. Manage Intake/Output

Infusion Care – F16
Actions performed to support solutions given through the vein.
F16.0.1. Assess Infusion Care
F16.0.2. Care Infusion Care
F16.0.3. Teach Infusion Care
F16.0.4. Manage Infusion Care

  Intravenous Care – F16.1
  Actions performed to administer an infusion through a vein.
  F16.1.1. Assess Intravenous Care
  F16.1.2. Care Intravenous Care
  F16.1.3. Teach Intravenous Care
  F16.1.4. Manage Intravenous Care

(Continued)

TABLE 14.14. CLINICAL CARE CLASSIFICATION OF 198 NURSING INTERVENTIONS (VERSION 2.0): CODED WITH DEFINITIONS, FOUR ACTION TYPES, AND CLASSIFIED BY 21 CARE COMPONENTS[a,b] **(CONTINUED)**

Venous Catheter Care – F16.2
Actions performed to control the use of infusion equipment.
F16.2.1. Assess Venous Catheter Care
F16.2.2. Care Venous Catheter Care
F16.2.3. Teach Venous Catheter Care
F16.2.4. Manage Venous Catheter Care

G. – HEALTH BEHAVIOR COMPONENT:
Cluster of elements that involve actions to sustain, maintain, or regain health.
Community Special Services – G17
Actions performed to provide advice or information about special community services.
G17.0.1. Assess Community Special Services
G17.0.2. Care Community Special Services
G17.0.3. Teach Community Special Services
G17.0.4. Manage Community Special Services
  Adult Day Center – G17.1
  Actions performed to direct the provision of a day program for adults in a specific location.
  G17.1.1. Assess Adult Day Center
  G17.1.2. Care Adult Day Center
  G17.1.3. Teach Adult Day Center
  G17.1.4. Manage Adult Day Center
  Hospice – G17.2
  Actions performed to support the provision of offering and/or providing care for terminally ill persons.
  G17.2.1. Assess Hospice
  G17.2.2. Care Hospice
  G17.2.3. Teach Hospice
  G17.2.4. Manage Hospice
  Meals-on-Wheels – G17.3
  Actions performed to direct the provision of community program of meals delivered to the home.
  G17.3.1. Assess Meals-on-Wheels
  G17.3.2. Care Meals-on-Wheels
  G17.3.3. Teach Meals-on-Wheels
  G17.3.4. Manage Meals-on-Wheels
Compliance Care – G18
Actions performed to encourage conformity in therapeutic recommendations.
G18.0.1. Assess Compliance Care
G18.0.2. Care Compliance Care
G18.0.3. Teach Compliance Care
G18.0.4. Manage Compliance Care
  Compliance with Diet – G18.1
  Actions performed to encourage conformity to food or fluid intake.
  G18.1.1. Assess Compliance with Diet
  G18.1.2. Care Compliance with Diet
  G18.1.3. Teach Compliance with Diet
  G18.1.4. Manage Compliance with Diet
  Compliance with Fluid Volume – G18.2
  Actions performed to encourage conformity to therapeutic intake of liquids.

  G18.2.1. Assess Compliance with Fluid Volume
  G18.2.2. Care Compliance with Fluid Volume
  G18.2.3. Teach Compliance with Fluid Volume
  G18.2.4. Manage Compliance with Fluid Volume
  Compliance with Medical Regimen – G18.3
  Actions performed to encourage conformity to physician's plan of care.
  G18.3.1. Assess Compliance with Medical Regimen
  G18.3.2. Care Compliance with Medical Regimen
  G18.3.3. Teach Compliance with Medical Regimen
  G18.3.4. Manage Compliance with Medical Regimen
  Compliance with Medication Regimen – G18.4
  Actions performed to encourage conformity to follow prescribed course of medicinal substances.
  G18.4.1. Assess Compliance with Medication Regimen
  G18.4.2. Care Compliance with Medication Regimen
  G18.4.3. Teach Compliance with Medication Regimen
  G18.4.4. Manage Compliance with Medication Regimen
  Compliance with Safety Precaution – G18.5
  Actions performed to encourage conformity with measures to protect self or others from injury, danger, or loss.
  G18.5.1. Assess Compliance with Safety Precautions
  G18.5.2. Care Compliance with Safety Precautions
  G18.5.3. Teach Compliance with Safety Precautions
  G18.5.4. Manage Compliance with Safety Precautions
  Compliance with Therapeutic Regimen – G18.6
  Actions performed to encourage conformity with the health team's plan of care.
  G18.6.1. Assess Compliance with Therapeutic Regimen
  G18.6.2. Care Compliance with Therapeutic Regimen
  G18.6.3. Teach Compliance with Therapeutic Regimen
  G18.6.4. Manage Compliance with Therapeutic Regimen
Nursing Contact – G19
Actions performed to communicate with another nurse.
G19.0.1. Assess Nursing Contact
G19.0.2. Care Nursing Contact
G19.0.3. Teach Nursing Contact
G19.0.4. Manage Nursing Contact
  Bill of Rights – G19.1
  Statements related to entitlements during an episode of illness.
  G19.1.1. Assess Bill of Rights
  G19.1.2. Care Bill of Rights
  G19.1.3. Teach Bill of Rights
  G19.1.4. Manage Bill of Rights
  Nursing Care Coordination – G19.2
  Actions performed to synthesize all plans of care by a nurse.
  G19.2.1. Assess Nursing Care Coordination
  G19.2.2. Care Nursing Care Coordination
  G19.2.3. Teach Nursing Care Coordination
  G19.2.4. Manage Nursing Care Coordination
  Nursing Status Report – G19.3
  Actions performed to document patient condition by a nurse.
  G19.3.1. Assess Nursing Status Report

(Continued)

TABLE 14.14. (CONTINUED)

G19.3.2. Care Nursing Status Report
G19.3.3. Teach Nursing Status Report
G19.3.4. Manage Nursing Status Report
Physician Contact – G20
Actions performed to communicate with a physician.
G20.0.1. Assess Physician Contact
G20.0.2. Care Physician Contact
G20.0.3. Teach Physician Contact
G20.0.4. Manage Physician Contact
  Medical Regimen Orders – G20.1
  Actions performed to support the physician's plan of
    treatment.
  G20.1.1. Assess Medical Regimen
  G20.1.2. Care Medical Regimen
  G20.1.3. Teach Medical Regimen
  G20.1.4. Manage Medical Regimen
  Physician Status Report – G20.2
  Actions performed to document patient condition by a
    physician.
  G20.2.1. Assess Physician Status Report
  G20.2.2. Care Physician Status Report
  G20.2.3. Teach Physician Status Report
  G20.2.4. Manage Physician Status Report
Professional/Ancillary Services – G21
Actions performed to support the duties performed by
  health team members.
G21.0.1. Assess Professional/Ancillary Services
G21.0.2. Care Professional/Ancillary Services
G21.0.3. Teach Professional/Ancillary Services
G21.0.4. Manage Professional/Ancillary Services
  Health Aide Service – G21.1
  Actions performed to support care services by a health aide.
  G21.1.1. Assess Health Aide Service
  G21.1.2. Care Health Aide Service
  G21.1.3. Teach Health Aide Service
  G21.1.4. Manage Health Aide Service
  Medical Social Worker Service – G21.2
  Actions performed to provide advice or instruction by a
    medical social worker.
  G21.2.1. Assess Medical Social Worker Service
  G21.2.2. Care Medical Social Worker Service
  G21.2.3. Teach Medical Social Worker Service
  G21.2.4. Manage Medical Social Worker Service
  Nurse Specialist Service – G21.3
  Actions performed to provide advice or instruction by an
    advanced practice nurse or nurse practitioner.
  G21.3.1. Assess Nurse Specialist Service
  G21.3.2. Care Nurse Specialist Service
  G21.3.3. Teach Nurse Specialist Service
  G21.3.4. Manage Nurse Specialist Service
  Occupational Therapist Service – G21.4
  Actions performed to provide advice or instruction by an
    occupational therapist.
  G21.4.1. Assess Occupational Therapist Service
  G21.4.2. Care Occupational Therapist Service

  G21.4.3. Teach Occupational Therapist Service
  G21.4.4. Manage Occupational Therapist Service
  Physical Therapist Service – G21.5
  Actions performed to provide advice or instruction by a
    physical therapist.
  G21.5.1. Assess Physical Therapist Service
  G21.5.2. Care Physical Therapist Service
  G21.5.3. Teach Physical Therapist Service
  G21.5.4. Manage Physical Therapist Service
  Speech Therapist Service – G21.6
  Actions performed to provide advice or instruction by a
    speech therapist.
  G21.6.1. Assess Speech Therapist Service
  G21.6.2. Care Speech Therapist Service
  G21.6.3. Teach Speech Therapist Service
  G21.6.4. Manage Speech Therapist Service

H. – MEDICATION COMPONENT:
Cluster of elements that involve medicinal substances.
Chemotherapy Care – H22
Actions performed to control and monitor antineoplastic
  agents.
H22.0.1. Assess Chemotherapy Care
H22.0.2. Care Chemotherapy Care
H22.0.3. Teach Chemotherapy Care
H22.0.4. Manage Chemotherapy Care
Injection Administration – H23
Actions performed to dispense a medication by a hypodermic.
H23.0.1. Assess Injection Administration
H23.0.2. Care Injection Administration
H23.0.3. Teach Injection Administration
H23.0.4. Manage Injection Administration
  Insulin Injection – H23.1
  Actions performed to administer a hypodermic
    administration of insulin.
  H23.1.1. Assess Insulin Injection
  H23.1.2. Care Insulin Injection
  H23.1.3. Teach Insulin Injection
  H23.1.4. Manage Insulin Injection
  Vitamin B12 Injection – H23.2
  Actions performed to administer a hypodermic
    administration of vitamin B12.
  H23.2.1. Assess Vitamin B12 Injection
  H23.2.2. Care Vitamin B12 Injection
  H23.2.3. Teach Vitamin B12 Injection
  H23.2.4. Manage Vitamin B12 Injection
Medication Care – H24
Actions performed to direct the dispensing of prescribed
  drugs.
H24.0.1. Assess Medication Care
H24.0.2. Care Medication Care
H24.0.3. Teach Medication Care
H24.0.4. Manage Medication Care
  Medication Actions – H24.1
  Actions performed to support and monitor the use of
    medicinal substances.

(Continued)

TABLE 14.14. CLINICAL CARE CLASSIFICATION OF 198 NURSING INTERVENTIONS (VERSION 2.0): CODED WITH DEFINITIONS, FOUR ACTION TYPES, AND CLASSIFIED BY 21 CARE COMPONENTS[a,b] (CONTINUED)

H24.1.1. Assess Medication Actions
H24.1.2. Care Medication Actions
H24.1.3. Teach Medication Actions
H24.1.3. Manage Medication Actions
Medication Pre-fill Preparation – H24.2
Actions performed to ensure the continued supply of prescribed drugs.
H24.2.1. Assess Medication Pre-fill Preparation
H24.2.2. Care Medication Pre-fill Preparation
H24.2.3. Teach Medication Pre-fill Preparation
H24.2.4. Manage Medication Pre-fill Preparation
Medication Side Effects – H24.3
Actions performed to control untoward reaction or conditions to prescribed drugs.
H24.3.1. Assess Medication Side Effects
H24.3.2. Care Medication Side Effects
H24.3.3. Teach Medication Side Effects
H24.3.4. Manage Medication Side Effects
Medication Treatment – H23.4
Actions performed to administer drugs or remedies regardless of route.
H24.4.1. Assess Medication Treatment
H24.4.2. Care Medication Treatment
H24.4.3. Teach Medication Treatment
H24.4.4. Manage Medication Treatment
Radiation Therapy Care – H25
Actions performed to control and monitor radiation therapy.
H25.0.1. Assess Radiation Therapy Care
H25.0.2. Care Radiation Therapy Care
H25.0.3. Teach Radiation Therapy Care
H25.0.4. Manage Radiation Therapy Care

I. – METABOLIC COMPONENT:
Cluster of elements that involve the endocrine and immunological processes.
Allergic Reaction Care – I26.0
Actions performed to reduce symptoms or precautions to reduce allergies.
I26.0.1. Assess Allergic Reaction Care
I26.0.2. Care Allergic Reaction Care
I26.0.3. Teach Allergic Reaction Care
I26.0.4. Manage Allergic Reaction Care
Diabetic Care – I27
Actions performed to support the control of diabetic conditions.
I27.0.1. Assess Diabetic Care
I27.0.2. Care Diabetic Care
I27.0.3. Teach Diabetic Care
I27.0.4. Manage Diabetic Care
Immunological Care – I65
Actions preformed to protect against a particular disease.
I65.0.1. Assess Immunological Care
I65.0.2. Care Immunological Care
I65.0.3. Teach Immunological Care
I65.0.4. Manage Immunological Care

J. – NUTRITIONAL COMPONENT:
Cluster of elements that involve the intake of food and nutrients.
Enteral Tube Care – J28
Actions performed to control the use of an enteral drainage tube.
J28.0.1. Assess Enteral Tube Care
J28.0.2. Care Enteral Tube Care
J28.0.3. Teach Enteral Tube Care
J28.0.4. Manage Enteral Tube Care
Enteral Tube Insertion – J28.1
Actions performed to support the placement of an enteral drainage tube.
J28.1.1. Assess Enteral Tube Insertion
J28.1.2. Care Enteral Tube Insertion
J28.1.3. Teach Enteral Tube Insertion
J28.1.4. Manage Enteral Tube Insertion
Enteral Tube Irrigation – J28.2
Actions performed to flush or wash out an enteral tube.
J28.2.1. Assess Enteral Tube Irrigation
J28.2.2. Care Enteral Tube Irrigation
J28.2.3. Teach Enteral Tube Irrigation
J28.2.4. Manage Enteral Tube Irrigation
Nutrition Care – J29
Actions performed to support the intake of food and nutrients.
J29.0.1. Assess Nutrition Care
J29.0.2. Care Nutrition Care
J29.0.3. Teach Nutrition Care
J29.0.4. Manage Nutrition Care
Feeding Technique – J29.2
Actions performed to provide special measures to provide nourishment.
J29.2.1. Assess Feeding Technique
J29.2.2. Care Feeding Technique
J29.2.3. Teach Feeding Technique
J29.2.4. Manage Feeding Technique
Regular Diet – J29.3
Actions performed to support the ingestion of food and nutrients from established nutrition standards.
J29.3.1. Assess Regular Diet
J29.3.2. Care Regular Diet
J29.3.3. Teach Regular Diet
J29.3.4. Manage Regular Diet
Special Diet – J29.4
Actions performed to support the ingestion of food and nutrients prescribed for a specific purpose.
J29.4.1. Assess Special Diet
J29.4.2. Care Special Diet
J29.4.3. Teach Special Diet
J29.4.4. Manage Special Diet
Enteral Feeding – J29.5
Actions performed to provide nourishment through a gastrointestinal route.

(Continued)

TABLE 14.14. (CONTINUED)

J29.5.1. Assess Enteral Feeding
J29.5.2. Care Enteral Feeding
J29.5.3. Teach Enteral Feeding
J29.5.4. Manage Enteral Feeding
Parenteral Feeding – J29.6
Actions performed to provide nourishment through intravenous or subcutaneous routes.
J29.6.1. Assess Parenteral Feeding
J29.6.2. Care Parenteral Feeding
J29.6.3. Teach Parenteral Feeding
J29.6.4. Manage Parenteral Feeding
Breast-feeding Support – J66
Actions performed to provide nourishment of an infant at the breast.
J66.0.1. Assess Breast-feeding Support
J66.0.2. Care Breast-feeding Support
J66.0.3. Teach Breast-feeding Support
J66.0.4. Manage Breast-feeding Support
Weight Control – J67
Actions performed to control obesity or debilitation.
J67.0.1. Assess Weight Control
J67.0.2. Care Weight Control
J67.0.3. Teach Weight Control
J67.0.4. Manage Weight Control

K. – PHYSICAL REGULATION COMPONENT
Cluster of elements that involve bodily processes.
Infection Control – K30
Actions performed to contain a communicable disease.
K30.0.1. Assess Infection Control
K30.0.2. Care Infection Control
K30.0.3. Teach Infection Control
K30.0.4. Manage Infection Control
  Universal Precautions – K30.1
  Practices to prevent the spread of infections and infectious diseases.
  K30.1.1. Assess Universal Precautions
  K30.1.2. Care Universal Precautions
  K30.1.3. Teach Universal Precautions
  K30.1.4. Manage Universal Precautions
Physical Health Care – K31
Actions performed to support somatic problems.
K31.0.1. Assess Physical Health Care
K31.0.2. Care Physical Health Care
K31.0.3. Teach Physical Health Care
K31.0.4. Manage Physical Health Care
  Health History – K31.1
  Actions performed to obtain information about past illness and health status.
  K31.1.1. Assess Health History
  K31.1.2. Care Health History
  K31.1.3. Teach Health History
  K31.1.4. Manage Health History
  Health Promotion – K31.2
  Actions performed to encourage behaviors to enhance health state.

K31.2.1. Assess Health Promotion
K31.2.2. Care Health Promotion
K31.2.3. Teach Health Promotion
K31.2.4. Manage Health Promotion
  Physical Examination – K31.3
  Actions performed to observe somatic events.
  K31.3.1. Assess Physical Examination
  K31.3.2. Care Physical Examination
  K31.3.3. Teach Physical Examination
  K31.3.4. Manage Physical Examination
  Clinical Measurements – K31.4
  Actions performed to conduct procedures to evaluate somatic events.
  K31.4.1. Assess Clinical Measurements
  K31.4.2. Care Clinical Measurements
  K31.4.3. Teach Clinical Measurements
  K31.4.4. Manage Clinical Measurements
Specimen Care – K32
Actions performed to direct the collection and/or the examination of a bodily specimen.
K32.0.1. Assess Specimen Care
K32.0.2. Care Specimen Care
K32.0.3. Teach Specimen Care
K32.0.4. Manage Specimen Care
  Blood Specimen Care – K32.1
  Actions performed to collect and/or examine a sample of blood.
  K32.1.1. Assess Blood Specimen Care
  K32.1.2. Care Blood Specimen Care
  K32.1.3. Teach Blood Specimen Care
  K32.1.4. Manage Blood Specimen Care
  Stool Specimen Care – K32.2
  Actions performed to collect and/or examine a sample of feces.
  K32.2.1. Assess Stool Specimen Care
  K32.2.2. Care Stool Specimen Care
  K32.2.3. Teach Stool Specimen Care
  K32.2.4. Manage Stool Specimen Care
  Urine Specimen Care – K32.3
  Actions performed to collect and/or examine a sample of urine.
  K32.3.1. Assess Urine Specimen Care
  K32.3.2. Care Urine Specimen Care
  K32.3.3. Teach Urine Specimen Care
  K32.3.4. Manage Urine Specimen Care
  Sputum Specimen Care – K32.5
  Actions performed to collect and/or examine a sample of sputum.
  K32.5.1. Assess Sputum Specimen Care
  K32.5.2. Care Sputum Specimen Care
  K32.5.3. Teach Sputum Specimen Care
  K32.5.4. Manage Sputum Specimen Care
Vital Signs – K33
Actions performed to measure temperature, respiration, pulse, and blood pressure.

(Continued)

TABLE 14.14. CLINICAL CARE CLASSIFICATION OF 198 NURSING INTERVENTIONS (VERSION 2.0): CODED WITH DEFINITIONS, FOUR ACTION TYPES, AND CLASSIFIED BY 21 CARE COMPONENTS[a,b] (CONTINUED)

K33.0.1. Assess Vital Signs
K33.0.2. Care Vital Signs
K33.0.3. Teach Vital Signs
K33.0.4. Manage Vital Signs
Blood Pressure – K33.1
Actions performed to measure the diastolic and systolic pressure of the blood.
K33.1.1. Assess Blood Pressure
K33.1.2. Care Blood Pressure
K33.1.3. Teach Blood Pressure
K33.1.4. Manage Blood Pressure
Temperature – K33.2
Actions performed to measure the body temperature.
K33.2.1. Assess Temperature
K33.2.2. Care Temperature
K33.2.3. Teach Temperature
K33.2.4. Manage Temperature
Pulse – K33.3
Actions performed to measure rhythmical beats of the heart.
K33.3.1. Assess Pulse
K33.3.2. Care Pulse
K33 3.3. Teach Pulse
K33.3.4. Manage Pulse
Respiration – K33.4
Actions performed to measure the function of breathing.
K33.4.1. Assess Respiration
K33.4.2. Care Respiration
K33.4.3. Teach Respiration
K33 4.4. Manage Respiration

L. – RESPIRATORY COMPONENT:
Cluster of elements that involve breathing and the pulmonary system.
Oxygen Therapy Care – L35
Actions performed to support the administration of oxygen treatment.
L35.0.1. Assess Oxygen Therapy Care
L35.0.2. Care Oxygen Therapy Care
L35.0.3. Teach Oxygen Therapy Care
L35.0.4. Manage Oxygen Therapy Care
Pulmonary Care – L36
Actions performed to support pulmonary hygiene.
L36.0.1. Assess Pulmonary Care
L36.0.2. Care Pulmonary Care
L36.0.3. Teach Pulmonary Care
L36.0.4. Manage Pulmonary Care
Breathing Exercises – L36.1
Actions performed to provide therapy on respiratory or lung exertion.
L36.1.1. Assess Breathing Exercises
L36.1.2. Care Breathing Exercises
L36.1.3. Teach Breathing Exercises
L36.1.4. Manage Breathing Exercises
Chest Physiotherapy – L36.2
Actions performed to provide exercises to provide postural drainage of lungs.

L36.2.1. Assess Chest Physiotherapy
L36.2.2. Care Chest Physiotherapy
L36.2.3. Teach Chest Physiotherapy
L36.2.4. Manage Chest Physiotherapy
Inhalation Therapy – L36.3
Actions performed to support breathing treatments.
L36.3.1. Assess Inhalation Therapy
L36.3.2. Care Inhalation Therapy
L36.3.3. Teach Inhalation Therapy
L36.3.4. Manage Inhalation Therapy
Ventilator Care – L36.4
Actions performed to control and monitor the use of a ventilator.
L36.4.1. Assess Ventilator Care
L36.4.2. Care Ventilator Care
L36.4.3. Teach Ventilator Care
L36.4.4. Manage Ventilator Care
Tracheostomy Care – L37
Actions performed to support a tracheostomy.
L37.0.1. Assess Tracheostomy Care
L37.0.2. Care Tracheostomy Care
L37.0.3. Teach Tracheostomy Care
L37.0.4. Manage Tracheostomy Care

M. – ROLE RELATIONSHIP COMPONENT:
Cluster of elements involving interpersonal, work, social, family, and sexual interactions.
Communication Care – M38
Actions performed to exchange verbal information.
M38.0.1. Assess Communication Care
M38.0.2. Care Communication Care
M38.0.3. Teach Communication Care
M38.0.4. Manage Communication Care
Psychosocial Care – M39
Actions performed to support the study of psychological and social factors.
M39.0.1. Assess Psychosocial Care
M39.0.2. Care Psychosocial Care
M39.0.3. Teach Psychosocial Care
M39.0.4. Manage Psychosocial Care
Home Situation Analysis – M39.1
Actions performed to analyze the living environment.
M39.1.1. Assess Home Situation Analysis
M39.1.2. Care Home Situation Analysis
M39.1.3. Teach Home Situation Analysis
M39.1.4. Manage Home Situation Analysis
Interpersonal Dynamics Analysis – M39.2
Actions performed to support the analysis of the driving forces in a relationship between people.
M39.2.1. Assess Interpersonal Dynamics Analysis
M39.2.2. Care Interpersonal Dynamics Analysis
M39.2.3. Teach Interpersonal Dynamics Analysis
M39.4.4. Manage Interpersonal Dynamics Analysis
Family Process Analysis – M39.3
Actions performed to support the change and/or modification of a related group.

(Continued)

TABLE 14.14. (CONTINUED)

M39.3.1. Assess Family Process Analysis
M39.3.2. Care Family Process Analysis
M39.3.3. Teach Family Process Analysis
M39.3.4. Manage Family Process Analysis
Sexual Behavior Analysis – M39.4
Actions performed to support the change and/or modification of a person's sexual response.
M39.4.1. Assess Sexual Behavior Analysis
M39.4.2. Care Sexual Behavior Analysis
M39.4.3. Teach Sexual Behavior Analysis
M39.4.4. Manage Sexual Behavior Analysis
Social Network Analysis – M39.5
Actions performed to improve the quantity or quality of personal relationships.
M39.5.1. Assess Social Network Analysis
M39.5.2. Care Social Network Analysis
M39.5.3. Teach Social Network Analysis
M39.5.4. Manage Social Network Analysis

N. – SAFETY COMPONENT:
Cluster of elements that involve prevention of injury, danger, loss, or abuse.
Substance Abuse Control – N40
Actions performed to control situations to avoid, detect, or minimize harm.
N40.0.1. Assess Substance Abuse Control
N40.0.2. Care Substance Abuse Control
N40.0.3. Teach Substance Abuse Control
N40.0.4. Manage Substance Abuse Control
Tobacco Abuse Control – N40.1
Actions performed to avoid, minimize, or control the use of tobacco.
N40.1.1. Assess Tobacco Abuse Control
N40.1.2. Care Tobacco Abuse Control
N40.1.3. Teach Tobacco Abuse Control
N40.1.4. Manage Tobacco Abuse Control
Alcohol Abuse Control – N40.2
Actions performed to avoid, minimize, or control the use of distilled liquors.
N40.2.1. Assess Alcohol Abuse Control
N40.2.2. Care Alcohol Abuse Control
N40.2.3. Teach Alcohol Abuse Control
N40.2.4. Manage Alcohol Abuse Control
Drug Abuse Control – N40.3
Actions performed to avoid, minimize, or control the use of any habit-forming medication.
N40.3.1. Assess Drug Abuse Control
N40.3.2. Care Drug Abuse Control
N40.3.3. Teach Drug Abuse Control
N40.3.4. Manage Drug Abuse Control
Emergency Care – N41
Actions performed to support a sudden or unexpected occurrence.
N41.0.1. Assess Emergency Care
N41.0.2. Care Emergency Care
N41 0.3. Teach Emergency Care
N41.0.4. Manage Emergency Care

Safety Precautions – N42
Actions performed to advance measures to avoid danger or harm.
N42.0.1. Assess Safety Precautions
N42.0.2. Care Safety Precautions
N42 0.3. Teach Safety Precautions
N42.0.4. Manage Safety Precautions
Environmental Safety – N42.1
Precautions recommended to prevent or reduce environmental injury.
N42.1.1. Assess Environmental Safety
N42.1.2. Care Environmental Safety
N42.1.3. Teach Environmental Safety
N42.1.4. Manage Environmental Safety
Equipment Safety – N42.2
Precautions recommended to prevent or reduce equipment injury.
N42.2.1. Assess Equipment Safety
N42.2.2. Care Equipment Safety
N42.2.3. Teach Equipment Safety
N42.2.4. Manage Equipment Safety
Individual Safety – N42.3
Precautions to reduce individual injury.
N42.3.1. Assess Individual Safety
N42.3.2. Care Individual Safety
N42.3.3. Teach Individual Safety
N42.4.4. Manage Individual Safety
Violence Control – N68
Actions performed to control behaviors that may cause harm to oneself or others.
N68.0.1. Assess Violence Control
N68.0.2. Care Violence Control
N68.0.3. Teach Violence Control
N68.0.4. Manage Violence Control

O. – SELF-CARE COMPONENT:
Cluster of elements that involve the ability to carry out activities to maintain oneself.
Personal Care – O43
Actions performed to care for oneself.
O43.0.1. Assess Personal Care
O43.0.2. Care Personal Care
O43.0.3. Teach Personal Care
O43.0.4. Manage Personal Care
Activities of Daily Living (ADLs) – O43.1
Actions performed to support personal activities to maintain oneself.
O43.1.1. Assess Activities of Daily Living (ADLs)
O43.1.2. Care Activities of Daily Living (ADLs)
O43.1.3. Teach Activities of Daily Living (ADLs)
O43.1.4. Manage Activities of Daily Living (ADLs)
Instrumental Activities of Daily Living (IADLs) – O43.2
Complex activities performed to support basic life skills.
O43.2.1. Assess Instrumental Activities of Daily Living (IADLs)
O43.2.2. Care Instrumental Activities of Daily Living (IADLs)
O43.2.3. Teach Instrumental Activities of Daily Living (IADLs)
O53.2.4. Manage Instrumental Activities of Daily Living (IADLs)

(Continued)

TABLE 14.14. CLINICAL CARE CLASSIFICATION OF 198 NURSING INTERVENTIONS (VERSION 2.0): CODED WITH DEFINITIONS, FOUR ACTION TYPES, AND CLASSIFIED BY 21 CARE COMPONENTS[a,b] (CONTINUED)

P. – SELF-CONCEPT COMPONENT:
Cluster of elements that involve an individual's mental image of oneself.
Mental Health Care – P45
Actions taken to promote emotional well-being.
P45.0.1. Assess Mental Health
P45.0.2. Care Mental Health
P45.0.3. Teach Mental Health Care
P45.0.4. Manage Mental Health Care
  Mental Health History – P45.1
  Actions performed to obtain information about past or present emotional well-being.
  P45.1.1. Assess Mental Health History
  P45.1.2. Care Mental Health History
  P45.1.3. Teach Mental Health History
  P45.1.4. Manage Mental Health History
  Mental Health Promotion – P45.2
  Actions performed to encourage or further emotional well-being.
  P45.2.1. Assess Mental Health Promotion
  P45.2.2. Care Mental Health Promotion
  P45.2.3. Teach Mental Health Promotion
  P45.2.4. Manage Mental Health Promotion
  Mental Health Screening – P45.3
  Actions performed to systematically examine the emotional well-being.
  P45.3.1. Assess Mental Health Screening
  P45.3.2. Care Mental Health Screening
  P45.3.3. Teach Mental Health Screening
  P45.3.4. Manage Mental Health Screening
  Mental Health Treatment – P45.4
  Actions performed to support protocols used to treat emotional problems.
  P45.4.1. Assess Mental Health Treatment
  P45.4.2. Care Mental Health Treatment
  P45.4.3. Teach Mental Health Treatment
  P45.4.4. Manage Mental Health Treatment

Q. – SENSORY COMPONENT:
Cluster of elements that involve the senses, including pain.
Pain Control – Q47
Actions performed to support responses to injury or damage.
Q47.0.1. Assess Pain Control
Q47.0.2. Care Pain Control
Q47.0.3. Teach Pain Control
Q47.0.4. Manage Pain Control
  Acute Pain Control – Q47.1
  Actions performed to control physical suffering, hurting, or distress.
  Q47.1.1. Assess Acute Pain Control
  Q47.1.2. Care Acute Pain Control
  Q47.1.3. Teach Acute Pain Control
  Q47.1.4. Manage Acute Pain Control

  Chronic Pain Control – Q47.2
  Actions performed to control physical suffering, hurting, or distress that continues longer than expected.
  Q47.2.1. Assess Chronic Pain Control
  Q47.2.2. Care Chronic Pain Control
  Q47.2.3. Teach Chronic Pain Control
  Q47.2.4. Manage Chronic Pain Control
Comfort Care – Q48
Actions performed to enhance or improve well-being.
Q48.0.1. Assess Comfort Care
Q48.0.2. Care Comfort Care
Q48.0.3. Teach Comfort Care
Q48.0.4. Manage Comfort Care
Ear Care – Q49
Actions performed to support ear problems.
Q49.0.1. Assess Ear Care
Q49.0.2. Care Ear Care
Q49.0.3. Teach Ear Care
Q49.0.4. Manage Ear Care
  Hearing Aid Care – 49.1
  Actions performed to control the use of a hearing aid.
  Q49.1.1. Assess Hearing Aid Care
  Q49.1.2. Care Hearing Aid Care
  Q49.1.3. Teach Hearing Aid Care
  Q49.1.4. Manage Hearing Aid Care
  Wax Removal – Q49.2
  Actions performed to remove cerumen from ear.
  Q49.2.1. Assess Wax Removal
  Q49.2.2. Care Wax Removal
  Q49.2.3. Teach Wax Removal
  Q49.2.4. Manage Wax Removal
Eye Care – Q50
Actions performed to support eye problems.
Q50.0.1. Assess Eye Care
Q50.0.2. Care Eye Care
Q50.0.3. Teach Eye Care
Q50.0.4. Manage Eye Care
  Cataract Care – Q50.1
  Actions performed to control cataract conditions.
  Q50.1.1. Assess Cataract Care
  Q50.1.2. Care Cataract Care
  Q50.1.3. Teach Cataract Care
  Q50.1.4. Manage Cataract Care
  Vision Care – Q50.2
  Actions performed to control vision problems.
  Q50.2.1. Assess Vision Care
  Q50.2.2. Care Vision Care
  Q50.2.3. Teach Vision Care
  Q50.2.4. Manage Vision Care

R. – SKIN INTEGRITY COMPONENT:
Cluster of elements that involve the mucous membrane, corneal, integumentary, or subcutaneous structures of the body.

(Continued)

TABLE 14.14. (CONTINUED)

Pressure Ulcer Care – R51

Actions performed to prevent, detect, and treat skin integrity breakdown caused by pressure.

R51.0.1. Assess Pressure Ulcer Care
R51.0.2. Care Pressure Ulcer Care
R51.0.3. Teach Pressure Ulcer Care
R51.0.4. Manage Pressure Ulcer Care

  Pressure Ulcer Stage 1 Care – R51.1

  Actions performed to prevent, detect, and treat Stage 1 skin breakdown.

  R51.1.1. Assess Pressure Ulcer Stage 1 Care
  R51.1.2. Care Pressure Ulcer Stage 1 Care
  R51.1.3. Teach Pressure Ulcer Stage 1 Care
  R51.1.4. Manage Pressure Ulcer Stage 1 Care

  Pressure Ulcer Stage 2 Care – R51.2

  Actions performed to prevent, detect, and treat Stage 2 skin breakdown.

  R51.2.1. Assess Pressure Ulcer Stage 2 Care
  R51.2.2. Care Pressure Ulcer Stage 2 Care
  R51.2.3. Teach Pressure Ulcer Stage 2 Care
  R51.2.4. Manage Pressure Ulcer Stage 2 Care

  Pressure Ulcer Stage 3 Care – R51.3

  Actions performed to prevent, detect, and treat Stage 3 skin breakdown.

  R51.3.1. Assess Pressure Ulcer Stage 3 Care
  R51.3.2. Care Pressure Ulcer Stage 3 Care
  R51.3.3. Teach Pressure Ulcer Stage 3 Care
  R51.3.4. Manage Pressure Ulcer Stage 3 Care

  Pressure Ulcer Stage 4 Care – R51.4

  Actions performed to prevent, detect, and treat Stage 4 skin breakdown.

  R51.4.1. Assess Pressure Ulcer Stage 4 Care
  R51.4.2. Care Pressure Ulcer Stage 4 Care
  R51.4.3. Teach Pressure Ulcer Stage 4 Care
  R51.4.4. Manage Pressure Ulcer Stage 4 Care

Mouth Care – R53

Actions performed to support oral cavity problems.

R53.0.1. Assess Mouth Care
R53.0.2. Care Mouth Care
R53.0.3. Teach Mouth Care
R53.0.4. Manage Mouth Care

  Denture Care – R53.1

  Actions performed to control the use of artificial teeth.

  R53.1.1. Assess Denture Care
  R53.1.2. Care Denture Care
  R53.1.3. Teach Denture Care
  R53.1.4. Manage Denture Care

Skin Care – R54

Actions to control the integument/skin.

R54.0.1. Assess Skin Care
R54.0.2. Care Skin Care
R54.0.3. Teach Skin Care
R54.0.4. Manage Skin Care

  Skin Breakdown Control – R54.1

  Actions performed to support integument/skin problems.

  R54.1.1. Assess Skin Breakdown Control
  R54.1.2. Care Skin Breakdown Control
  R54.1.3. Teach Skin Breakdown Control
  R54.1.4. Manage Skin Breakdown Control

Wound Care – R55

Actions performed to support open skin areas.

R55.0.1. Assess Wound Care
R55.0.2. Care Wound Care
R55.0.3. Teach Wound Care
R55.0.4. Manage Wound Care

  Drainage Tube Care – R55.1

  Actions performed to support drainage from tubes.

  R55.1.1. Assess Drainage Tube Care
  R55.1.2. Care Drainage Tube Care
  R55.1.3. Teach Drainage Tube Care
  R55.1.4. Manage Drainage Tube Care

  Dressing Change – R55.2

  Actions performed to remove and replace a new bandage to a wound.

  R55.2.1. Assess Dressing Change
  R55.2.2. Care Dressing Change
  R55.2.3. Teach Dressing Change
  R55.2.4. Manage Dressing Change

  Incision Care – R55.3

  Actions performed to support a surgical wound.

  R55.3.1. Assess Incision Care
  R55.3.2. Care Incision Care
  R55.3.3. Teach Incision Care
  R55.3.4. Manage Incision Care

S. – TISSUE PERFUSION COMPONENT:

Cluster of elements that involve the oxygenation of tissues, including the circulatory and neurovascular systems.

Foot Care – S56

Actions performed to support foot problems.

S56.0.1. Assess Foot Care
S56.0.2. Care Foot Care
S56.0.3. Teach Foot Care
S56.0.4. Manage Foot Car

Perineal Care – S57

Actions performed to support perineal problems.

S57.0.1. Assess Perineal Care
S57.0.2. Care Perineal Care
S57.0.3. Teach Perineal Care
S57.0.4. Manage Perineal Care

Edema Control – S69

Actions performed to control excess fluid in tissue.

S69.0.1. Assess Edema Control
S69.0.2. Care Edema Control
S69.0.3. Teach Edema Control
S69.0.4. Manage Edema Control

Circulatory Care – S70

Actions performed to support the circulation of the blood (blood vessels).

S70.0.1. Assess Circulatory Care
S70.0.2. Care Circulatory Care
S70.0.3. Teach Circulatory Care
S70.0.4. Manage Circulatory Care

(Continued)

TABLE 14.14. CLINICAL CARE CLASSIFICATION OF 198 NURSING INTERVENTIONS (VERSION 2.0): CODED WITH DEFINITIONS, FOUR ACTION TYPES, AND CLASSIFIED BY 21 CARE COMPONENTS[a,b] (CONTINUED)

Neurovascular Care – S71
Actions performed to control problems of the nerves and vascular systems.
S71.0.1. Assess Neurovascular Care
S71.0.2. Care Neurovascular Care
S71.0.3. Teach Neurovascular Care
S71.0.4. Manage Neurovascular Care

T. – URINARY ELIMINATION COMPONENT:
Cluster of elements that involve the genitourinary system.
Bladder Care – T58
Actions performed to control urinary drainage problems.
T58.0.1. Assess Bladder Care
T58.0.2. Care Bladder Care
T58.0.3. Teach Bladder Care
T58.0.4. Manage Bladder Care
  Bladder Instillation – T58.1
  Actions performed to pour liquid through a catheter into the bladder.
  T58.1.1. Assess Bladder Instillation
  T58.1.2. Care Bladder Instillation
  T58.1.3. Teach Bladder Instillation
  T58.1.4. Manage Bladder Instillation
  Bladder Training – T58.2
  Actions performed to provide instruction on the training care of urinary drainage.
  T58.2.1. Assess Bladder Training
  T58.2.2. Care Bladder Training
  T58.2.3. Teach Bladder Training
  T58.2.4. Manage Bladder Training
Dialysis Care – T59
Actions performed to support dialysis treatments.
T59.0.1. Assess Dialysis Care
T59.0.2. Care Dialysis Care
T59.0.3. Teach Dialysis Care
T59.0.4. Manage Dialysis Care
Urinary Catheter Care – T60
Actions performed to control the use of a urinary catheter.
T60.0.1. Assess Urinary Catheter Care
T60.0.2. Care Urinary Catheter Care
T60.0.3. Teach Urinary Catheter Care
T60.0.4. Manage Urinary Catheter Care
  Urinary Catheter Insertion – T60.1
  Actions performed to place a urinary catheter in bladder.
  T60.1.1. Assess Urinary Catheter Insertion
  T60.1.2. Care Urinary Catheter Insertion
  T60.1.3. Teach Urinary Catheter Insertion
  T60.1.4. Manage Urinary Catheter Insertion
  Urinary Catheter Irrigation – T60.2
  Actions performed to flush a urinary catheter.
  T60.2.1. Assess Urinary Catheter Irrigation
  T60.2.2. Care Urinary Catheter Irrigation
  T60.2.3. Teach Urinary Catheter Irrigation
  T60.2.4. Manage Urinary Catheter Irrigation
Urinary Incontinence Care – T72
Actions performed to control the inability to retain and/or involuntary retain urine.

T72.0.1. Assess Urinary Incontinence Care
T72.0.2. Care Urinary Incontinence Care
T72.0.3. Teach Urinary Incontinence Care
T72.0.4. Manage Urinary Incontinence Care
Renal Care – T73
Actions performed to control problems pertaining to the kidney.
T73.0.1. Assess Renal Care
T73.0.2. Care Renal Care
T73.0.3. Teach Renal Care
T73.0.4. Manage Renal Care

U. – LIFE CYCLE COMPONENT:
Cluster of elements that involve the life span of individuals.
Reproductive Care – U74
Actions performed to support the production of an offspring/child.
U74.0.1. Assess Reproductive Care
U74.0.2. Care Reproductive Care
U74.0.3. Teach Reproductive Care
U74.0.4. Manage Reproductive Care
  Fertility Care – U74.1
  Actions performed to increase conception of an offspring/child.
  U74.1.1. Assess Fertility Care
  U74.1.2. Care Fertility Care
  U74.1.3. Teach Fertility Care
  U74.1.4. Manage Fertility Care
  Infertility Care – U74.2
  Actions performed to support conception of the infertile client of an offspring/child.
  U74.2.1. Assess Infertility Care
  U74.2.2. Care Infertility Care
  U74.2.3. Teach Infertility Care
  U74.2.4. Manage Infertility Care
  Contraception Care – U74.3
  Actions performed to prevent conception of an offspring/child.
  U74.3.1. Assess Contraception Care
  U74.3.2. Care Contraception Care
  U74.3.3. Teach Contraception Care
  U74.3.4. Manage Contraception Care
Perinatal Care – U75
Actions performed to support perineal problems.
U75.0.1. Assess Perinatal Care
U75.0.2. Care Perinatal Care
U75.0.3. Teach Perinatal Care
U75.0.4. Manage Perinatal Care
  Pregnancy Care – U75.1
  Actions performed to support the gestation period of the formation of an offspring/child (being with child).
  U75.1.1. Assess Pregnancy Care
  U75.1.2. Care Pregnancy Care
  U75.1.3. Teach Pregnancy Care
  U75.1.4. Manage Pregnancy Care

(Continued)

TABLE 14.14. (CONTINUED)

Labor Care – U75.2
Actions performed to support the bringing forth of an offspring/child.
U75.2.1. Assess Labor Care
U75.2.2. Care Labor Care
U75.2.3. Teach Labor Care
U75.2.4. Manage Labor Care
Delivery Care – U75.3
Actions performed to support the expulsion of an offspring/child at birth.
U75.3.1. Assess Delivery Care
U75.3.2. Care Delivery Care
U75.3.3. Teach Delivery Care
U75.3.4. Manage Delivery Care
Postpartum Care – U75.4
Actions performed to support the time period immediately after the delivery of an offspring/child.
U75.4.1. Assess Postpartum Care
U75.4.2. Care Postpartum Care
U75.4.3. Teach Postpartum Care
U75.4.4. Manage Postpartum Care
Growth & Development Care – U76
Actions performed to support normal standards of performing developmental skills and behavior of an individual of any age group.
U76.0.1. Assess Growth & Development Care
U76.0.2. Care Growth & Development Care
U76.0.3. Teach Growth & Development Care
U76.0.4. Manage Growth & Development Care
Newborn Care – U76.1 (first 30 days)
Actions performed to support normal standards of performing developmental skills and behavior of an individual of a typical newborn for the first 30 days of life.
U76.1.1. Assess Newborn Care
U76.1.2. Care Newborn Care
U76.1.3. Teach Newborn Care
U76.1.4. Manage Newborn Care
Infant Care – U76.2 (31 days through 11 months)

Actions performed to support normal standards of performing developmental skills and behavior of a typical infant 31 days through 11 months of age.
U76.2.1. Assess Infant Care
U76.2.2. Care Infant Care
U76.2.3. Teach Infant Care
U76.2.4. Manage Infant Care
Child Care – U76.3 (1 year through 11 years)
Actions performed to support normal standards of performing developmental skills and behavior of a typical child 1 year through 11 years of age.
U76.3.1. Assess Child Care
U76.3.2. Care Child Care
U76.3.3. Teach Child Care
U76.3.4. Manage Child Care
Adolescent Care – U76.4 (12 years through 20 years)
Actions performed to support normal standards of performing developmental skills and behavior of a typical adolescent 12 years through 20 years of age.
U76.4.1. Assess Adolescent Care
U76.4.2. Care Adolescent Care
U76.4.3. Teach Adolescent Care
U76.4.4. Manage Adolescent Care
Adult Care – U76.5 (21 years through 64 years)
Actions performed to support normal standards of performing developmental skills and behavior of a typical adult 21 years through 64 years of age.
U76.5.1. Assess Adult Care
U76.5.2. Care Adult Care
U76.5.3. Teach Adult Care
U76.5.4. Manage Adult Care
Older Adult Care – U76.6 (65 years and over)
Actions performed to support normal standards of performing developmental skills and behavior of typical older adult 65 years and over.
U76.6.1. Assess Older Adult Care
U76.6.2. Care Older Adult Care
U76.6.3. Teach Older Adult Care
U76.6.4. Manage Older Adult Care

[a]Clinical Care Classification of Nursing Interventions (Version 2.0) includes 12 New Major Categories and 24 Subcategories. See Appendix Table A.3 for revisions from Home Health Care Classification (Version 1.0).
[b]The Clinical Care Classification System is copyrighted and placed in the Public Domain, and cannot be sold, but is used with written permission.

© V. K. Saba—Revised 1992, 1994, 2002, 2004, 2006

REFERENCES

American Nurses Association. (1998). *Standards of clinical nursing practice* (2nd ed.). Washington, DC: ANA.

Holzemer, W. L., Henry, S. B., Dawson, C., Sousa, K., Bain, C., & Hsieh, S.-F. (1997). An evaluation of the utility of the home health care classification for categorizing patient problems and nursing interventions from the hospital setting. In U. Gerdin, M. Tallberg, & P. Wainwright (Eds.), *NI '99: Nursing informatics: The impact of nursing knowledge on health care informatics* (pp. 21–26). Stockholm, Sweden: IOS Press.

North American Nursing Diagnosis Association. (1991). *Taxonomy I: Revised-1991*. St. Louis, MO: NANDA.

North American Nursing Diagnosis Association. (1992). *NANDA nursing diagnoses: Definitions and classification 1992–1993*. St. Louis, MO: NANDA.

North American Nursing Diagnosis Association. (2001). *NANDA nursing diagnoses: Definitions and classification 2001–2002*. St. Louis, MO: NANDA.

Saba, V. K. (1994). Twenty nursing diagnoses home health care components. In R. M. Carroll-Johnson & M. Paquette (Eds.), *Classification of nursing diagnoses: Proceedings of the Tenth Conference* (p. 301). Philadelphia: J. B. Lippincott.

Saba, V. K. (1995). A new paradigm for computer-based nursing information systems: Twenty care components. In R. A. Greenes, H. E. Peterson, & D. J. Proti (Eds.), *MEDINFO '95 Proceedings* (pp. 1404–1406). Edmonton, Canada: IMIA.

Saba, V. K., & Sparks, S. M. (1998). Twenty care components: An educational strategy to teach nursing science. In B. Cesnik, A. T. McCray, & J. R. Scherrer (Eds.), *Medinfo '98: Proceedings of the Ninth World Congress on Medical Informatics* (pp. 756–759). Amsterdan, The Netherlands: IOS Press.

World Health Organization. (1992). *ICD-10: International Statistical Classification of Diseases and Related Health Problems: Tenth Revision: Volume 1*. Geneva, Switzerland: WHO.

APPENDICES

CLINICAL CARE CLASSIFICATION CARE COMPONENTS, NURSING DIAGNOSES, AND NURSING INTERVENTIONS (VERSION 2.0) REVISIONS FROM HOME HEALTH CARE CLASSIFICATION (VERSION 1.0)

Approved by HHCC Scientific Advisory Board as of September 22, 2002, and Published as CCC January 2003.

TABLE A.1. CLINICAL CARE CLASSIFICATION CARE COMPONENTS (VERSION 2.0) REVISIONS FROM HOME HEALTH CARE CLASSIFICATION (VERSION 1.0)

Format is based on HHCC (Version 1.0):
ADD Code/Term = Single Entry Represents New Code and Term (ALL CAPS)
DELETE Code/Term = Single Entry Represents Retired Code/Term (Lowercase)
ADD Term = Single Entry Represents Expansion of a Term with a New Word
DELETE Code with ADD Code = Double Entry Represents Revised Code
DELETE Term with ADD Term = Double Entry Represents Revised Term

DELETE Term	B – Bowel Elimination Component
ADD Term	B – BOWEL/GASTRIC COMPONENT
ADD Code/Term	U – LIFE CYCLE COMPONENT

TABLE A.2. CLINICAL CARE CLASSIFICATION OF NURSING DIAGNOSES (VERSION 2.0) REVISIONS FROM HOME HEALTH CARE CLASSIFICATION (VERSION 1.0)

Format is based on HHCC (Version 1.0):
ADD Code/Term = Single Entry Represents New Code and Term (ALL CAPS)
DELETE Code/Term = Single Entry Represents Retired Code/Term (Lowercase)
ADD Term = Single Entry Represents Expansion of a Term with a New Word
DELETE Code with ADD Code = Double Entry Represents Revised Code
DELETE Term with ADD Term = Double Entry Represents Revised Term

ADD Code/Term	A01.7 – SLEEP DEPRIVATION
ADD Code/Term	B51 – NAUSEA
ADD Code/Term	D07.1 – CONFUSION
ADD Code/Term	D09.1 – MEMORY IMPAIRMENT

(Continued)

TABLE A.2. CLINICAL CARE CLASSIFICATION OF NURSING DIAGNOSES (VERSION 2.0) REVISIONS FROM HOME HEALTH CARE CLASSIFICATION (VERSION 1.0) (CONTINUED)

ADD Code/Term	E52 – COMMUNITY COPING IMPAIRMENT
DELETE Code	G16 – Growth & Development Alteration
ADD Code	U61 – GROWTH & DEVELOPMENT ALTERATION
ADD Code/Term	G17.1 – FAILURE TO THRIVE
DELETE Term	K25.1 – Dysreflexia
ADD Term	K25.1 – AUTONOMIC DYSREFLEXIA
ADD Code/Term	K25.7 – INTRACRANIAL ADAPTIVE CAPACITY IMPAIRMENT
ADD Code/Term	L56 – VENTILATORY WEANING IMPAIRMENT
ADD Code/Term	M27.4 – CAREGIVER ROLE STRAIN
DELETE Code	M30– Grieving
ADD Code	E53 – GRIEVING
DELETE Code	M30.1 – Anticipatory Grieving
ADD Code	E53.1 – ANTICIPATORY GRIEVING
DELETE Code	M30.2 – Dysfunctional Grieving
ADD Code	E53.2 – DYSFUNCTIONAL GRIEVING
ADD Code/Term	M32.3 – RELOCATION STRESS SYNDROME
ADD Code/Term	N34.1 – SUICIDE RISK
ADD Code/Term	N34.2 – SELF-MUTILATION RISK
ADD Code/Term	N57 – PERIOPERATIVE INJURY RISK
ADD Code/Term	N57.1 – PERIOPERATIVE POSITIONING INJURY
ADD Code/Term	N57.2 – SURGICAL RECOVERY DELAY
ADD Code/Term	N58 – SUBSTANCE ABUSE
ADD Code/Term	N58.1 – TOBACCO ABUSE
ADD Code/Term	N58.2 – ALCOHOL ABUSE
ADD Code/Term	N58.3 – DRUG ABUSE
DELETE Code	O37 – Infant Feeding Pattern Impairment
ADD Code	J54 – INFANT FEEDING PATTERN IMPAIRMENT
DELETE Code	O37.1 – Breastfeeding Impairment
ADD Code	J55 – BREASTFEEDING IMPAIRMENT
ADD Code/Term	R46.5 – LATEX ALLERGY RESPONSE
ADD Code/Term	U59 – REPRODUCTIVE RISK
ADD Code/Term	U59.1 – FERTILITY RISK
ADD Code/Term	U59.2 – INFERTILITY RISK
ADD Code/Term	U59.3 – CONTRACEPTION RISK
ADD Code/Term	U60 – PERINATAL RISK
ADD Code/Term	U60.1 – PREGNANCY RISK
ADD Code/Term	U60.2 – LABOR RISK
ADD Code/Term	U60.3 – DELIVERY RISK
ADD Code/Term	U60.4 – POSTPARTUM RISK
ADD Code/Term	U61.1 – NEWBORN BEHAVIOR ALTERATION (First 30 Days)
ADD Code/Term	U61.2 – INFANT BEHAVIOR ALTERATION (31 Days Through 11 Months)
ADD Code/Term	U61.3 – CHILD BEHAVIOR ALTERATION (1 Year Through 11 Years)
ADD Code/Term	U61.4 – ADOLESCENT BEHAVIOR ALTERATION (12 Years Through 20 Years)
ADD Code/Term	U61.5 – ADULT BEHAVIOR ALTERATION (21 Years Through 64 Years)
ADD Code/Term	U61.6 – OLDER ADULT BEHAVIOR ALTERATION (65 Years & Older)

TABLE A.3. CLINICAL CARE CLASSIFICATION OF NURSING INTERVENTIONS (VERSION 2.0) REVISIONS FROM HOME HEALTH CARE CLASSIFICATION (VERSION 1.0)

Format is based on HHCC (Version 1.0):

ADD Code/Term = Single Entry Represents New Code and Term (All CAPS)

DELETE Code/Term = Single Entry Represents Retired Code/Term (Lowercase)

ADD Term = Single Entry Represents Expansion of a Term with a New Word

DELETE Code with ADD Code = Double Entry Represents Revised Code

DELETE Term with ADD Term = Double Entry Represents Revised Term

DELETE Code	A01.1 – Cardiac Rehabilitation
ADD Code	C08.1 – CARDIAC REHABILITATION
DELETE Term	A05 – Rehabilitation Care
ADD Term	A05 – MUSCULOSKELETAL CARE
ADD Code/Term	B06.4 – DIARRHEA CARE
ADD Code/Term	B62 – GASTRIC CARE
ADD Code/Term	B62.1 – NAUSEA CARE
ADD Code/Term	D63 – WANDERING CONTROL
ADD Code/Term	D64 – MEMORY LOSS CARE
ADD Code/Term	E12.3 – CRISIS THERAPY
DELETE Term	F15.1 – Hydration Status
ADD Term	F15.1 – HYDRATION CONTROL
DELETE Term	G17 – Community Special Programs
ADD Term	G17 – COMMUNITY SPECIAL SERVICES
DELETE Code/Term	G17.4 – Other Community Special Programs
DELETE Term	G18.3 – Compliance with Medical Regime
ADD Term	G18.3 – COMPLIANCE WITH MEDICAL REGIMEN
DELETE Term	G18.4 – Compliance with Medication Regime
ADD Term	G18.4 – COMPLIANCE WITH MEDICATION REGIMEN
DELETE Term	G18.6 – Compliance with Therapeutic Regime
ADD Term	G18.6 – COMPLIANCE WITH THERAPEUTIC REGIMEN
DELETE Term	G20.1 – Medical Regime Orders
ADD Term	G20.1 – MEDICAL REGIMEN ORDERS
DELETE Code/Term	G21.7 – Other Ancillary Service
DELETE Code/Term	G21.8 – Other Professional Service
DELETE	H24 – Medication Administration
ADD Term	H24 – MEDICATION CARE
ADD Code/Term	H24.4 – MEDICATION TREATMENT
DELETE Term	I26 – Allergic Reaction Care
ADD Term	I26 – ALLERGIC REACTION CONTROL
ADD Code/Term	I65 – IMMUNOLOGICAL CARE
DELETE Term	J28 – Gastronomy/Nasogastric Care
ADD Term	J28 – ENTERAL TUBE CARE
DELETE Term	J28.1 – Gastronomy/Nasogastric Tube Insertion
ADD Term	J28.1 – ENTERAL TUBE INSERTION
DELETE Term	J28.2 – Gastronomy/Nasogastric Tube Irrigation
ADD Term	J28.2 – ENTERAL TUBE IRRIGATION
DELETE Term	J29.1 – Enteral/Parenteral Feeding
ADD Code/Term	J29.5 – ENTERAL FEEDING
ADD Code/Term	J29.6 – PARENTERAL FEEDING
ADD Code/Term	J66 – BREASTFEEDING SUPPORT
DELETE Term	K31.4 – Physical Measurements

(Continued)

TABLE A.3. CLINICAL CARE CLASSIFICATION OF NURSING INTERVENTIONS (VERSION 2.0) REVISIONS FROM HOME HEALTH CARE CLASSIFICATION (VERSION 1.0) (CONTINUED)

ADD Term	K31.4 – CLINICAL MEASUREMENTS
DELETE Term	K32 – Specimen Analysis
ADD	K32 – SPECIMEN CARE
DELETE Term	K32.1 – Blood Specimen Analysis
ADD Term	K32.1 – BLOOD SPECIMEN CARE
DELETE Term	K32.2 – Stool Specimen Analysis
ADD Term	K32.2 – STOOL SPECIMEN CARE
DELETE Term	K32.3 – Urine Specimen Analysis
ADD Term	K32.3 – URINE SPECIMEN CARE
DELETE Code/Term	K32.4 – Other Specimen Analysis
ADD Code/Term	K32.5 – SPUTUM SPECIMEN CARE
DELETE Code	K34 – Weight Control
ADD Code	J67 – WEIGHT CONROL
DELETE Term	L36 – Respiratory Care
ADD Term	L36 – PULMONARY CARE
DELETE Term	M39 – Psychosocial Analysis
ADD Term	M39 – PSYCHOSOCIAL CARE
ADD Code/Term	M39.3 – FAMILY PROCESS ANALYSIS
ADD Code/Term	M39.4 – SEXUAL BEHAVIOR ANALYSIS
ADD Code/Term	M39.5 – SOCIAL NETWORK ANALYSIS
DELETE Term	N40 – Abuse Control
ADD Term	N40 – SUBSTANCE ABUSE CONTROL
ADD Code/Term	N40.1 – TOBACCO ABUSE CONTROL
ADD Code/Term	N40.2 – ALCOHOL ABUSE CONTROL
ADD Code/Term	N40.3 – DRUG ABUSE CONTROL
DELETE Code	O44 – Bedbound Care
ADD Code	A61 – BEDBOUND CARE
DELETE Code	O44.1 – Positioning Therapy
ADD Code	A61.1 – POSITIONING THERAPY
DELETE Code	P46 – Violence Control
ADD	N68 – VIOLENCE CONTROL
ADD Code/Term	Q47.1 – ACUTE PAIN CONTROL
ADD Code/Term	Q47.2 – CHRONIC PAIN CONTROL
ADD Code/Term	Q50.2 – VISION CARE
DELETE Term	R51 – Decubitus Care
ADD Term	R51 – PRESSURE ULCER CARE
DELETE Term	R51.1 – Decubitus Stage 1
ADD Term	R51.1 – PRESSURE ULCER STAGE 1 CARE
DELETE Term	R51.2 – Decubitus Stage 2
ADD Term	R51.2 – PRESSURE ULCER STAGE 2 CARE
DELETE Term	R51.3 – Decubitus Stage 3
ADD Term	R51.3 – PRESSURE ULCER STAGE 3 CARE
DELETE Term	R51.4 – Decubitus Stage 4
ADD Term	R51.4 – PRESSURE ULCER STAGE 4 CARE
DELETE Code	R52 – Edema Control
ADD Code	S69 – EDEMA CONTROL
ADD Code/Term	S70 – CIRCULATORY CARE
ADD Code/Term	S71 – NEUROVASCULAR CARE
ADD Code/Term	T72 – URINARY INCONTINENCE CARE
ADD Core/Term	T73 – RENAL CARE

(Continued)

TABLE A.3. (CONTINUED)

ADD Code/Term	U74 – REPRODUCTIVE CARE
ADD Code/Term	U74.1 – FERTILITY CARE
ADD Code/Term	U74.2 – INFERTILITY CARE
ADD Code/Term	U74.3 – CONTRACEPTION CARE
ADD Code/Term	U75 – PERINATAL CARE
ADD Code/Term	U75.1 – PREGNANCY CARE
ADD Code/Term	U75.2 – LABOR CARE
ADD Code/Term	U75.3 – DELIVERY CARE
ADD Code/Term	U75.4 – POSTPARTUM CARE
ADD Code/Term	U76 – GROWTH & DEVELOPMENT CARE
ADD Code/Term	U76.1 – NEWBORN CARE (First 30 Days)
ADD Code/Term	U76.2 – INFANT CARE (31 Days Through 11 Months)
ADD Code/Term	U76.3 – CHILD CARE (1 Year Through 11 Years)
ADD Code/Term	U76.4 – ADOLESCENT CARE (12 Years Through 20 Years)
ADD Code/Term	U76.5 – ADULT CARE (21 Years Through 64 Years)
ADD Code/Term	U76.6 – OLDER ADULT CARE (65 Years and Over)

Appendix B

SABACARE, INC.

Permission Form

Date: _____

To: Dr. Virginia K. Saba, Director SabaCare, Inc.

_____ [name of entity] ("the Company") requests permission to nonexclusive world rights in all languages and in all editions and formats–printed hardcopy and/or electronic version– to the Clinical Care Classification (CCC) System terminologies for use in its products. The CCC System (formerly known as the Home Health Care Classification (HHCC) System) consists of two terminologies: (1) CCC of Nursing Diagnoses and Outcomes and (2) the CCC of Nursing Interventions and Actions, both of which are classified by 21 Care Components. The CCC is copyrighted as TX 6-100-481.

OBLIGATIONS OF THE COMPANY:

1. The CCC System will be used only with computer applications developed by the Company.
2. The CCC System will not be sold or transferred as a derivative product by the Company.
3. The CCC System will not be separately sold or copyrighted by the Company, and the Company will not charge usage fees or royalties from its customers specifically for use of the CCC System.
4. The Company will give full credit to the CCC System in its product collateral and in any copyright registration.
5. The Company will share with Dr. Saba any new concepts (nursing diagnoses/outcomes or nursing interventions/actions) identified while deploying CCC.

Company Name:_____

Address:

_____

City:_____

State:_____ **Zip:**_____

Signature:_____
(Authorized Representative of the Company)

Title:_____

Date:_____

APPROVAL OF REQUEST:

The foregoing permission is hereby granted.

Date of Approval:_____

Approved By: _____

© V. K. Saba—Revised 2006

NTIS ORDER FORM

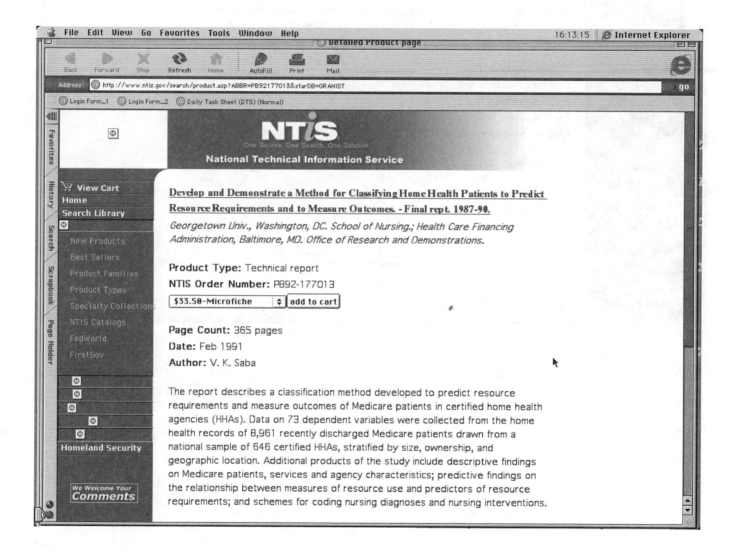

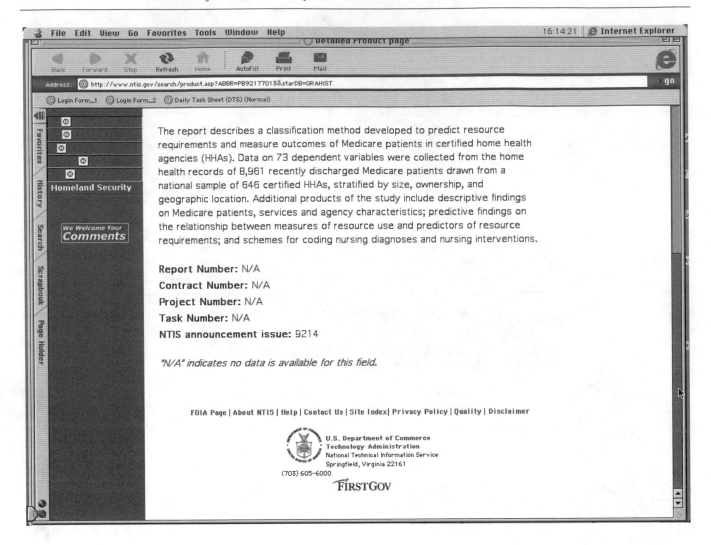

The report describes a classification method developed to predict resource requirements and measure outcomes of Medicare patients in certified home health agencies (HHAs). Data on 73 dependent variables were collected from the home health records of 8,961 recently discharged Medicare patients drawn from a national sample of 646 certified HHAs, stratified by size, ownership, and geographic location. Additional products of the study include descriptive findings on Medicare patients, services and agency characteristics; predictive findings on the relationship between measures of resource use and predictors of resource requirements; and schemes for coding nursing diagnoses and nursing interventions.

Report Number: N/A
Contract Number: N/A
Project Number: N/A
Task Number: N/A
NTIS announcement issue: 9214

"N/A" indicates no data is available for this field.

FOIA Page | About NTIS | Help | Contact Us | Site Index | Privacy Policy | Quality | Disclaimer

U.S. Department of Commerce
Technology Administration
National Technical Information Service
Springfield, Virginia 22161
(703) 605-6000

FIRSTGOV

INDEX

INDEX

In this index, the letters "f", "t" and "e" denote figures, tables and exhibits, respectively.